Diagnostic Imaging of Kidney: Tools and Techniques

Diagnostic Imaging of Kidney: Tools and Techniques

Edited by Eliza Harris

STATES
ACADEMIC PRESS
www.statesacademicpress.com

States Academic Press,
109 South 5th Street,
Brooklyn, NY 11249, USA

Visit us on the World Wide Web at:
www.statesacademicpress.com

ISBN: 978-1-63989-150-4

Cataloging-in-Publication Data

Diagnostic imaging of kidney : tools and techniques / edited by Eliza Harris.
p. cm.
Includes bibliographical references and index.
ISBN 978-1-63989-150-4
1. Kidneys--Imaging. 2. Diagnostic imaging. 3. Imaging systems.
4. Imaging systems in medicine. I. Harris, Eliza.

RC904.5.I42 D53 2022
616.610 757--dc23

Table of Contents

Preface

I am honored to present to you this unique book which encompasses the most up-to-date data in the field. I was extremely pleased to get this opportunity of editing the work of experts from across the globe. I have also written papers in this field and researched the various aspects revolving around the progress of the discipline. I have tried to unify my knowledge along with that of stalwarts from every corner of the world, to produce a text which not only benefits the readers but also facilitates the growth of the field.

Diagnostic imaging of the kidneys is used to analyze the kidneys and their function. Several imaging techniques are used for diagnostic imaging such as MRI, ultrasound and CT scan. The medical imaging technique which makes use of strong magnetic fields, radio waves and magnetic field gradients for the purpose of producing images of the organs in the body is known as magnetic resonance imaging (MRI). It helps to detect and characterize renal lesions. MRI of the kidneys is used in cases wherein a person's renal system is compromised, or suffers from contrast allergy. It is also used to avoid radiation exposure to people such as pregnant women and small children. In cases where the CT scan results are nondiagnostic, MRI can be used as a problem solving modality. This book elucidates the concepts and innovative models around prospective developments with respect to the diagnostic imaging of the kidneys. It presents studies on the tools and techniques used within this field in the most comprehensible and easy to understand language. This book includes contributions of experts and scientists which will provide innovative insights into this field.

Finally, I would like to thank all the contributing authors for their valuable time and contributions. This book would not have been possible without their efforts. I would also like to thank my friends and family for their constant support.

Editor

1

Analysis Protocol for Renal Sodium (^{23}Na) MR Imaging

James T. Grist, Esben Søvsø Szocska Hansen, Frank G. Zöllner, and Christoffer Laustsen

Abstract

The signal acquired in sodium (^{23}Na) MR imaging is proportional to the concentration of sodium in a voxel, and it is possible to convert between the two using external calibration phantoms. Postprocessing, and subsequent analysis, of sodium renal images is a simple task that can be performed with readily available software. Here we describe the process of conversion between sodium signal and concentration, estimation of the corticomedullary sodium gradient and the procedure used for quadrupolar relaxation analysis.

This chapter is based upon work from the COST Action PARENCHIMA, a community-driven network funded by the European Cooperation in Science and Technology (COST) program of the European Union, which aims to improve the reproducibility and standardization of renal MRI biomarkers. This analysis protocol chapter is complemented by two separate chapters describing the basic concept and experimental procedure.

Key words Magnetic resonance imaging (MRI), Kidney, Rats, ^{23}Na, Sodium

1 Introduction

The signal acquired in sodium (^{23}Na) MR imaging is proportional to the concentration of sodium in a voxel, and it is possible to convert between the two using external calibration phantoms. To calculate sodium concentration maps, an imaging volume including the tissue of interest and external calibration phantoms is required, using a gradient echo (GRE) sequence for data acquisition. T_2^* relaxation maps can be calculated from multiecho GRE data acquired in the same acquisition. Theoretical considerations and acquisition protocols are detailed in the chapters by Grist JT et al. "Sodium (^{23}Na) MRI of the Kidney: Basic Concept" and "Sodium (^{23}Na) MRI of the Kidney: Experimental Protocol." Creation of sodium concentration maps can be performed with several commercially available software packages (*see* **Note 1**). In general, a linear fit is performed between the mean signal intensity of each calibration phantoms and a region of noise. The fitting coefficients are used to convert sodium signal to sodium concentration. This chapter focuses on how to do this, conceptually.

This analysis protocol chapter is complemented by two separate chapters describing the basic concept and experimental procedure, which are part of this book.

2 Materials

2.1 Software Requirements

1. To calculate parameter maps: A programming environment capable of applying fitting models, such as Python (www.python.org), Octave (www.gnu.org/software/octave) or MATLAB (The MathWorks, Natick, MA, USA) with a curve fitting capability. The method described in this chapter provides a detailed description for a solution in MATLAB, but can be adopted to other platforms.
2. Optional: A image processing software such as Fiji (www.fiji.sc) or Horos (www.horosproject.org).

2.2 Source Data: Format Requirements and Quality Check

2.2.1 Input Requirements

To be able to calculate sodium concentration maps, images including sodium calibration phantoms acquired during an experiment are required, as well as the known absolute concentration of sodium in the calibration phantoms.

2.2.2 Data Exclusion

When sodium imaging is acquired, it commonly has a low signal-to-noise ratio (SNR). In order to construct accurate sodium T_2* maps, it is important to ensure that the signal of kidneys is greater than that of the background noise, else a poor fit will occur. Therefore, data with SNR lower than a threshold (e.g., SNR $<$ 5) should be discarded.

This step should be avoided for concentration mapping, as a region of noise is required to calculate an assumed 0 mmol/L signal value.

2.2.3 SNR Check for T_2* Mapping

To check SNR in renal sodium imaging in MATLAB (NB: example code for SNR measurements assumes a single slice and absolute value data):

1. Draw an ROI, using the "roipoly" command, over a region of background noise free of artefacts.

```
Region = poly2mat(roipoly(mat2gray(image_slice)));
Masked_Region = Region .* image_slice;
```

2. Calculate the standard deviation of the noise using the "std" command.

```
NoiseSTD = std(Masked_Region(Masked_Region >0));
```

3. Divide the original image by 0.66 multiplied by the standard deviation of the noise to produce SNR maps.

```
Image_SNR = image_slice ./ (sqrt(2)*NoiseSTD);
```

4. SNR maps can then be used to form a mask to remove signal less than a predefined SNR value (e.g., 5).

```
Image_SNR(Image_SNR<5) = 0;
Image_SNR(Image_SNR>1) = 1;
Masked_Image_Slice = Image_slice .* Image_SNR
```

2.2.4 Dual Flip Angle B_1 Mapping for Sodium Concentration Mapping

Furthermore, if local send and receive RF coils are used, B_1 mapping to correct for signal inhomogeneity due to coil profiles can be performed (*see* **Note 2**).

3 Methods

3.1 Sodium Concentration Mapping

The mean signal from phantoms in the images can be derived using regions of interest (ROIs). Furthermore, a mean image noise value should be defined on a slice by slice basis using signal outside of the body.

Once the mean signal of each phantom, as well as noise, has been calculated, a linear fit should be performed between the known concentration values and the phantom/noise signal (assuming noise represents 0 mmol/L sodium).

The coefficients derived from the fit (offset and slope) can then be used to convert each voxel in the image from signal intensity to concentration using Eq. 1, below.

$$\text{Sodium concentration}\left(\text{mmolL}^{-1}\right) = \frac{\text{signal} - \text{offset}}{\text{slope}} \tag{1}$$

3.1.1 Algorithm for Sodium Concentration Mapping

1. Define region of noise on a slice-by-slice basis using either automated (selecting voxels in a specific region of each image) or via ROI placement on a slice-by-slice basis.
2. Calculate the mean of each noise region and store this value in a vector (e.g., *meannoise*).
3. Segment sodium calibration phantoms using ROIs and calculate the mean signal for each phantom.
4. Perform concentration mapping by calculating a linear fit between the noise, phantom signals, and the known

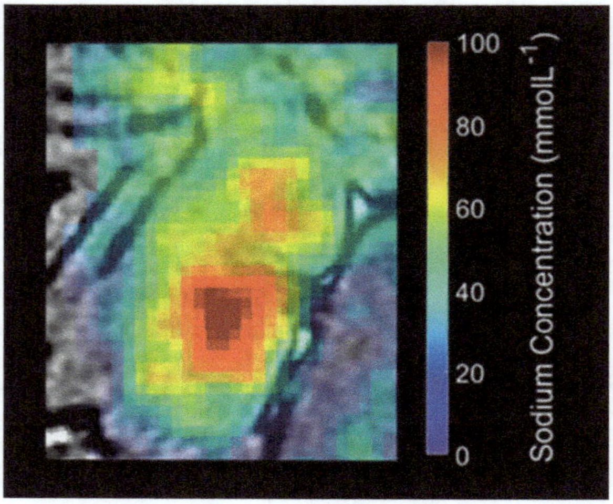

Fig. 1 Example images of sodium signal in the healthy porcine kidney, acquired at 3T, demonstrating increase sodium signal in the medulla, in comparison to the cortex

concentrations of the phantoms (example code presented below) on a slice by slice basis

3.1.2 Example Matlab Code

```
for zslice = 1:Number_Of_Z_Slices
      fitting = polyfit([0,conc1,conc2],[meannoise(zslice),
Phantom1, Phantom2],1);
    slope = fitting(1);
    offset = fitting(2);
    Image(:,:,zslice) = (Image(:,:,zslice) - offset)./slope;
End
```

Example sodium concentration mapping data of the porcine kidney can be seen in Fig. 1.

3.1.3 Biexponential T_{2^*} Mapping

In order to map the biexponential T_2^* of the kidney (separating the restricted quadrupolar spins and the freely moving spins), a more complicated process of signal fitting is required. Utilizing multi-echo GRE data, acquired in the same imaging acquisition, a non-linear fitting routine is employed to determine the behavior of the sodium signal, as described in Eq. 2.

$$s(\mathrm{TE}) = \left(a\, e^{-\frac{\mathrm{TE}}{\mathrm{T}^*_{2,\mathrm{Short}}}} + b\, e^{-\frac{\mathrm{TE}}{\mathrm{T}^*_{2,\mathrm{Long}}}} \right) \quad (2)$$

where a and b are the relative pool sizes, and $\mathrm{T}^*_{2,\mathrm{Short}}$ and $\mathrm{T}^*_{2,\mathrm{Long}}$ are the pool T_2^* constants (ms), with the constraints that $a + b = 1$, and $\mathrm{T}^*_{2,\mathrm{Short}} > \mathrm{T}^*_{2,\mathrm{Long}}$. Assuming five or more data sets are acquired, the following MATLAB code can be used to fit the above curve. An example fit is shown in Fig. 2.

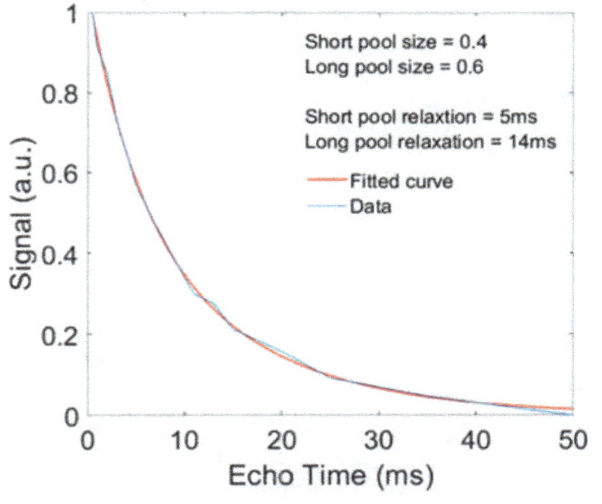

Fig. 2 Example fit of biexponential data acquired from an agar phantom

3.1.4 Algorithm for T2 Mapping*

1. Perform SNR thresholding as detailed in Subheading 2.2.3.
2. Loop biexponential curve-fitting code (example Matlab code presented below) over all SNR masked regions in the image. The fit algorithm used here is trust region reflective.
3. Store data either as DICOM, proprietary (e.g., .mat), or text files.

3.1.5 Example Matlab Fitting Code

```
%% List of echo times acquired during imaging
TE_List = [TE1, TE2, TE3,...];
%% Setting up fit options
fopts = fitoptions('Method','NonlinearLeastSquares',...
                  'Lower',[0,0,0,5],...
                  'Upper',[1,1,5,55]
                  'StartPoint',[0.2 1,10]);
% Fit curve equation
ft = fittype('a*exp(-x/b) + (1-a)*exp(-x/c),'coefficients',
{'a', 'T21','T22'},'independent','x','options',fopts);
%% Pre-allocation of memory to speed up fitting
ShortPoolSize(xvoxel,yvoxel,zvoxel) = ...
 zeros(size(Imaging_Data,1),size(imageing_Data,2),size(Ima-
ging_Data,3));
LongPoolSize(xvoxel,yvoxel,zvoxel) = ...
 zeros(size(Imaging_Data,1),size(imageing_Data,2),size(Ima-
ging_Data,3));
ShortPoolRelaxation(xvoxel,yvoxel,zvoxel) = ...
 zeros(size(Imaging_Data,1),size(imageing_Data,2),size(Ima-
ging_Data,3));
LongPoolRelaxation(xvoxel,yvoxel,zvoxel) = ...
 zeros(size(Imaging_Data,1),size(imageing_Data,2),size(Ima-
ging_Data,3));
```

```
%% Fitting loop core
for zslice = 1:Number_Of_Z_Slices
   for yvoxel = 1:Number_Of_Y_Voxels
      for xvoxel = 1:Number_Of_X_Voxels
         if (Masked_Image_Slice ~= 0)
            % Extract data vector for one pixel
            Data_Vector = Imaging_Data (xvoxel,yvoxel,zlice,:);
            % Do curve fitting for one voxel
            [Fit,gof] = fit(TE_List,Data_Vector, ft);
            % Store results
            ShortPoolSize(xvoxel,yvoxel,zvoxel) = Fit.a;
            LongPoolSize(xvoxel,yvoxel,zvoxel) = 1 - Fit.a;
            ShortPoolRelaxation(xvoxel,yvoxel,zvoxel) = Fit.b;
            LongPoolRelaxation(xvoxel,yvoxel,zvoxel) = Fit.c
         end
      end
   end
end
```

If data are acquired at higher magnetic field strengths ($B_0 \geq 3T$), it is advisable to alter the pool constraints for the parameter *fopts* to reflect the shorter $T^*_{2,\text{Short}}$ and $T^*_{2,\text{Long}}$ components.

3.2 Visual Display

There is no current consensus on the best colour map to use when displaying sodium concentration images. T_1- or T_2-weighted images acquired in the same slice position can provide guidance for the interpretation as well as base layer for presenting the images as a set of fused images, *see* Fig. 1.

An example display option for MATLAB is described below:

1. Display the parameter map, which is a matrix with floating point numbers, as an image (in MATLAB: imagesc (ShortPoolRelaxation)).
2. Remove axis labels and ensure the axis are scaled equally, so that pixels are square and not rectangular (in MATLAB: axis off; axis equal;).
3. Select the color map and display a color bar (in MATLAB: colormap(hot(256)); colorbar;).
4. Set the display range for the color coding, for example, for short and long T_2* [0 5] and [5 60], respectively; (in MATLAB: caxis([0 5]);).

3.3 Quantification

In order to obtain quantitative medulla and cortex values from sodium concentration maps, the kidney can be segmented using either concentric objects or semiautomated ROI placement [1, 2]. To assess the corticomedullary sodium gradient, a linear fit can be performed across concentration values derived from the

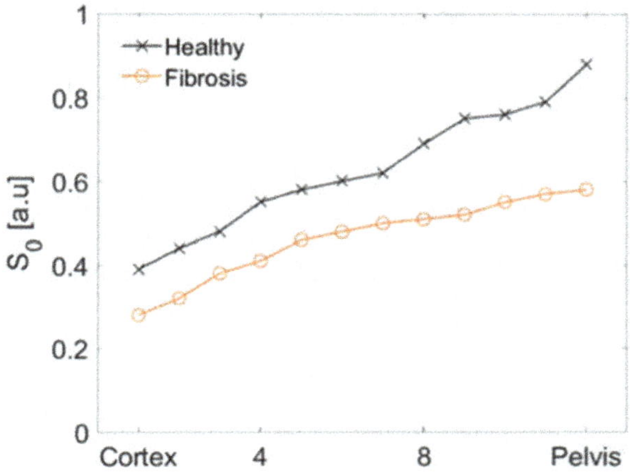

Fig. 3 Example corticomedullary sodium gradient, healthy (black) and impaired rodent kidney (orange)

Table 1
Example sodium concentration values from renal compartments, derived from post-sacrifice kidneys [5]

Tissue type	Total sodium concentration (mmol/L)
Cortex	29 ± 7
Outer-medullar	75 ± 20
Inner-medullar	161 ± 29

concentric objects method, providing the slope of the gradient. An example corticomedullary sodium gradient in both healthy and fibrosis impaired rodent kidney can be seen in Fig. 3.

3.4 Results Validation

3.4.1 Comparison with Tissue Values from Biopsy

Further validation of imaging derived results can be performed using biopsy derived tissue samples, using methods such as flame photometry, mass spectrometry, or *ex vivo* spectroscopy.

3.4.2 Comparison with Reference Values from the Literature

If biopsy derived results cannot be obtained, for example due to longitudinal studies, obtained values for both tissue segmentation can be compared against reference values, shown in Table 1.

4 Notes

1. Processing is typically performed in software packages such as MATLAB (The MathWorks, MA) or open source platforms as python programming language (python.org). The data can either

be processed as DICOM images or if available as the raw data format from the scanner (dicomstandard.org/using/cds/). Finalizing the data in the DICOM format pipelines the data for further analysis and comparison to conventional MRI images.

2. The linear proportionality of the NMR signal to the spin density allows for the absolute quantification of the Total Sodium Concentration (TSC) on the basis of a known concentration reference. However, TSC measurements are distorted by hardware-dependent influences and by typical ^{23}Na-NMR properties. This can be determined and corrected with the help of B_1 mapping methods [3]. Mapping methods which allow short TE are the double-angle and the phase-sensitive method [4].

Acknowledgments

This chapter is based upon work from COST Action PARENCH IMA, supported by European Cooperation in Science and Technology (COST). COST (www.cost.eu) is a funding agency for research and innovation networks. COST Actions help connect research initiatives across Europe and enable scientists to enrich their ideas by sharing them with their peers. This boosts their research, career, and innovation.

PARENCHIMA (renalmri.org) is a community-driven Action in the COST program of the European Union, which unites more than 200 experts in renal MRI from 30 countries with the aim to improve the reproducibility and standardization of renal MRI biomarkers.

References

1. Milani B, Ansaloni A, Sousa-Guimaraes S et al (2017) Reduction of cortical oxygenation in chronic kidney disease: evidence obtained with a new analysis method of blood oxygenation level-dependent magnetic resonance imaging. Nephrol Dial Transplant 32(12):2097–2105
2. Mikheev A, Lim RP (2016) A semi-automated "blanket" method for renal segmentation from non-contrast T1-weighted MR images. MAGMA 29:197–206
3. Gatzeva-topalova PZ, Warner LR, Pardi A, Carlos M (2011) Quantitative sodium imaging with a flexible twisted projection pulse sequence. Magn Reson Med 18:1492–1501
4. Morrell GR, Schabel MC (2010) An analysis of the accuracy of magnetic resonance flip angle measurement methods. Phys Med Biol 55:6157–6174
5. Saikia TC (1964) Composition of the renal cortex and medulla of rats during water diuresis and antidiuresis. J Clin Invest 51:1145–1151

2

Denoising for Improved Parametric MRI of the Kidney: Protocol for Nonlocal Means Filtering

Ludger Starke, Karsten Tabelow, Thoralf Niendorf, and Andreas Pohlmann

Abstract

In order to tackle the challenges caused by the variability in estimated MRI parameters (e.g., T_2* and T_2) due to low SNR a number of strategies can be followed. One approach is postprocessing of the acquired data with a filter. The basic idea is that MR images possess a local spatial structure that is characterized by equal, or at least similar, noise-free signal values in vicinities of a location. Then, local averaging of the signal reduces the noise component of the signal. In contrast, nonlocal means filtering defines the weights for averaging not only within the local vicinity, bur it compares the image intensities between *all* voxels to define "nonlocal" weights. Furthermore, it generally compares not only single-voxel intensities but small spatial patches of the data to better account for extended similar patterns. Here we describe how to use an open source NLM filter tool to denoise 2D MR image series of the kidney used for parametric mapping of the relaxation times T_2* and T_2.

This chapter is based upon work from the COST Action PARENCHIMA, a community-driven network funded by the European Cooperation in Science and Technology (COST) program of the European Union, which aims to improve the reproducibility and standardization of renal MRI biomarkers.

Key words Magnetic resonance imaging (MRI), Kidney, Mice, Rats, Parametric mapping, T_2, T_2*, Diffusion

1 Introduction

Mapping of the transverse relaxation times T_2* and T_2 (or relaxation rates $R_2^* = 1/T_2^*$ and $R_2 = 1/T_2$) requires series of MR images with different echo times TE: The maps are obtained by fitting the exponential model curve $S(\mathrm{TE}) = S_0 \exp(-\mathrm{TE}/T_2^{(*)})$ to the signal intensities of each image pixel with increasing TE. This approach is inherently associated with decreasing signal-to-noise ratio (SNR) for the image volumes obtained for longer echo times. Similarly, there is a substantial signal attenuation and SNR reduction in diffusion-weighted MRI versus images acquired without diffusion-sensitizing gradients. Low SNR basically poses two general problems: First, it leads to a variability for the parameter estimates in the quantitative maps or derived model parameters. Second, it induces a systematic bias for the estimated parameter maps [1]. Please *see* Polzehl and Tabelow [2] for an elaboration of the issues and possible solutions.

In order to tackle the challenges caused by the variability in the estimated parameters due to low SNR a number of strategies can be followed. The obvious one is hardware related and includes improvements on the MR scanner side, such as dedicated RF coils or the use of cryogenically cooled RF probes [3]. Then, SNR is increased by reducing the variability of the measurement. Since the magnitude of the MR signal is directly related to the voxel volume [4], SNR increase can be achieved by reducing the spatial resolution of the image acquisition. This is obviously a very unfavorable solution. Alternatively, signal variability can be reduced by averaging of the signal over multiple acquisitions. This approach comes at the cost of prolonged acquisition times. Acceleration techniques like parallel imaging [5, 6] or compressed sensing [7] allow for more signal averaging within the same time span. Image postprocessing provides another alternative for reducing the variability of the data. Within this chapter, we specifically consider a class of methods that post-processes the acquired data, that is, smoothing. The basic idea is that MR images (like all images) possess a local spatial structure that is characterized by equal, or at least similar, noise-free signal values in vicinities of a location. Then, local averaging of the signal reduces the noise component of the signal. The simplest approach is the application of a Gaussian filter which performs a local averaging with weights defined by a (Gaussian) kernel function and a bandwidth. Due to its simple mathematical formulation it can be performed very fast on data volumes independent of the spatial dimensionality of the data. However, it comes with the blurring of the images, which is evident at edges between different tissues, especially hindering the analysis of fine structures within the volumes.

Alternatively, adaptive smoothing methods have been developed that aim to take the local properties of the specific data at hand into account. The specific methods are based on different methodologies, like anisotropic diffusion [8–11], nonlocal means [12], penalization techniques [13, 14] wavelet filtering [15], model-based methods [16, 17], the propagation-separation approach [18, 19], or other local techniques [20, 21]. Many of these techniques have been applied to diffusion-weighted MRI data but are also applicable for relaxometry measurements. Depending on the specific method and the input data at adaptive smoothing is performed on each image volume separately or uses the combined information from all available raw data. In contrast to nonadaptive filters such as the Gaussian filter, these methods typically require longer computation times and the choice of one or more smoothing parameters. Furthermore, in a similar way as the Gaussian filter induced blurring of images, adaptive filters might impose artifacts depending on their assumptions on the data like a cartoonesque appearance due to a step-function reconstruction of the images.

Here, we specifically consider the nonlocal means (NLM) filter [22, 23], which is of proven value for MRI. In contrast to defining the weights for averaging within the local vicinity of a location depending on the spatial distance only, it compares the image intensities between *all* voxels to define "nonlocal" weights for averaging intensities. Furthermore, it generally compares not only single-voxel intensities but small spatial patches of the data to better account for extended similar patterns. It is related to the bilateral filtering [24], where the *local* weights are refined by a factor related to local intensity differences; nonlocal means can thus be considered as a bilateral filter with infinite spatial bandwidth making it nonlocal. The filter can be applied to images in two dimensions but also in 3D or for multispectral [25] such as multiecho imaging techniques used in MR relaxometry.

Advantages of the application of the NLM filter are manifold: As a purely postprocessing method it does not require special hardware or sophisticated image acquisition techniques but can be applied offline. Many implementations and extensions of the original algorithm as open-source software are freely available. Examples are provided under: https://sites.google.com/site/pierrickcoupe/softwares/denoising-for-medical-imaging/dwi-denoising/dwi-denoising-software. Most of the implementations require MATLAB. Although smoothing parameters need to be tuned, default settings provide a very good starting point. Images processed with the NLM filter exhibit an improved SNR, show no extra blurring of the edges and preserve effective spatial resolution. Occasional and slight introduction of large-scale structures along the coordinate axis is a recognized limitation of the NLM filter because the comparison of spatial patches is in favor of these directions.

In this protocol we describe the application of a purpose-build implementation of the NLM filter for 2D MRI relaxometry data (*see* **Note 1** for implementation details). The open source tool comes in two versions: (1) each echo time is filtered independently (*2D-NLM*) (2) similarities between image patches are estimated jointly for the complete stack of echo images (*stackNLM*). While the first is a straightforward block-wise implementation of the NLM filter, the second proposes a novel method exploiting the redundancy of information in MR relaxometry data (*see* **Note 1** for implementation details). Both filters reduce the noise level in low SNR relaxometry data with version 2 offering slightly superior results (*see* **Note 2** for a detailed example). Additionally, application of the MATLAB Image Processing toolbox function imnlmfilt is described. This function performs similar to 2D-NLM while being considerably faster. To complete the preprocessing of MRI relaxometry data, correction of the Rician noise bias is described.

This chapter is part of the book Pohlmann A, Niendorf T (eds) (2020) Preclinical MRI of the Kidney—Methods and Protocols. Springer, New York.

2 Materials

2.1 Software Requirements

The processing steps outlined in this protocol require the following:

1. The software development environments *MATLAB®* (The MathWorks, Natick, Massachusetts, USA; mathworks.com) or *Octave* (gnu.org/software/octave).
2. The MATLAB/Octave implementation of the NLM filter downloadable from github.com/LudgerS/MRIRelaxometryNLM
3. Optional: The MATLAB Image Processing Toolbox release R2018b or newer.
4. A MATLAB/Octave tool for noise bias correction downloadable from github.com/LudgerS/MRInoiseBiasCorrection. This tool includes detailed documentation to facilitate adaptation for other software development environments or use with multichannel coil data.
5. A tool for data import. This tool will depend on the data format:

   DICOM data—MATLAB contains a build in function to import dicom data: dicomread. For Octave support is offered by the following package octave.sourceforge.io/dicom/.

   Bruker data—Bruker also offers a toolbox to import data into MATLAB directly. To obtain Bruker's *pvtools* contact Bruker software support (mri-software-support@bruker.com).

2.2 Data Requirements

1. The following protocol assumes that a pure noise scan was acquired to reliable estimate the data noise level.
2. *See* **Note 3** for comments on noise scan acquisition.

3 Methods

3.1 Data Import

These steps should be executed for both the relaxometry data and the noise scan data. In the following sections it is assumed that the relaxometry data was stored in variable relaxData and the noise scan in variable noiseData.

3.1.1 DICOM Data

1. To import dicom data execute the command

```
data = dicomread(filePath);
```

where 'filePath' is a string containing the relative or absolute path of the .dcm file.

3.1.2 Bruker Data

For a Linux or MacOS system, substitute the file separator \ by /.

1. Ensure that pvtools is on the search path:

```
addpath(genpath(...\pvtools))
```

where '...\pvtools' specifies the path of the pvtools folder.

2. Store the path to the scan you want to load in variable scanFolder.
3. Read the visu_pars parameter file:

```
visuPars = readBrukerParamFile([scanFolder, '\visu_pars']);
```

4. Load the Paravision reconstruction:

```
[data, ~] = readBruker2dseq([scanFolder, '\pdata\1\2dseq'], visuPars);
```

3.2 Correct Data Scaling

The data scaling needs to be corrected in some cases depending on the data format and vendor if the relaxometry data and noise scan were acquired with different numbers of averages. For example, in Bruker data, the individual averages are simply added instead of computing the mean (*see* **Note 4** for a procedure to test the scaling convention). Assuming the noise scan was acquired with a single average and the relaxometry data with NA averages, use the following processing step:

1. `relaxData = relaxData/NA`

3.3 Noise Level Estimation

We assume the availability of a pure noise scan. In this case the complete noise data constitutes a background region. Assuming that the noise scan was acquired with a single average and the relaxometry data with NA averages, the noise level can be computed as

1. `sigma = std(noiseData(:))/(0.6551*sqrt(NA));`

The factor 0.6551 accounts for the different standard deviations in background and high SNR regions in MR magnitude images [1, 26, 27]. For data from multichannel coils *see* **Note 5**.

3.4 Application of the NLM Filter

3.4.1 Filtering of Individual Echoes with 2D-NLM

To apply the provided NLM filter implementation, use a loop over all echo times. It is assumed that the relaxometry images are two dimensional and that the echoes are stored along the third dimension of relaxData.

1. Set the parameters of the filter (*see* **Note 6** for an explanation of choices)

```
params.centerDistance = 1; % distance between individual blocks
params.blockRadius = 1; % size of the blocks;
params.searchRadius = 10; % determines the number of searched blocks
params.beta = 0.5; % adjusts the filter strength
```

2. Prealocate memory for the filtered data

```
filteredData = zeros(size(relaxData));
```

3. Apply the filter to every echo individually

```
for ii = 1:size(relaxData, 3)
filteredData(:,:,ii) = nlmFilter2D(relaxData(:,:,ii), sigma, params);
end
```

3.4.2 Filtering Using stackNLM

1. Set the paramters of the filter (*see* **Note 4** for an explanation of choices)

```
params.centerDistance = 1; % distance between individual blocks
params.blockRadius = 1; % size of the blocks;
params.searchRadius = 10; % determines the number of searched blocks
params.beta = 0.3; % adjusts the filter strength
```

2. Directly apply the filter to all echoes

```
filteredData(:,:,ii) = stackNlmFilter(relaxData, sigma, params);
```

3.4.3 Filtering Using MATLAB's Imnlmfilt

MATLAB's imnlmfilt works on 2D images. Again a loop over the echo times is used:

1. Prealocate memory for the filtered data

```
filteredData = zeros(size(relaxData));
```

2. Apply the filter to every echo individually

```
for ii = 1:size(relaxData, 3)
filteredData(:,:,ii) = imnlmfilt(relaxData(:,:,ii),
degreeOfSmoothing, sigma);
end
```

3.5 Bias Correction

To correct the Rician noise bias, the MRInoiseBiasCorrection toolbox is used. Importantly, the noise level sigma of the original data and not that of the filtered image needs to be given as an input parameter.

1. Ensure that the toolbox is on the search path

```
addpath(...\MRInoiseBiasCorrection)
```

where '...\MRInoiseBiasCorrection' specifies the path of the toolbox folder.

2. Apply the noise bias correction

```
correctedImage = correctNoiseBias(imageData,
sigma, 1);
```

The last argument specifies the number of channels in the RF coil.

4 Notes

1. The provided tool follows the block-wise implementation of the NLM filter outlined by Coupé et al. for 3D data [28]. The noise level σ is expected to be provided by separate means such as the noise scan described in this protocol. The filtering parameter h is set to $\sqrt{2\beta\sigma^2 n}$, where n is the number of pixels in the compared blocks and β a parameter which can be controlled by the user (*see* **Note 5**). Noise bias correction was not integrated into the filter but is recommended as a subsequent step.
2. We present an example application to showcase the potential of the NLM filter for T_2* relaxometry. For this purpose the kidney of an ex vivo rat phantom was scanned with a multiecho gradient-echo (MGE) sequence (TR = 50 ms, TE = 2.14 ms, 2.47 ms echo spacing, ten echoes, [38.2 × 48.5] mm^2 FOV, 1 mm slice thickness, [202 × 256] image matrix, 80 repetitions, one average per repetition). The average of all 80 repetitions was used as a reference measurement. T_2* maps were computed from unfiltered data and data filtered following the protocols of Subheading 3.4.1 (2D-NLM) and Subheading 3.4.2 (stackNLM).

   Figure 1 shows maps for a single repetition (NA = 1), the average of four repetitions (NA = 4) and the reference data

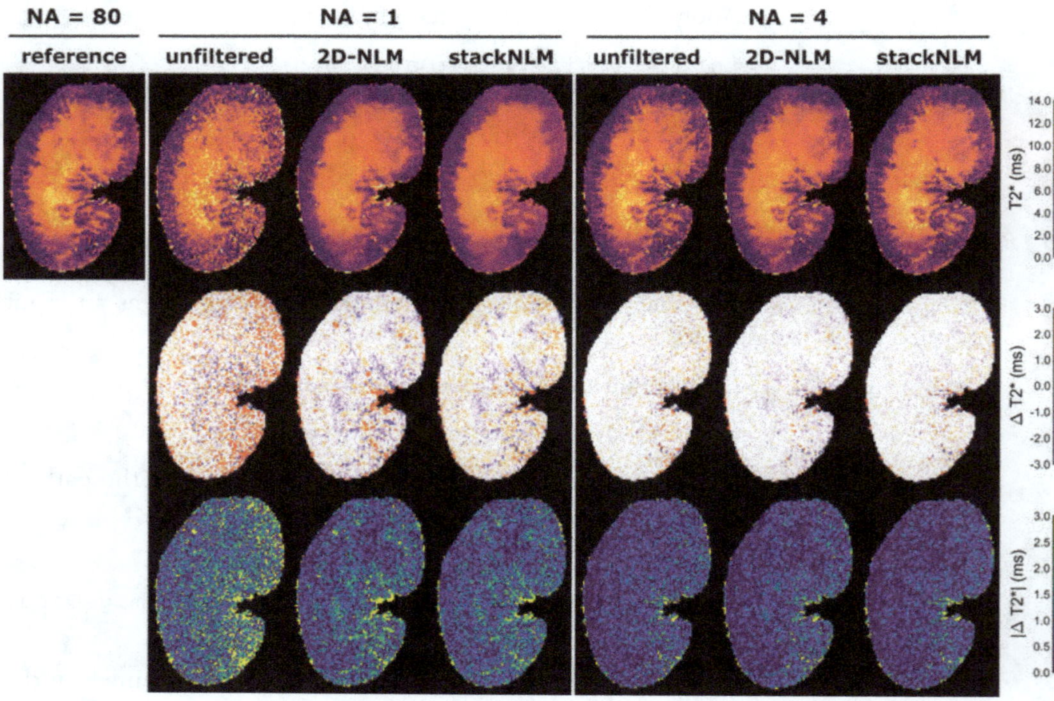

Fig. 1 Filtered and unfiltered kidney T_2* maps acquired in an ex vivo rat phantom. The reference was computed from unfiltered data and NA denotes the number of averages. The second row shows the T_2* deviation from the reference while the third row shows the magnitude of the T_2* deviation

with 80 averages. Maps showing the deviation from the reference (ΔT_2*) and the magnitude deviation ($|\Delta T_2$*$|$) highlight the strongly reduced noise level in filtered images for NA = 1. No bias is introduced and edges are preserved. The filter working on the complete stack of echoes (stackNLM) is more robust regarding outliers. For NA = 4 only very little improvement is achieved due to the already good data quality, yet also no artifacts are introduced.

The root-mean-square deviations (RMSD) of the T_2* maps from the reference support this visual assessment (Fig. 2a). At low SNR (low number of averages) the filtered data outperform the maps computed without filtering. The improvement exceeds the gain achieved by doubling the measurement time. At higher SNR filtered and unfiltered data perform similarly. stackNLM consistently performs better than 2D-NLM. Figure 2b shows selected echoes for NA = 1 and the reference. Here the improved performance of stackNLM becomes obvious for data acquired with TE = 19.4 ms where signal is recovered with sharper detail.

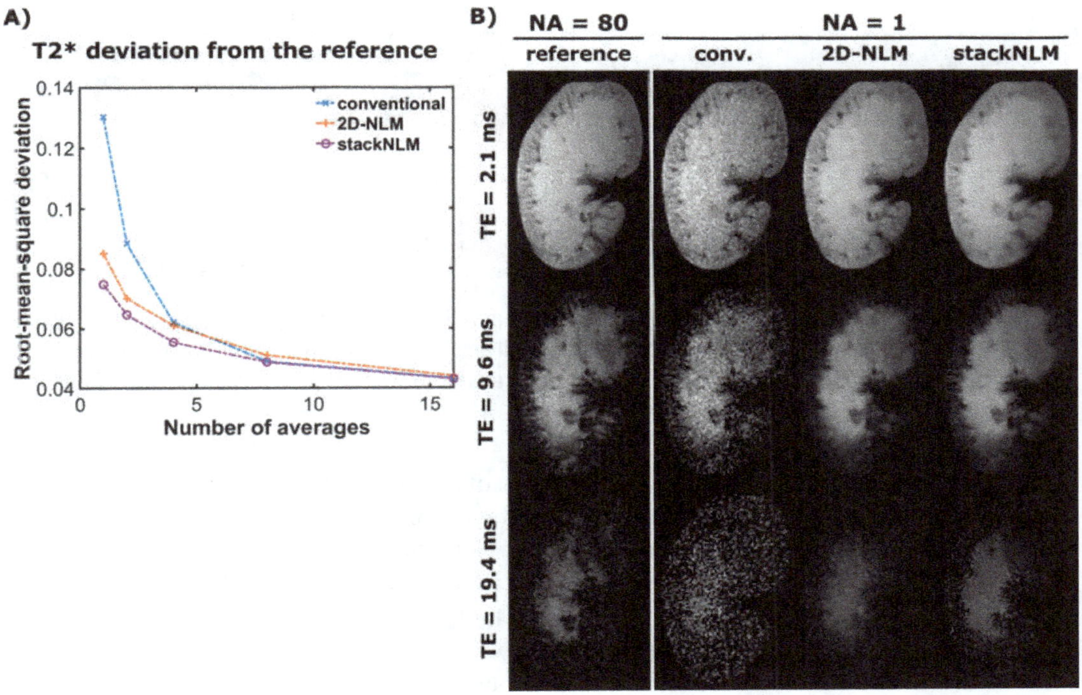

Fig. 2 (**a**) Root-mean-square deviation (RMSD) from the reference (NA = 80, unfiltered) for T_2* maps computed from filtered and unfiltered data. (**b**) Image data for selected echo times (TE). The scaling is set individually for each row

Figure 3 shows an in vivo example for both T_2* and T_2 data. Here little filtering is performed for the high SNR T_2* data, whereas the T_2 map is effectively denoised.

3. A pure noise scan is acquired by setting the excitation flip angle and reference power to zero so that no excitation occurs and pure noise is acquired. The receiver gain needs to be set identical to all other scans for which the noise level should be determined. The number of averages can be reduced to one, as the resulting change in noise level is easily compensated. Alternatively, the output of the RF power supply can be disconnected following the system adjustments.

4. To determine the employed convention of averaging, acquire high SNR phantom data with varying numbers of averages while keeping all other parameters fixed. Import the data as described in Subheading 3.1. If all scans show the same signal magnitude, the scaling step described in Subheading 3.2 should be omitted. However if for example doubling the number of averages also doubles the signal amplitude, rescaling should be performed.

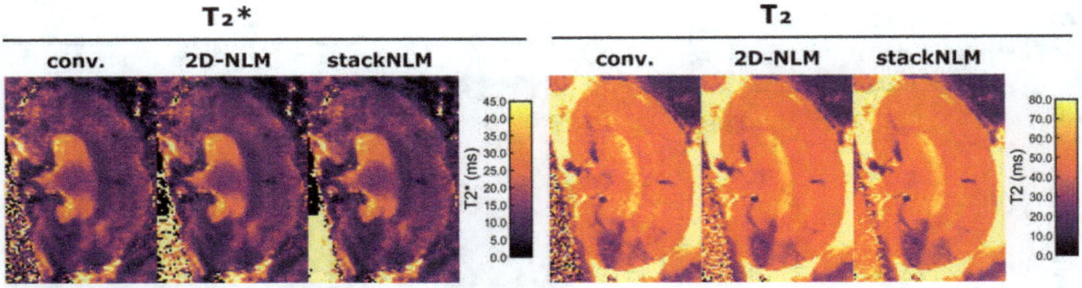

Fig. 3 Filtered and unfiltered T_2 and T_2* maps acquired in a rat in vivo. In this experimental set-up (a healthy naive rat kidney being imaged using a dedicated 9.4T small animal MR system) the SNR is sufficiently high for the denoising to have only minor denoisng effect. The parameter β was set to 0.4 for the stackNLM filter to increase the smoothing effect

5. Assuming a sum-of-squares reconstruction, the factor 0.6551 should be replaced by 0.6824, 0.6953, 0.7014 or 0.7043 for 2, 4, 8 or 16 receive element coil data [29].
6. The block-wise NLM filter compares overlapping square image patches or blocks. The larger the distance between block centers (params.centerDistance), the fewer blocks are in the image. Reducing the number of blocks will accelerate the filter but might lead to artifacts in the vicinity of contrast edges. params.blockRadius determines the size of the blocks and must always be larger than params.centerDistance to ensure overlap. The block is a square patch of area $(\text{params.centerDistance} + 1)^2$. Increasing the size of blocks will improve performance in homogeneous areas but prevent the filter from finding similar blocks in areas with small features. params.searchRadius specifies the number of compared image blocks: each block is compared with the adjacent $(\text{params.searchRadius} + 1)^2$ blocks to determine the corresponding filter weights. In the ideal case the algorithm would always search the complete image for similar blocks; however, the computational cost to do so would be prohibitive while the benefit diminishes fast with increasing search radius. params.beta specifies the parameter β introduced in **Note 1**. While theoretical considerations suggest a value close to 1, the optimal value of β is known to vary with the noise level [28]. Increasing the value of β will increase the smoothing effect. The proposed values of 0.5 for 2D-NLM and 0.3 for stackNLM were found to perform well over a wide range of noise levels.

Acknowledgments

This work was funded, in part (S.W. and A.P.; DFG WA2804, DFG PO1869), by the Deutsche Forschungsgemeinschaft and, in part (Thoralf Niendorf and Andreas Pohlmann), by the German Research Foundation (Gefoerdert durch die Deutsche Forschungsgemeinschaft (DFG), Projektnummer 394046635, SFB 1365, RE NOPROTECTION . Funded by the Deutsche Forschungsgemeinschaft (DFG, German Research Foundation), Project number 394046635, SFB 1365, RENOPROTECTION).
This chapter is based upon work from COST Action PARENCH IMA, supported by European Cooperation in Science and Technology (COST). COST (www.cost.eu) is a funding agency for research and innovation networks. COST Actions help connect research initiatives across Europe and enable scientists to enrich their ideas by sharing them with their peers. This boosts their research, career, and innovation.
PARENCHIMA (renalmri.org) is a community-driven Action in the COST program of the European Union, which unites more than 200 experts in renal MRI from 30 countries with the aim to improve the reproducibility and standardization of renal MRI biomarkers.

References

1. Gudbjartsson H, Patz S (1995) The Rician distribution of noisy MRI data. Magn Reson Med 34:910–914
2. Polzehl J, Tabelow K (2016) Low SNR in diffusion MRI models. J Am Stat Assoc 111 (516):1480–1490
3. Niendorf T, Pohlmann A, Reimann HM et al (2015) Advancing cardiovascular, neurovascular, and renal magnetic resonance imaging in small rodents using cryogenic radiofrequency coil technology. Front Pharmacol 6:255
4. Edelstein W, Glover G, Hardy C, Redington R (1986) The intrinsic signal-to-noise ratio in NMR imaging. Magn Reson Med 3 (4):604–618
5. Pruessmann KP, Weiger M et al (1999) SENSE: sensitivity encoding for fast MRI. Magn Reson Med 42(5):952–962
6. Griswold MA, Jakob PM et al (2002) Generalized autocalibrating partially parallel acquisitions (GRAPPA). Magn Reson Med 47 (6):1202–1210
7. Lustig M, Donoho D, Pauly JM (2007) Sparse MRI: the application of compressed sensing for rapid MR imaging. Magn Reson Med 58:1182–1195
8. Ding Z, Gore J, Anderson A (2005) Reduction of noise in diffusion tensor images using anisotropic smoothing. Magn Reson Med 53 (2):485–490
9. Parker G, Schnabel J, Symms M, Werring D, Barker G (2000) Nonlinear smoothing for reduction of systematic and random errors in diffusion tensor imaging. J Magn Reson Imaging 11:702–710
10. Xu Q, Anderson AW, Gore JC, Ding Z (2010) Efficient anisotropic filtering of diffusion tensor images. Magn Reson Imaging 28 (2):200–211
11. Duits R, Franken E (2011) Left-invariant diffusions on the space of positions and orientations and their application to crossing-preserving smoothing of HARDI images. Int J Comput Vis 92(3):231–264
12. Manjón JV, Thacker NA, Lull JJ, Garcia-Martí G, Martí-Bonmatí L, Robles M (2009) Multicomponent MR image denoising. Int J Biomed Imaging 2009:756897
13. McGraw T, Vemuri B, Özarslan E, Chen Y, Mareci T (2009) Variational denoising of diffusion weighted MRI. Inverse Probl Imaging 3:625–648

14. Haldar JP (2014) Low-rank modeling of local k-space neighborhoods (LORAKS) for constrained MRI. IEEE Trans Med Imaging 33 (3):668–681
15. Lohmann G, Bohn S, Müller K, Trampel R, Turner R (2010) Image restoration and spatial resolution in 7-Tesla magnetic resonance imaging. Magn Reson Med 64(1):15–22
16. Fletcher PT (2004) Statistical variability in nonlinear spaces: application to shape analysis and DT-MRI, Ph.D. thesis. University of North Carolina at Chapel Hill, Chapel Hill, NC
17. Tabelow K, Polzehl J, Spokoiny V, Voss HU (2008) Diffusion tensor imaging: structural adaptive smoothing. Neuroimage 39:1763–1773
18. Becker SMA, Tabelow K, Voss HU, Anwander A, Heidemann RM, Polzehl J (2012) Position-orientation adaptive smoothing of diffusion weighted magnetic resonance data (POAS). Med Image Anal 16 (6):1142–1155
19. Becker SMA, Tabelow K, Mohammadi S, Weiskopf N, Polzehl J (2014) Adaptive smoothing of multi-shell diffusion-weighted magnetic resonance data by msPOAS. Neuroimage 95:90–105
20. Aja-Fernández S, Niethammer M, Kubicki M, Shenton ME, Westin C-F (2008) Restoration of DWI data using a Rician LMMSE estimator. IEEE Trans Med Imaging 27:1389–1403
21. Tristán-Vega A, Aja-Fernández S (2010) DWI filtering using joint information for DTI and HARDI. Med Image Anal 14(2):205–218
22. Buades A, Coll B, Morel J (2005) A non-local algorithm for image denoising. In: IEEE Computer Society conference on computer vision and pattern recognition (CVPR'05), San Diego, CA, vol 2. IEEE Computer Society, Washington, DC, pp 60–65
23. Wiest-Daesslé N, Prima S, Coupe P, Morrissey SP, Barillot C (2007) Nonlocal means variants for denoising of diffusion-weighted and diffusion tensor MRI. MICCAI 10(2):344–351
24. Tomasi C, Manduchi R (1998) Bilateral filtering for gray and color images. In: Proceedings of the sixth international conference on computer vision (ICCV '98). IEEE Computer Society, Washington, DC
25. Bouhrara M, Bonny J-M, Ashinsky BG, Maring MC, Spencer RG (2017) Noise estimation and reduction in multispectral magnetic resonance images. IEEE Trans Med Imaging 36 (1):181–193
26. National Electrical Manufacturers Association (2001) Determination of signal-to-noise ratio (SNR) in diagnostic magnetic resonance imaging. NEMA standards publication MS 1–200. NEMA, Arlington, VA
27. Henkelman RM (1985) Measurement of signal intensities in the presence of noise in MR images. Med Phys 12(2):232–233
28. Coupe P, Yger P, Prima S, Hellier P, Kervrann C, Barillot C (2008) An optimized blockwise nonlocal means denoising filter for 3-D magnetic resonance images. IEEE Trans Med Imaging 27(4):425–441
29. Constantinides CD, Atalar E, McVeigh ER (1997) Signal-to-noise measurements in magnitude images from NMR phased arrays. Magn Reson Med 38(5):852–857

3

Analysis Protocol for Dynamic Contrast Enhanced (DCE) MRI of Renal Perfusion and Filtration

Frank G. Zöllner, Walter Dastrù, Pietro Irrera, Dario Livio Longo, Kevin M. Bennett, Scott C. Beeman, G. Larry Bretthorst, and Joel R. Garbow

Abstract

Here we present an analysis protocol for dynamic contrast enhanced magnetic resonance imaging (DCE-MRI) data of the kidneys. It covers comprehensive steps to facilitate signal to contrast agent concentration mapping via T_1 mapping and the calculation of renal perfusion and filtration parametric maps using model-free approaches, model free analysis using deconvolution, the Toft's model and a Bayesian approach.

This chapter is based upon work from the COST Action PARENCHIMA, a community-driven network funded by the European Cooperation in Science and Technology (COST) program of the European Union, which aims to improve the reproducibility and standardization of renal MRI biomarkers. This analysis protocol chapter is complemented by two separate chapters describing the basic concept and experimental procedure.

Keywords Magnetic resonance imaging (MRI), Dynamic contrast enhanced (DCE), Contrast agent, Kidney, Mice, Rats, Deconvolution, Toft's model, T_1 mapping, Perfusion, Filtration

1 Introduction

Contrast enhanced imaging is based on the use of endogenous tracers (or contrast agents) with para- or ferromagnetic properties and was proposed in the mid-1980s. The aim was to measure or derive the tissue perfusion and capillary permeability from the signal changes caused by the tracer. Based on the employed imaging technique, this concept is called dynamic susceptibility contrast (DSC) or dynamic contrast-enhanced (DCE) MRI whereby the first is used in conjunction with T_2-weighted imaging techniques whereas the latter is used in T_1-weighted imaging. During such DCE-MRI exams a signal time curve (STC) is recorded that reflects the passage of the tracer through tissue and therefore also the perfusion and filtration of the renal tissue. To analyze the tracer kinetics and the STC various approaches were proposed comprising semiquantitative, model-free, and model based approaches which will be outlined in this chapter [1–6].

Theoretical considerations and acquisition protocols are detailed in the chapters by Pedersen M et al. "Dynamic Contrast Enhancement (DCE) MRI–Derived Renal Perfusion and Filtration: Basic Concepts" and by Irrera P et al. "Dynamic Contrast Enhanced (DCE) MRI-Derived Renal Perfusion and Filtration: Experimental Protocol."

A typical workflow for analyzing DCE-MRI data and for calculating parametric maps of renal perfusion and filtration comprises the segmentation of the kidney and the delineation of the arterial input function (AIF), calculation of T_1 maps to convert voxel-wise STCs to concentration time curves (CTC), model selection, and eventually the calculation of perfusion and filtration parameters [7–10]. There are several existing software packages that can calculate renal perfusion and filtration from a dynamic contrast enhanced MRI scan. However, none of the packages provide a complete solution so that the user has to select the package(s) that fit(s) his needs most.

This analysis protocol chapter is complemented by two separate chapters describing the basic concept and experimental procedure, which are part of this book.

This chapter is part of the book Pohlmann A, Niendorf T (eds) (2020) Preclinical MRI of the Kidney—Methods and Protocols. Springer, New York.

2 Materials

2.1 Software Requirements

The methods described in this chapter require the following software tools:

1. A recent version of the DICOM workstation OsiriX (www.pixmeo.com) or Horos (https://horosproject.org/).
2. UMMPerfusion Plugin version 1.5.3 (http://www.opossumm.de/redmine/projects/ummperfusion).
3. Bayesian Data-Analysis Toolbox (a working manual of the entire Bayesian Data-Analysis Toolbox, including server- and client-side installation and operation instructions, descriptions and operating instructions for software packages and an overview of Bayesian Probability Theory can be found at: http://bayes.wustl.edu/Manual/BayesManual.pdf). Information on server-side and client-side configurations may be found below in **Notes 1** and **2**.

2.2 Source Data: Format Requirements and Quality Check

2.2.1 Input Requirements

To analyze preclinical data with UMMPerfusion, the image data need to be converted into DICOM prior to the analysis [11, 12]. It is recommended to convert DICOM to NIFTI first, then use the NIFTI images for all processing within ROCKETSHIP [13]. Data can be imported into DCE@ur-Lab from DICOM format, Bruker Biospin MRI data format (http://www.bruker.com/products/mr/mri.html), as well as from binary unformatted data [14]. MITK-model fit can import various data formats like DICOM or NIFTI [15].

2.2.2 Prequality Check

Visual inspection is required to check that all slices are aligned as time advances. Slices with clear motion artifacts should be removed. More robustly, data with slight movements can be recovered by coregistration images to suitable baseline image(s).

3 Methods

3.1 Segmentation

For the calculation of whole kidney GFR it is necessary to segment the kidneys and to determine their volume.

3.2 T_1 Mapping

According to the software chosen for performing the analysis the series of images acquired may be converted to a convenient format (e.g., DICOM).

The calculations should be performed only on the pixels obtained from renal segmentation (*see* Subheading 3.1).

More detailed descriptions of T_1 mapping calculations are described in the chapter by Garteiser P et al. "Analysis Protocols for MRI Mapping of Renal T_1."

3.2.1 VTR Analysis

For the analysis of the VTR images a pixel-by-pixel fitting procedure is used to fit the intensities of every renal pixel in the images as a function of TR against the following signal equation

$$S = A + S_o\left(1 - e^{-\mathrm{TR}/T_1}\right) \tag{1}$$

where TR is the repetition time, A is a bias intensity, and S_0 is the intensity once reached a plateau.

For every pixel a T_1 value can be obtained according to the fitting of Eq. 1 (an example of T_1 map fitting within the Bruker Paravision® software is shown in Fig. 1).

3.2.2 VFA Analysis

For the analysis of the VFA images a pixel by pixel fitting procedure is used to fit the intensities of every renal pixel in the images as a function of FA against the following signal equation

$$S = A + S_o\left[\frac{\sin \mathrm{FA} \times \left(1 - e^{-\mathrm{TR}/T_1}\right)}{1 - \cos \mathrm{FA} \times e^{-\mathrm{TR}/T_1}}\right] \tag{2}$$

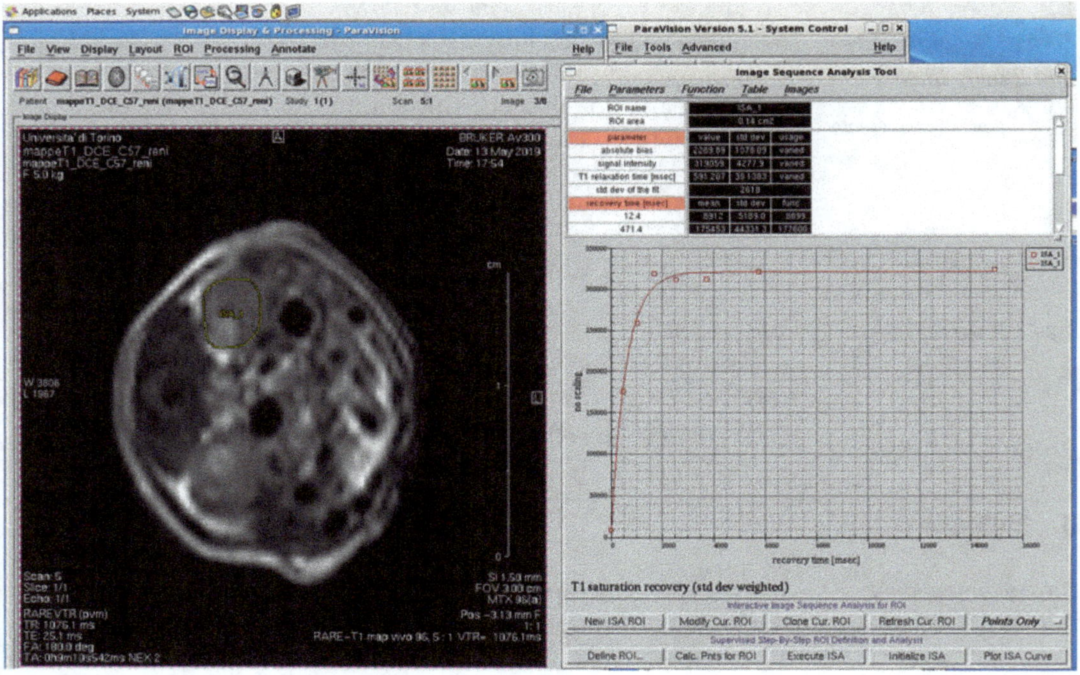

Fig. 1 T_1 map fitting under the VTR scheme performed within the Bruker Paravision 5.1® software for a selected ROI

where FA is the flip angle, TR is the repetition time, A is a bias intensity and S_0 is the intensity reached a plateau.

For every pixel a T_1 value can be obtained according to the fitting of Eq. 2.

3.3 Model Selection and Quantification

Several methods for DCE-MRI analysis have been proposed, with different mathematical representation of physiologic system interpretation through kinetic modeling [1]. Due to the large number of these methods and models, herein we describe only those that are mostly used and that can be easily exploited due to the availability of free software for these analyses. Among them we will consider deconvolution approaches (*see* Subheading 3.4) and extended Toft's model (*see* Subheading 3.5). In addition, a description on how to select the best model based on Bayesian approaches according to the acquired data is also provided (*see* Subheading 3.6).

3.4 Deconvolution Approach

The following steps are based on the UMMPerfusion plugin [12] and the DICOM workstation OsiriX.

1. Open the dataset in the Osirix 4D-viewer (*see* **Note 3**):
2. OsiriX will check if the data selected are a 4D data set (3D spatial plus 1D temporal), however, sometimes this internal check fails. Therefore, an intermediate step might be

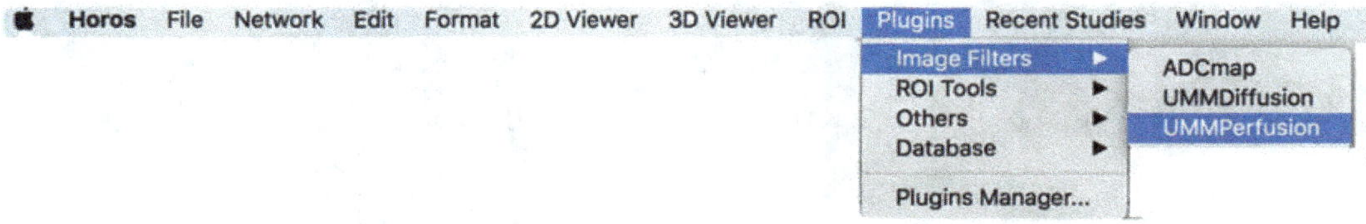

Fig. 2 Selecting the UMMPerfusion plugin from the plugin menu of OsiriX

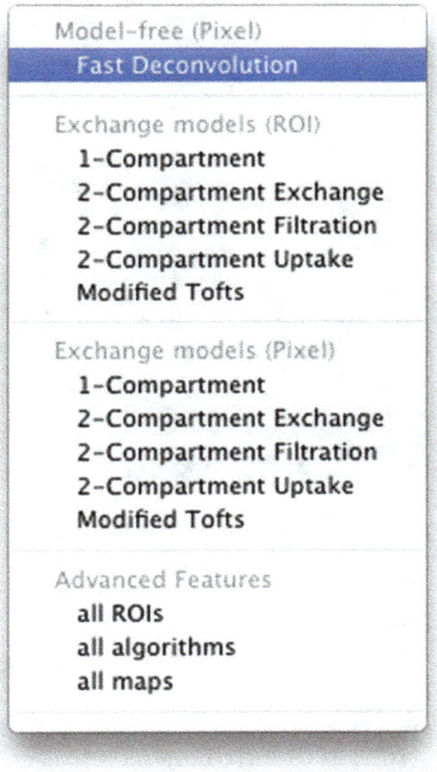

Fig. 3 UMMperfusion drop down menu to select a perfusion model

necessary to load the data into the UMMPerfusion plugin. To do so, select the series in the database window. Press the Alt-Key and click the 2D-viewer's icon at the same time. A window will open. Select/click on the 4D-viewer button, the series will appear within the 4D viewer, although it was not designed for it initially.

3. Start the plugin via the Osirix plugin menu (*see* Fig. 2):

   Plugins → image filter → UMMPerfusion

4. Select algorithm from the tool bar (*see* Fig. 3).

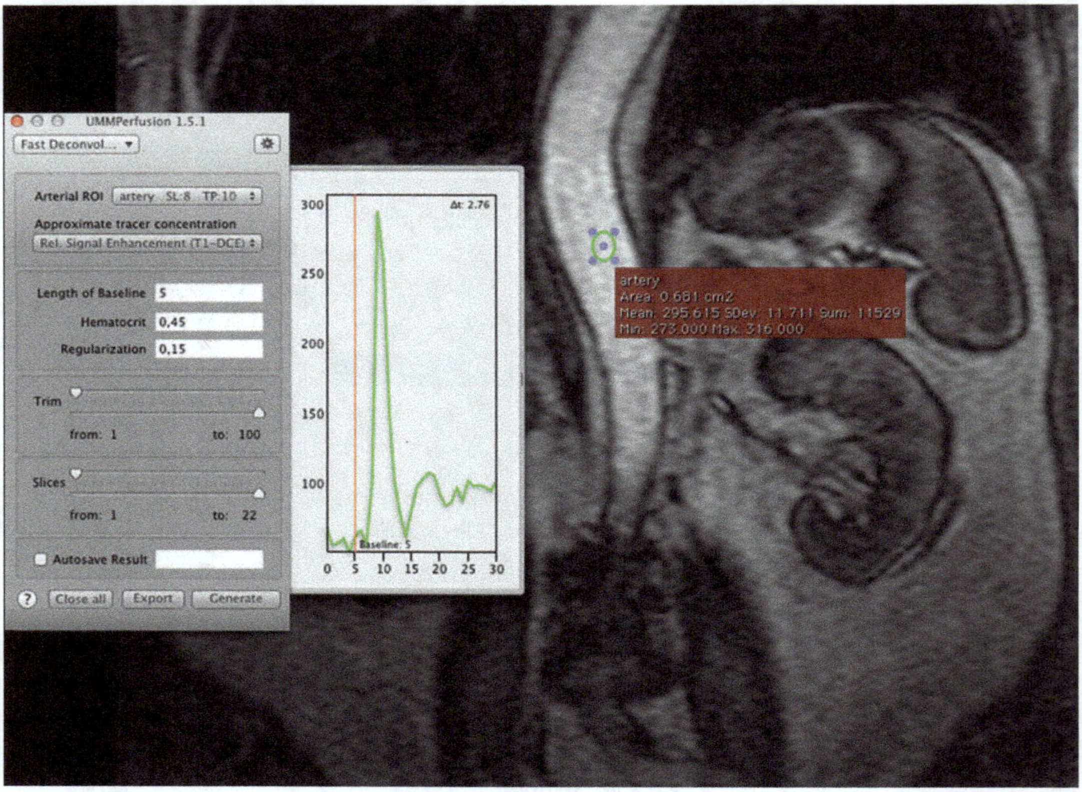

Fig. 4 Example of placing a ROI to select the AIF. The AIF is displayed as a chart next to the plugin

5. Place a ROI on a clearly visible artery in order to receive an arterial input function.
6. For ensuring correct results all algorithms require an arterial input function (AIF). This function is defined by using the Osirix ROI-tool and by placing/designating a "region of interest" (ROI) on the abdominal artery. An oval is used as a standard, however all ROI-tools offered by Osirix are supported by UMMPerfusion.
7. Upon placing a ROI, a chart will appear on the right-hand side of the plugin window, depicting the arterial input function. The aif-color corresponds to the current ROI border color, whereas the vertical line, the base line will always be in red. When a ROI is created, it will be attached to the popup-menu. If several ROIs have been created within this dataset, the desired ROI has to be assigned to its determined position. If only one pixel shall be the source of the AIF, the ROI-Brush-Tool with the size of 1px is to be used in order to specify the smallest ROI possible (Fig. 4).

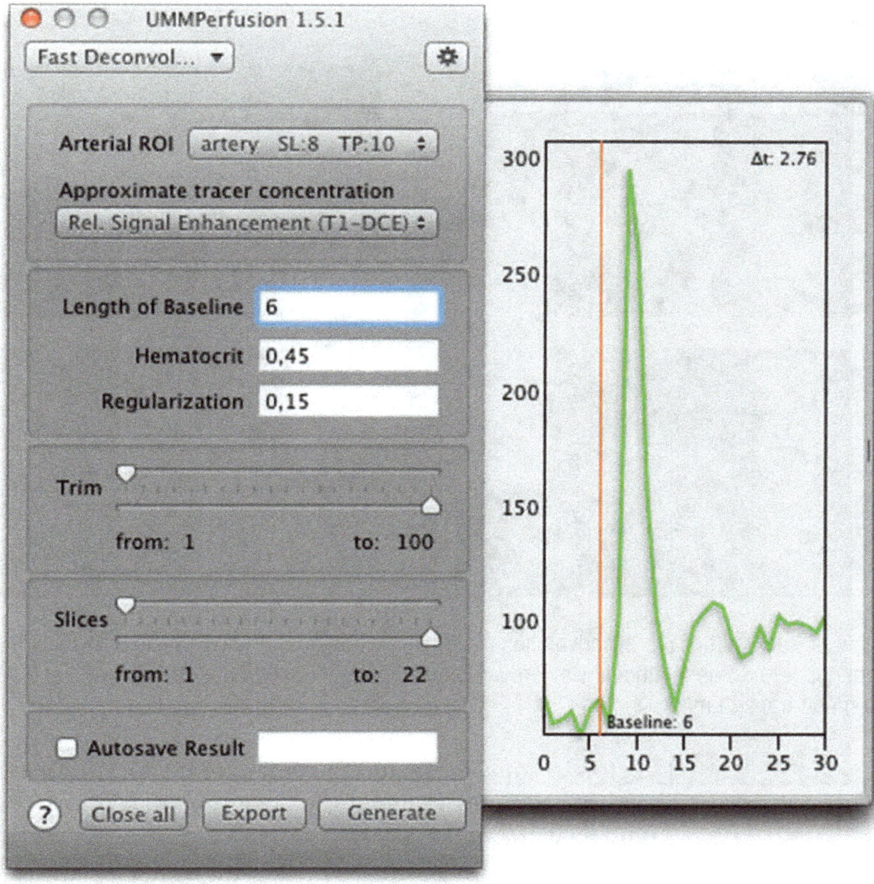

Fig. 5 Selection of the baseline

8. Make sure that the desired ROI is selected in the popup menu called "Arterial."
9. A good ROI selection can be recognized by a large peak on the chart to the right of the plugin-window.
10. Drag the baseline to a desired position or simply enter the value in the respective text field.
11. The length of baseline represents the number of images during a certain period of time that are used for signal normalization. For attaining correct results, the baseline should be chosen in a way that the tracer is not yet visible at that point of time. The easiest way to set the baseline is to drag the baseline with the mouse to its desired timeframe in the AIF-chart. The value can alternatively be inserted into the baseline textfield (*see* **Note 4**, and Fig. 5).
12. Set limits to the relevant scope by using the trim-sliders if necessary.

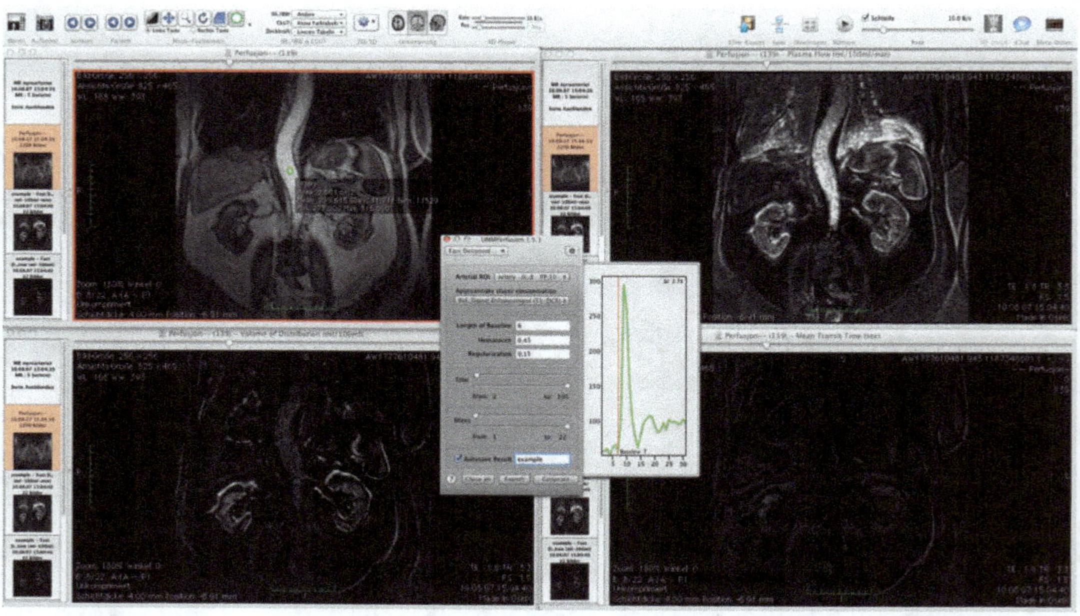

Fig. 6 Example of the result of the deconvolution model implemented in UMMPerfusion. Besides the original DCE-MRI data (top left), three additional viewers are opened presenting parametric maps of blood flow, blood volume, and mean transit time

13. Before hitting the generate-button, there is the opportunity to activate the autosave-checkbox to automatically save the results and to generate a report.
14. The calculation begins after using the generate-button.
15. As a result, three new views/viewers are created in which the calculated data are presented. Each viewer shows one parametric map calculated by the deconvolution approach: blood flow (perfusion) in ml/100 ml/min, the blood volume (ml/100 ml) and the mean transit time (s) (Fig. 6).
16. If the autosave function has not been activated before using the generate button, it is still possible to save the results as well as the report after the calculation. In this case, use the export button next to the generate-button.

3.5 Toft's Model

Three open source packages for renal perfusion and filtration quantification implement the Toft's model, namely, UMMPerfusion [12], ROCKETSHIP [13], MITK-model fit [15], and DCE@urLAB [14]. In the following, the processing steps are given for UMMPerfusion; however, the other three tools can be used in exchange. For details on using them please refer to the respective documentation.

1. Open the dataset in the Osirix 4D-viewer.

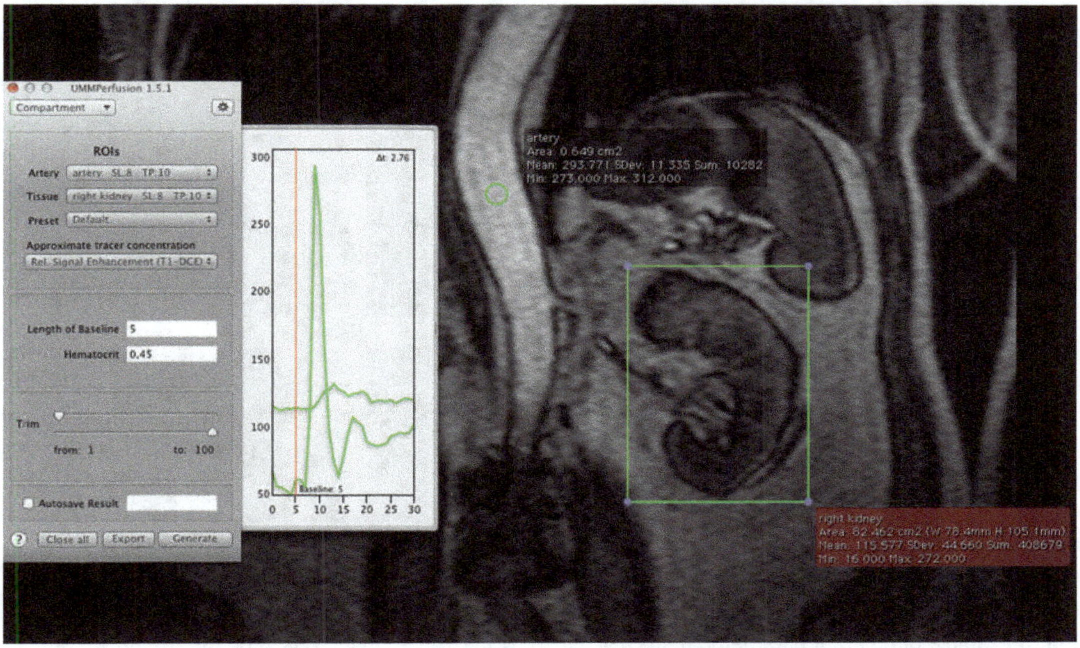

Fig. 7 Example of rectangular ROI placed tight around the kidney. Within this ROI, a voxel-wise fit of the Toft's model is performed, all pixels outside the ROI are not considered

2. Start the plugin via the Osirix plugin menu:
   Plugins → image filter → UMMPerfusion.
3. Select algorithm from the tool bar.
   UMMperfusion implements the extended Toft's model. It can be calculated either ROI-based (*see* **Note 5**) or pixel-wise. The latter is described in the following.
4. Place a ROI on a clearly visible artery in order to receive an arterial input function. The recommended shape of the ROI is oval.
   Please *see* Subheading 3.4 for more details.
5. Place a rectangular ROI on the relevant tissue. When using the pixel-based compartment model algorithms, only a rectangular ROI shape is supported at the moment by UMMPerfusion.
6. The pixelwise calculation might require some time to calculate. To save time, the ROI should be accurately fitting around the tissue that is to be analyzed (*see* Fig. 7).
7. The arterial-ROI and the tissue-ROI do not have to be on the same slice.
8. Make sure that the desired arterial-ROI is selected in the popup menu called "Arterial."
9. Make sure that the desired tissue-ROI is selected in the popup menu called "Tissue."

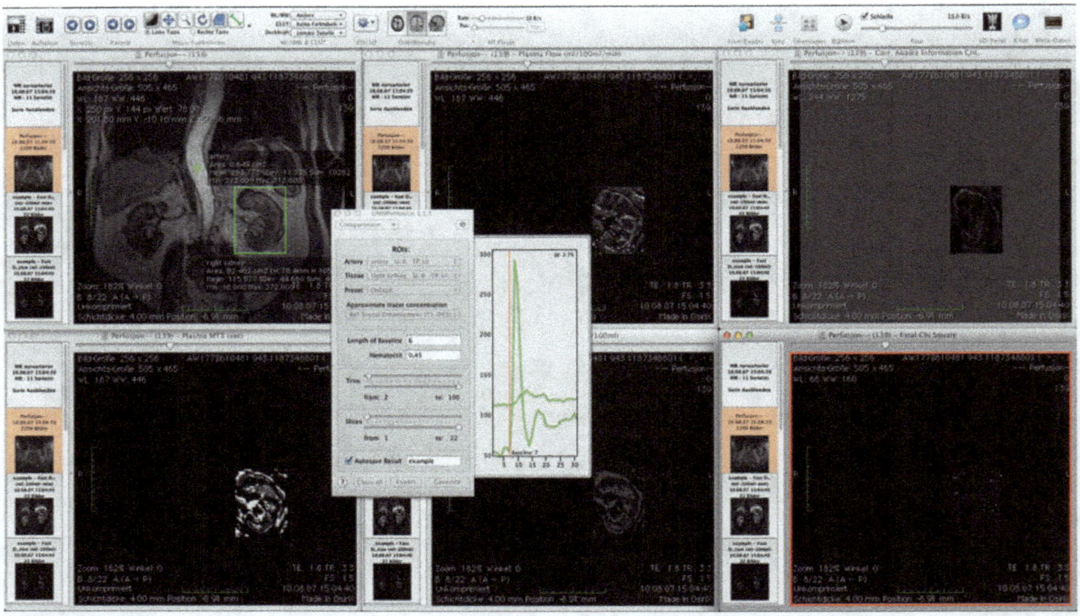

Fig. 8 Example of different parametric maps calculated by the Toft's model. Based on the ROI drawn around the kidney, only voxels within this ROI are used during model fit. Voxels outside the ROI are not taken into account

10. Select the tracer approximation, baseline, and spatiotemporal trimming of the data as described in Subheading 3.4.
11. The calculation begins after using the generate-button. A new window will appear, in which the desired viewers (parametric maps) can be chosen.
12. Upon approval with the OK button the selected viewers will appear and show the specified area (*see* Fig. 8).
13. If the autosave function has not been activated before using the generate button, it is still possible to save the results, as well as the report. In that case, use the export button next to the generate-button. The dataset's name will be appended on your specified name.

3.6 Bayesian Model Selection

3.6.1 Analyzing Regions of Interest Data Using the Enter ASCII Model Package

From the client-side Java interface:

1. Select the "enter ASCII Model" option under the "Package" menu.
2. Load your signal model.
   - Your own signal model can be loaded using the "User" button (links to the client-side .../Bayes/BayesAsciiModels folder, where you should store you model and parameter files).

- A prepackaged "System" model can be loaded using the "System" button (links to Server-side models).

3. Load ASCII data using widgets.
   - File → Load ASII → File.
   - Data file must be in ASCII format.
   - Data are typically in 2-column ASCII format (abscissa, ordinate), however, the software package allows both multicolumn abscissas and ordinates.
4. Build your model using the "Build" button.
5. OPTIONAL: If you believe that your data contains outliers, you can check the "Find Outliers" option under "Analysis Options."
6. Under the "Prior Viewer" tab, review your user-defined prior probability distributions and parameter ranges.
7. If you have multiple servers running the Bayesian Data-Analysis Toolbox, select the desired server for processing the analysis using the "Select" button.
8. OPTIONAL: You can check the status of the selected server using the "Status" button.
9. Run the analysis using the "Run" button.
10. You can monitor the status of the analysis using the Status button or the button bearing a picture of an eye at the bottom left of the window.
11. Once the analysis is complete, retrieve the results using the "Get Job" button or the job will be automatically retrieved when the job status is checked and the job is completed.

3.6.2 Model Selection and Analysis of Region of Interest Data Using the Enter ASCII Model Selection Package

From the client-side Java interface:

1. Select the "enter ASCII Model Selection" option under the "Package" menu.
2. Load all of the signal models that you would like to compare.
   - Your own signal models can be loaded using the "User" button (links to the client-side ../Bayes/BayesAsciiModels folder, where a model and parameter files are stored).
   - Prepackaged "System" models can be loaded using the "System" button (links to Server-side models).
3. Load your data.
   - File → Load ASII → File.
   - Data file must be in ASCII format.
   - Data are typically in 2-column ASCII format (abscissa, ordinate), however, the software package allows for

multicolumn data and abscissaes (See the Bayesian Data-Analysis Toolbox manual, Appendix A for details).

4. Build your models using the "Build" button.
5. OPTIONAL: If you believe that your data contain outliers, you can check the "Find Outliers" option under "Analysis Options."
6. Under the "Fortran/C Model Viewer" → "Parameters" tabs, review your user-defined prior probability distributions.
7. If you have multiple servers running the Bayesian Data-Analysis Toolbox, select desired server for processing the analysis using the "Select" button.
8. OPTIONAL: You can check the status of the selected server using the "Status" button.
9. Run the analysis using the "Run" button.
10. You can monitor the status of the analysis with the Button bearing a picture of an eye at the bottom left of the window, or using the status button.
11. Once the analysis is complete, retrieve the results using the "Get Job" button. The job is automatically retrieved when the job status is checked and the job is completed.

3.7 Voxel-Wise Image Analysis

3.7.1 Analyzing Image Data Using the Analyze Image Pixels Package

From the client-side Java interface:

1. Select the "Analyze Image Pixels" option under the "Package" menu.
2. Load your signal model.
   - Your own signal model can be loaded using the "User" button (links to the client-side ../Bayes/BayesAsciiModels folder, where you should store you model and parameter files).
   - A prepackaged "System" model can be loaded using the "System" button (links to Server-side models).
3. Load your data.
   - File → Load Image.
   - Select the file format of your data.
4. Load an abscissa file (your vector specifying the time at which data were collected, *b*-values, echo times, etc.).
5. Set the noise standard deviation of the data.
   - An acceptable approximation of the noise standard deviation for this purpose would be to draw an ROI in a region of no signal of an image and input the RMS value of this ROI. Tools to make this measurement are available in the main window once data have been loaded—Do not use the standard deviation of the data.

6. Compile your signal model using the “Build” button.
7. OPTIONAL: If you believe that your data contains outliers, you can check the “Find Outliers” option under “Analysis Options.”
8. OPTIONAL: If you want a much faster analysis, you can select the “Max Probability” option. The option comes at the cost of only returning the max probability parameter value. No posterior probability distribution information is available if you use this option.
9. Under the “Prior Viewer” tab, review the prior probability distributions.
10. If you have multiple servers running the Bayesian Data-Analysis Toolbox, select desired server for processing the analysis using the “Select” button.
11. OPTIONAL: You can check the status of the selected server using the “Status” button.
12. Run the analysis using the “Run” button.
13. You can monitor the status of the analysis with the status button or the button bearing a picture of an eye at the bottom left of the window.
14. Once the analysis is complete, retrieve the results using the “Get Job” button. The job is automatically retrieved when the job status is checked and the job is completed.

3.7.2 Model Selection and Analysis of Image Data Using the Image Model Selection Package

From the client-side Java interface:

1. Select the “Analyze Image Pixels” option under the “Package” menu.
2. Load all of the signal models that you would like to compare.
   - Your own signal models can be loaded using the “User” button (links to the client-side ../Bayes/BayesAsciiModels folder, where you should store you model and parameter files).
   - Prepackaged “System” models can be loaded using the “System” button (links to Server-side models).
3. Load your data.
   - File → Load Image.
   - Select the file format of your images.
4. Load an abscissa file (your vector specifying the time at which data were collected, *b*-values, echo times, etc.).
5. Set the noise standard deviation of the data.
   - An acceptable approximation of the noise standard deviation for this purpose would be to draw an ROI in a region of no

signal of an image and input the RMS value of this ROI. Tools to make this measurement are available in the main window once data have been loaded.

6. Build your signal models using the "Build" button.
7. Under the "Fortran/C Model Viewer" → "Parameters" tabs, review your user-defined prior probability distributions.
8. If you have multiple servers running the Bayesian Data-Analysis Toolbox, select desired server for processing the analysis using the "Select" button.
9. OPTIONAL: You can check the status of the selected server using the "Status" button.
10. Run the analysis using the "Run" button.
11. You can monitor the status of the analysis using the status button, or with the Button bearing a picture of an eye at the bottom left of the window.
12. Once the analysis is complete, retrieve the results using the "Get Job" button. The job is automatically retrieved when the job status is checked and the job is completed.

3.8 Results Validation

3.8.1 Evaluation of Analysis Errors and Variability Using Synthetic Data

UMMPerfusion has been in-house certified by the authors and comes with a set of simulated data to test the technical validity of the algorithms. Also, the other software packages provide example data for testing. The Bayesian Data-Analysis Toolbox provides an estimation of uncertainty, even for a single measurement and it has been validated with simulated data for which ground truth is known [4].

Table 1
Values of renal blood flow (RBF) reported in the literature for different animal models and field strengths

Animal model	RBF (ml/100 ml/min)	Field strength, T	Reference
Lewis rats		3	Zimmer et al. [16]
Healthy	542 ± 85		
AKI	407 ± 119		
SD rats		3	Sadick et al. [17]
Healthy	440 ± 86		
PKD	156 ± 40		
PCK	69 ± 23		
Swiss mice		7	Oostendorp et al. [18]
Healthy	481 ± 26		
AKI	451 ± 24		

AKI acute kidney injury, *PKD* polycystic kidney disease, *PCK* autosomal polycystic kidney disease

3.8.2 Comparison with Reference Values from the Literature

Table 1 surveys reference values from the literature for renal blood flow in small rodents. Please note that these values might vary versus those obtained by the reader following this chapter due to different AIF selection and acquisition parameters.

4 Notes

1. Recommended server configuration and server-side installation of the Bayesian Data-Analysis Toolbox: Multicore LinuxPC (32 or 64 cores); 32- or 64-bit processor; Operating system: Linux (CentOS 4.7 or higher) or Sun Solaris 9 or 10; Installing Fortran and C is strongly recommended (required to build and analyze data with your own signal model). Server-side installation instruction can be found at: http://bayesiananalysis.wustl.edu/install.html.
2. Recommended client-side configuration for the Bayesian Data-Analysis Toolbox: any operating system that can run Java 6 or higher. Note that the client machine only runs a Java graphical user interface that the sends and receives jobs from the server-side Bayesian Data-Analysis Toolbox. Through this interface, data can be loaded and visualized, mathematical models can be written in Fortran and tested, jobs can be sent to the server-side software for analysis, and completed jobs can be retrieved from the server-side Bayesian Data-Analysis Toolbox and visualized.
3. If T_1-mapping is available, please convert signal intensities to concentrations beforehand and save this back into DICOM files.
4. If concentration time curves are used, please select the option "Signal enhancement."
5. For examples to perform ROI based analysis with UMMperfusion please see http://www.opossumm.de/redmine/projects/ummperfusion/wiki/Tutorials__How_to_.

Acknowledgments

The Italian Ministry for Education and Research (MIUR) is gratefully acknowledged for yearly FOE funding to the Euro-BioImaging Multi-Modal Molecular Imaging Italian Node (MMMI).

This chapter is based upon work from COST Action PARENCH IMA, supported by European Cooperation in Science and Technology (COST). COST (www.cost.eu) is a funding agency for research and innovation networks. COST Actions help connect research initiatives across Europe and enable scientists to enrich their ideas by sharing them with their peers. This boosts their research, career, and innovation.

PARENCHIMA (renalmri.org) is a community-driven Action in the COST program of the European Union, which unites more than 200 experts in renal MRI from 30 countries with the aim to improve the reproducibility and standardization of renal MRI biomarkers.

References

1. Sourbron SP, Buckley DL (2013) Classic models for dynamic contrast-enhanced MRI. NMR Biomed 26(8):1004–1027. https://doi.org/10.1002/nbm.2940
2. Sourbron S, Dujardin M, Makkat S, Luypaert R (2007) Pixel-by-pixel deconvolution of bolus-tracking data: optimization and implementation. Phys Med Biol 52(2):429–447. https://doi.org/10.1088/0031-9155/52/2/009
3. Duan C, Kallehauge JF, Bretthorst GL, Tanderup K, Ackerman JJ, Garbow JR (2017) Are complex DCE-MRI models supported by clinical data? Magn Reson Med 77(3):1329–1339. https://doi.org/10.1002/mrm.26189
4. Beeman SC, Osei-Owusu P, Duan C, Engelbach J, Bretthorst GL, Ackerman JJH, Blumer KJ, Garbow JR (2015) Renal DCE-MRI model selection using Bayesian Probability Theory. Tomography 1(1):61–68. https://doi.org/10.18383/j.tom.2015.00133
5. Sourbron SP, Michaely HJ, Reiser MF, Schoenberg SO (2008) MRI-measurement of perfusion and glomerular filtration in the human kidney with a separable compartment model. Investig Radiol 43(1):40–48. https://doi.org/10.1097/RLI.0b013e31815597c5
6. Baumann D, Rudin M (2000) Quantitative assessment of rat kidney function by measuring the clearance of the contrast agent Gd(DOTA) using dynamic MRI. Magn Reson Imaging 18(5):587–595
7. Eikefjord E, Andersen E, Hodneland E, Hanson EA, Sourbron S, Svarstad E, Lundervold A, Rørvik JT (2017) Dynamic contrast-enhanced MRI measurement of renal function in healthy participants. Acta Radiol 58(6):748–757. https://doi.org/10.1177/0284185116666417
8. Ebrahimi B, Textor SC, Lerman LO (2014) Renal relevant radiology: renal functional magnetic resonance imaging. Clin J Am Soc Nephrol. https://doi.org/10.2215/CJN.02900313
9. Sourbron SPMH, Reiser MF, Schoenberg SO (2008) MRI-measurement of perfusion and glomerular filtration in the human kidney with a separable compartment model. Invest Radiol 43(1):40–48
10. Buckley DL, Shurrab AE, Cheung CM, Jones AP, Mamtora H, Kalra PA (2006) Measurement of single kidney function using dynamic contrast-enhanced MRI: comparison of two models in human subjects. J Magn Reson Imaging 24(5):1117–1123. https://doi.org/10.1002/jmri.20699
11. Zollner FG, Daab M, Sourbron SP, Schad LR, Schoenberg SO, Weisser G (2016) An open source software for analysis of dynamic contrast enhanced magnetic resonance images: UMM-Perfusion revisited. BMC Med Imaging 16:7. https://doi.org/10.1186/s12880-016-0109-0
12. Zollner FG, Weisser G, Reich M, Kaiser S, Schoenberg SO, Sourbron SP, Schad LR (2013) UMMPerfusion: an open source software tool towards quantitative MRI perfusion analysis in clinical routine. J Digit Imaging 26(2):344–352. https://doi.org/10.1007/s10278-012-9510-6
13. Barnes SR, Ng TS, Santa-Maria N, Montagne A, Zlokovic BV, Jacobs RE (2015) ROCKETSHIP: a flexible and modular software tool for the planning, processing and analysis of dynamic MRI studies. BMC Med Imaging 15:19. https://doi.org/10.1186/s12880-015-0062-3
14. Ortuno JE, Ledesma-Carbayo MJ, Simoes RV, Candiota AP, Arus C, Santos A (2013) DCE@urLAB: a dynamic contrast-enhanced MRI pharmacokinetic analysis tool for

preclinical data. BMC Bioinformatics 14:316. https://doi.org/10.1186/1471-2105-14-316

15. Debus C, Floca R, Ingrisch M, Kompan I, Maier-Hein K, Abdollahi A, Nolden M (2019) MITK-ModelFit: a generic open-source framework for model fits and their exploration in medical imaging - design, implementation and application on the example of DCE-MRI. BMC Bioinformatics 20(1):31. https://doi.org/10.1186/s12859-018-2588-1
16. Zimmer F, Zollner FG, Hoeger S, Klotz S, Tsagogiorgas C, Kramer BK, Schad LR (2013) Quantitative renal perfusion measurements in a rat model of acute kidney injury at 3T: testing inter- and intramethodical significance of ASL and DCE-MRI. PLoS One 8(1). https://doi.org/10.1371/journal.pone.0053849
17. Sadick M, Schock D, Kraenzlin B, Gretz N, Schoenberg SO, Michaely HJ (2009) Morphologic and dynamic renal imaging with assessment of glomerular filtration rate in a pcy-mouse model using a clinical 3.0 Tesla scanner. Investig Radiol 44(8):469–475. https://doi.org/10.1097/RLI.0b013e3181a8afa1
18. Oostendorp M, de Vries EE, Slenter JM, Peutz-Kootstra CJ, Snoeijs MG, Post MJ, van Heurn LW, Backes WH (2011) MRI of renal oxygenation and function after normothermic ischemia-reperfusion injury. NMR Biomed 24(2):194–200. https://doi.org/10.1002/nbm.1572

4

Analysis Methods for Hyperpolarized Carbon (^{13}C) MRI of the Kidney

Galen D. Reed, Natalie J. Korn, Christoffer Laustsen, and Cornelius von Morze

Abstract

Hyperpolarized ^{13}C MR is a novel medical imaging modality with substantially different signal dynamics as compared to conventional ^{1}H MR, thus requiring new methods for processing the data in order to access and quantify the embedded metabolic and functional information. Here we describe step-by-step analysis protocols for functional renal hyperpolarized ^{13}C imaging. These methods are useful for investigating renal blood flow and function as well as metabolic status of rodents in vivo under various experimental physiological conditions.

This chapter is based upon work from the COST Action PARENCHIMA, a community-driven network funded by the European Cooperation in Science and Technology (COST) program of the European Union, which aims to improve the reproducibility and standardization of renal MRI biomarkers. This analysis protocol chapter is complemented by two separate chapters describing the basic concept and experimental procedure.

Key words Magnetic resonance imaging (MRI), Kidney, Mice, Rats, Hyperpolarization, ^{13}C, Dynamic nuclear polarization (DNP)

1 Introduction

Hyperpolarized ^{13}C imaging experiments can yield a wide variety of metabolic, structural, and functional information which is extracted via analysis of time-varying NMR signals. The choice of analysis strategy depends on numerous factors, including the imaging agent, the organ of interest, the acquisition strategy, and imaging parameter being measured. In general, much of the image-formation pipelines are nearly identical to those for ^{1}H MRI; particularly, the steps of Fourier transforming k-space data, reconstructing under-sampled data using parallel imaging afforded by RF coil arrays, etc. are nearly identical and will not be discussed in detail here. Instead, we describe some of the applications more specific to hyperpolarized ^{13}C data analysis, and we guide the reader through details and attempt to point out pitfalls. We select a few applications which will be interesting for researchers studying renal physiology and function in a preclinical setting, and where available, we point to links to source code for image processing pipelines.

Beginning at the steps of image formation, there are some key attributes differentiating hyperpolarized from conventional MRI. One of the primary differences is the constant depolarization of the contrast agent during imaging. Image encoding requires radio frequency (RF) excitation of z polarization that is typically nonrenewable, meaning it does not recover with T_1 relaxation. Instead, T_1 relaxation imposes an exponential decay envelope which decreases the z polarization over time. In addition to potentially degrading image resolution, this window has the consequence that physiological parameters calculated from the time course of image pixel intensity may be biased, either by RF flip angle (θ) nonuniformity or by influence of relaxation times which are almost never known precisely beforehand in vivo. In some of the subsequent examples of this chapter, this effect is accounted for, or it may be compensated for through the use of acquisition-based signal compensation. However, a thorough error propagation of parameter estimation is extremely difficult as is the estimation of all ancillary parameters influencing the measurements. For instance, although precise flip angle knowledge is key to the estimation of virtually every parameter measured here, θ is typically estimated using an external reference phantom during imaging. Furthermore, it is extremely difficult to map out the transmitter profile due to the low natural ^{13}C abundance *in vivo*. In general, the nuances of hyperpolarized MRI may complicate image processing and could potentially bias parameters that are calculated from images if not properly taken into account.

This analysis protocol chapter is complemented by two separate chapters describing the basic concept and experimental procedure, which are part of this book.

2 Materials

2.1 Software Analysis Tools

There are numerous publicly shared, open-source MRI processing code written on the MATLAB platform which can be directly ported to the open source platform GNU Octave. Processing requiring nonlinear optimization, signal processing, image manipulations, or DICOM reading/writing will require installation of additional toolboxes. Octave and MATLAB provide excellent prototyping platforms since the file input/output interface for most vendors' raw data formats can be found on online repositories or via the vendor directly. For example, the files for reading the GE P-file format are distributed with the EPIC software development kit (SDK) software release via the MR collaboration community portal

[1]. Within this SDK is the set of MATLAB scripts in the folder read_MR that may be invoked as

```
[rawdata, header] = read_MR_rawdata(filename)
```

Where filename is the name of the raw file (P-file), and rawdata and header are the parsed outputs. The variable rawdata is parsed as

```
rawdata(yres, xres, phases, echoes, slices, receivers)
```

Note that GE P-files are stored on the scanner directory /usr/g/mrraw. An example 2D Fourier Transform reconstruction of a single slice, single coil image will look like

```
singleSliceImage = abs(fftnc(rawdata(:, :, 1, 1, sliceIndex,
coilIndex)));
```

Aside from vendor-specific items, the vast majority of publicly shared source code is on a github repository. To interact with this code base, git should be loaded on your localhost. On Mac, this can be done with the MacPorts utility (www.macports.org) via terminal command

```
sudo port install git
```

Note that all MacPorts-installed code can be conveniently updated via the single command sudo port selfupdate. The example code-base for this book chapter [2] can be cloned from the github repository by running the following in your terminal:

```
git clone https://github.com/galenreed/renalC13MRIBook.git
```

This will clone the repository and create a folder called renalC13MRIBook with subfolders and scripts that can be run and modified locally.

3 Methods

3.1 Quantitative Perfusion Imaging

Noninvasive determination of perfusion has been of significant interest in contrast-enhanced MRI and has numerous applications in oncology and cerebral blood flow mapping. Unlike contrast-enhanced MRI using gadolinium (Gd) based agents, hyperpolarized ^{13}C images contain no background signal contribution and thus have the desirable characteristic that their signal intensity is proportional to the agent concentration. Commonly used hyperpolarized ^{13}C perfusion targets are [^{13}C]urea [3], [^{13}C, ^{15}N]urea

[4], bis-1,1-(hydroxymethylcyclopropane-D_8) (commonly referred to as HP001) [5], and [^{13}C]tert-butanol [6]. These molecules differ greatly in their tissue permeability [7], biodistribution, and relaxation time-based contrast [4]. Furthermore, the endogenous nature of many hyperpolarized probes makes them highly attractive as a potential agent which may be delivered to patients with impaired renal function. Data for perfusion imaging typically consist of time- and space resolved magnitude images of nonexchanging molecular probes which are acquired with gradient echo (GRE) or steady state free precession (SSFP) pulse sequences. Since the initial tissue uptake is an important piece of the curve for data processing, data acquisition is typically initiated before or at the beginning of contrast agent injection, and temporal resolution should be adequate to encode the uptake and washout curves.

In this section, we walk through the processing script example_perfusion.m that contains the essential processing elements of data from this experiment. The goal this problem is to solve the convolution integral

$$C_{\mathrm{VOI}}(t) = F\int_0^{\infty} C_{\mathrm{a}}(\tau)R(t-\tau)\mathrm{d}\tau \tag{1}$$

for the product of the residue function $R(t)$ and flow rate F. This model uses the bolus tracking theory which is described in depth in ref. 8. In this approach, the concentration of the tracer in the tissue $C_{\mathrm{VOI}}(t)$ is modeled as a convolution integral with the arterial input function $C_{\mathrm{a}}(t)$ and the residue function. Since $C_{\mathrm{VOI}}(t)$ and $C_{\mathrm{a}}(t)$ are measured directly off the time course images, the $F{\cdot}R(t)$ can be estimated via deconvolution. The product $F{\cdot}R(t)$ serves as the tissue impulse response in this framework. The essential steps in the processing pipeline are as follows:

1. Delineate the arterial pixels. In the example code, a single coordinate from the center of the artery is stored in the array AIFPixels with a single index per slice. Note that this processing script creates a rectangular ROI centered around the pixel coordinate to reduce noise. The intensity of these pixels is used as the function $C_{\mathrm{a}}(t)$.
2. Create the matrix A which whose columns consist of $C_{\mathrm{a}}(t)$, where each subsequent column is translated one time point (see line 58 in example_perfusion.m and equation 11 in ref. 8). This is for discretizing the convolution integral in order to recast it as a matrix multiplication, which can then be inverted to measure the product $F{\cdot}R(t)$. *See* refs. 8–10 for details
3. Loop through all pixels within the image and create the temporal curve to create $C_{\mathrm{VOI}}(t)$
4. Invert the linear system to estimate $F{\cdot}R(t)$. The code example gives two examples of how to do this: the first uses Tikhonov

regularization, the second uses singular value decomposition (SVD)-based thresholding.

5. Compute the maximum of this function to obtain the flow rate, then normalize by Δt to recast the value in standard mL/mL/s units.

A few nuances of the computation are discussed. The tissue residue function $R(t)$ tends to have a monotonically decreasing shape and is often approximated as a single exponential decay in model-dependent deconvolution techniques. By definition, $R(0) = 1$, since it depends on the cumulative distribution of the tracer transit times in the tissue. Therefore, the flow F can be solved for once $R(t)$ is estimated.

$$F = \frac{\max(FR(t))}{\Delta t} \tag{2}$$

Note that the maximum operation is used rather than taking the value $R(t = 0)$ to account for possible imaging/infusion delays. Hyperpolarized ^{13}C images are proportional to the concentration which simplifies the estimation of $C_{vol}(t)$ and $C_a(t)$ since they can be directly measured from image ROIs. However, the polarization level constantly decreases post injection, so the signal proportionality is not constant over time. To compensate this effect, $R(t)$ has been modelled as a product $R_t(t)P(t)$, where $R_t(t)$ is the true residue function and $P(t)$ is an exponential decay which models the T_1 decay and RF depolarization [9]. Alternatively, an acquisition-based compensation using progressively increasing flip angles on subsequent time-points can be used to offset this signal decay over a fixed horizon [10]. As ref. 8 points out, it is highly important to handle noise amplification in this inversion by using techniques such as singular value decomposition- (SVD) based thresholding or regularization. Figure 1 shows the effects of Tikhonov regularization on the calculated flow images and highlights its importance. When no regularization is used, the estimated $F{\cdot}R(t)$ product shows large oscillations over the time course. Adding regularization not only smooths the time-course curve but also yields a residue function closely resembling the expected exponential decay.

3.2 Relaxation Mapping

Preliminary measurements of NMR relaxation times (T_1 and T_2) of hyperpolarized ^{13}C contrast agents show interesting in vivo renal tissue contrast. The T_2 of [1-^{13}C]lactate after injection of hyperpolarized [1-^{13}C]pyruvate has been shown to increase in tumor regions in preclinical models [11]. The T_2 of [^{13}C, ^{15}N]urea has been shown to greatly increase in the rat kidney [4], and this signal change has been linked to the glomerular filtration process [12]. Anatomically, an inward, cortex-to-medulla T_2 gradient is observed. This gradient becomes disrupted in diabetic nephropathy

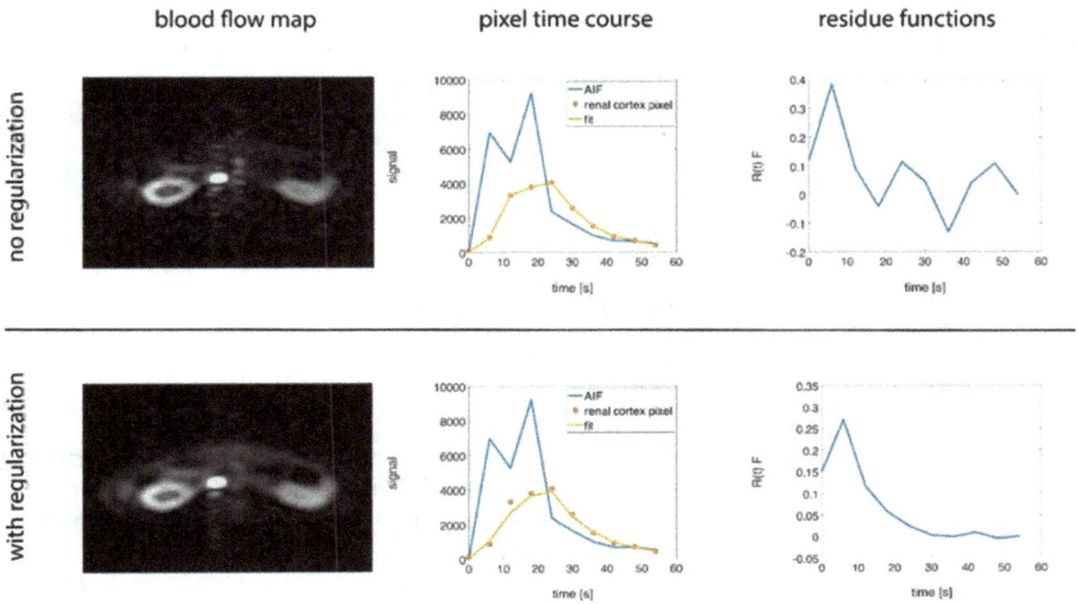

Fig. 1 Estimating blood flow from dynamic hyperpolarized [^{13}C]urea images of a rat kidney. The top and bottom panels show the problem solved with and without using regularization. The blood flow maps (left) are calculated from solving the deconvolution of the arterial input function (AIF) and the tissue uptake curves (center). Note that there is a dip in the AIF due to a chase infusion of saline. The curves on the right highlight the need for some degree of regularization. The top solution, derived without regularization, shows large-amplitude fluctuations, while the bottom curve, derived with regularization, shows a much cleaner curve more closely resembling an exponential decay. Regularization does slightly decrease curve fit/data consistency; this can be seen on the orange curves in the center plot, where the regularized curve (bottom) deviates slightly more from the nonregularized curves (top). However, it generally produces cleaner images with reduces noise sensitivity

[13] as well as in ischemic injury [14]. T_2 mapping is performed on magnitude images which are spatially and echo-time-resolved. Acquisitions are based on multiple spin-echo acquisitions that must be specifically tailored to the hyperpolarized experiment. To best utilize the nonrenewable magnetization, acquisitions start with a 90° excitation followed by a train of spin echo RF pulses and encoding gradients. Hyperpolarized ^{13}C T_2 values reported in the literature are long compared to those of ^{1}H, ranging from hundreds of milliseconds to several seconds. The effective T_2 measured can have some dependence on the inhomogeneity of the transmit field ($B_1{}^+$), but the dependency is not strong unless the deviation from 180° is very large [12].

Modeling multiexponential T_2, decay in NMR signals is typically performed by matching the signal to an expression of the form

$$S = S_0 + \sum_{i=i}^{n} a_i e^{-t/T_{2,i}} \tag{3}$$

where S_0 is a bias term, a_i is the signal amplitude of the ith T_2 component, and $T_{2,i}$ is the decay time constant. Typically, a_i and $T_{2,i}$ are all unknown beforehand and must be solved for. If SNR is sufficiently high, the bias term can be ignored. The T_2NNLS algorithm [15] casts the estimation of multiple T_2 decays as a matrix inversion problem:

$$\begin{pmatrix} S(\mathrm{TE}_1) \\ \vdots \\ S(\mathrm{TE}_n) \end{pmatrix} = \begin{pmatrix} e^{-\mathrm{TE}_1/T_{2,1}} & \cdots & e^{-\mathrm{TE}_1/T_{2,m}} \\ \vdots & \ddots & \vdots \\ e^{-\mathrm{TE}_n/T_{2,1}} & \cdots & e^{-\mathrm{TE}_n/T_{2,m}} \end{pmatrix} \begin{pmatrix} a_1 \\ \vdots \\ a_m \end{pmatrix} \quad (4)$$

Note that this is a standard problem of the form

$$y = Ax \quad (5)$$

where the matrix A is constructed from selecting m logarithmically spaced T_2 values from within a defined range, then computing an idealized T_2 decay curve sampled at each acquired echo time. These idealized single-exponential decays constitute the columns of the A matrix. The column vector x contains the amplitudes which are solved for, and y contains the measurements. Equation 5 is solved for using regularized, nonnegative least squares.

$$\underset{x}{\operatorname{argmin}} \quad \|Ax - y\|^2 + \lambda\|x\|^2 \quad (6)$$

Similar to the perfusion measurement, the use of the L2 norm for the regularization term is required as detecting multiple T_2 values that are different but close in value can be exceedingly susceptible to noise amplification.

In the example script example_t2nnls.m, the following steps are used to demonstrate the T_2 nonnegative least squares algorithm on rat kidney data:

1. Reconstruct spatially and echo-time-resolved magnitude images.
2. Is spatial resolution is sufficient to resolve respiratory motion, an image alignment via rigid translation may be applied [12].
3. Create a list of echo times (TElist in the script) corresponding to the TE of each image.
4. Create a T_2 axis which is a vector of logarithmically spaced T_2 values spanning the expected solution range.
5. Create the matrix A from Eqs. 4 and 5 as is performed in the script t2nnls.m (where the matrix is stored as the variable T2DecayMatrix).
6. Extract signal intensity of a single pixel over TEs ($S(\mathrm{TE})_1 \ldots S(\mathrm{TE})_n$).
7. Compute the best fit solution $S(T_2)$. This function can be created at each pixel. Figure 2 shows example $S(T_2)$

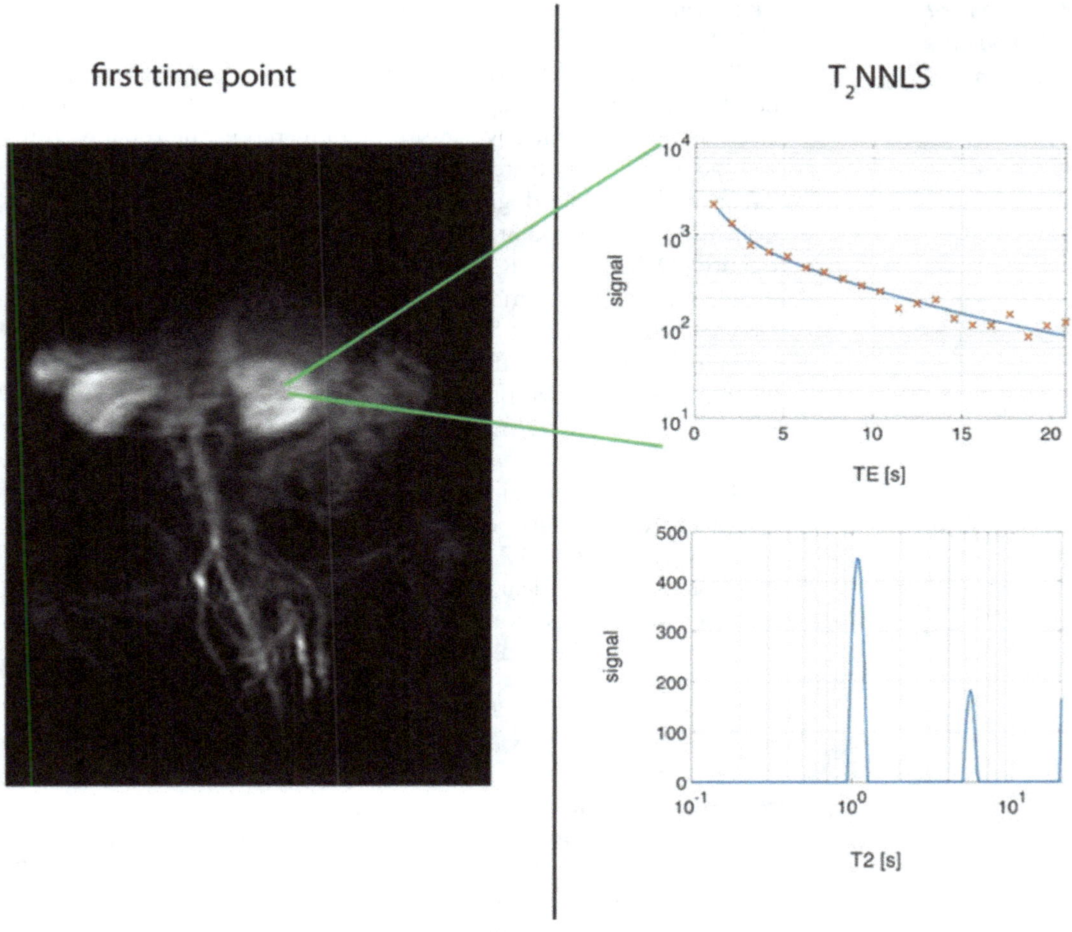

Fig. 2 Multiexponential analysis of a hyperpolarized T_2 mapping experiment. Left: coronal [^{13}C, ^{15}N]urea image of a rat at the earliest echo time (500 ms). Right, top: T_2 decay curve from a single pixel inside the kidney. Right, bottom: multiexponential analysis using the T2NNLS algorithm. Using L2 regularization penalty causes broadened peaks in the T_2 spectrum. Note that bias offsets are captured as signal at the high extremum of the T_2 domain. Hyperpolarized [^{13}C, ^{15}N]urea images of the rat kidney show two distinct decay modes representing the vascular and renal filtrate pools of the contrast agent

distributions calculated from a single pixel within the kidney calculated differing values of the regularization parameter.

8. $S(T_2)$ can be treated as a spectrum, so the signal intensity within some given T_2 bounds may be integrated to find the intensity within that range. Alternatively, the expectation value $\langle T_2 \rangle$ can be calculated by treating $S(T_2)$ as a probability distribution function and computing moments. This is demonstrated in Eq. 2, ref. 16 for estimating water content in vivo.

3.3 Glomerular Filtration Rate Estimation

A key component of renal function is the glomerular filtration rate (GFR), and nearly all hyperpolarized ^{13}C probes are sufficiently small to be freely filtered at the glomerulus. Molecules which are metabolically inert, not appreciably reabsorbed in the nephron, and have T_1 values sufficiently long to be detected in the renal medulla may be good targets for GFR measurement. Although urea is reabsorbed to some degree, there is a strong appeal of using this molecule as a hyperpolarized GFR marker due to its extremely low toxicity. Data for GFR estimation are spatially and temporally resolved magnitude images with spatial resolution sufficient to resolve the renal cortex from the medulla and temporal resolution sufficient to trace the medullary uptake curve with several data points. Since the current example uses data only from the uptake phase, the effects of transmitter-based depolarization are likely small.

GFR estimation using hyperpolarized ^{13}C imaging has been demonstrated by retrospectively processing datasets using the Baumann–Rudin model [17]. This technique was originally developed for measuring renal clearance of Gd agents in rats [18] and uses the time-varying signals from the renal cortex (C_{cortex}) and medulla (C_{medulla}) to estimate an effective exchange rate.

$$\frac{dC_{\text{medulla}}}{dt} = KC_{\text{cortex}}(t). \tag{7}$$

Here the constant K represents the one-way exchange rate from cortex to medulla. Although one-way exchange is an invalid assumption for probes that are reabsorbed, the model is assumed to hold true in the initial uptake phase. Solving Eq. 7 analytically requires initial conditions for the concentration variables which, therefore, requires an additional arterial input model parameter. To avoid this computational complexity, this model can instead be solved algebraically by normalizing the mean slope (dC_{medulla}/dt) during the uptake phase by the mean cortex signal and scaling by the medullary volume [19]. The script example_GFR.m demonstrates the following steps for calculating GFR from a dynamic set of [^{13}C]urea images

1. Time-dependent, magnitude images are reconstructed.
2. The renal cortical and medullary ROIs are delineated, and a mean taken over these ROIs is used to create $C_{\text{medulla}}(t)$ and $C_{\text{cortex}}(t)$.
3. The initial uptake period of the time domain is isolated (uptakeInds in the script).
4. A linear fit is performed on $C_{\text{medulla}}(t)$ to estimate its slope $\frac{dC_{\text{medulla}}}{dt}$ during the uptake period. These curves and the slope estimates are shown in Fig. 3.

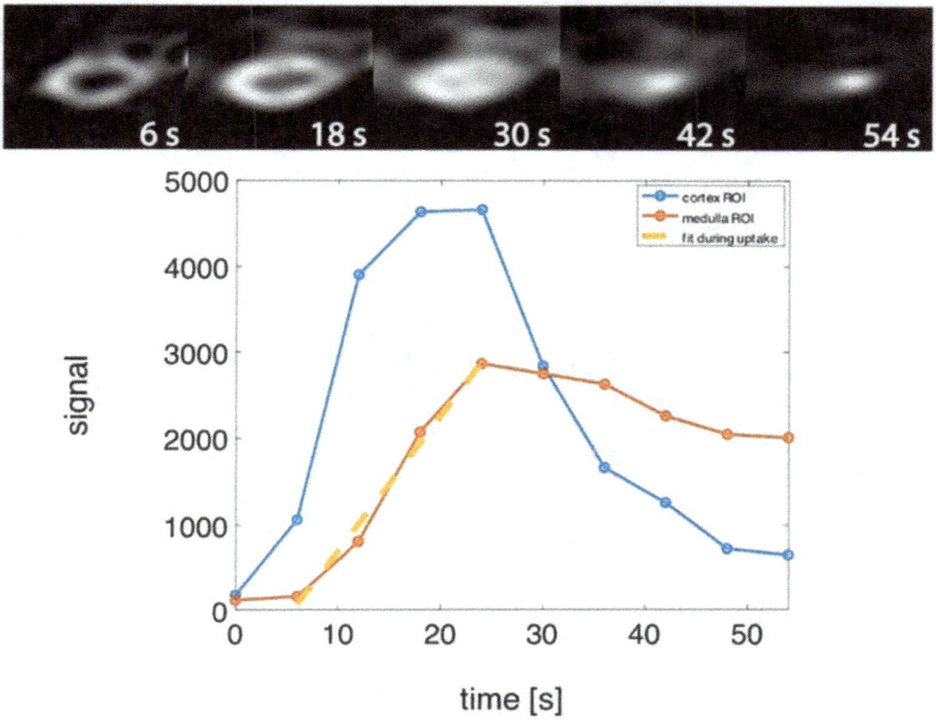

Fig. 3 Estimating glomerular filtration rate from dynamic ^{13}C urea images of a rat. The top frame shows every other time point of the acquisition, and the bottom plot gives the uptake curves from the renal cortex and medulla. The yellow trace shows the best linear fit of the medulla signal during uptake; the rate from this fit is used for GFR estimation

5. The parameter K from Eq. 7 is estimated via $K = \frac{dC_{\text{medulla}}}{dt} / \langle C_{\text{cortex}}(t) \rangle$, where $\langle C_{\text{cortex}}(t) \rangle$ is the mean value of $C_{\text{cortex}}(t)$ during the uptake phase.
6. The GFR can then be estimated as $\text{GFR} = K \cdot V_{\text{medulla}} \cdot 60$, where V_{medulla} is the medullary volume in mL, making GFR in mL/min.

3.4 Metabolic Rate Constant Estimation

The estimation of the metabolic flux from a hyperpolarized substrate to some metabolic products which are distinguished from the substrate via chemical shift is a topic of paramount interest. The metabolic conversion of hyperpolarized ^{13}C substrates can be an extremely complex process. For instance, the conversion of hyperpolarized [1-^{13}C]pyruvate to hyperpolarized [1-^{13}C]lactate depends on arterial input to the tissue, the monocarboxylate transporter-mediated transport into the cell where the substrate undergoes a Michaelis–Menten exchange with lactate. Therefore, the net conversion of the substrate depends not only on the rate of each transport step but also the availability of the enzyme and cofactor, and the size of the steady-state lactate pool [20]. Using hyperpolarized ^{13}C NMR to capture this effect requires fitting signal amplitudes of data acquired from a spectroscopic readout. The data may be spatially resolved, but frequently a "slice dynamic" acquisition is used which greatly simplifies setting up the acquisition protocol and maximizes the probability of detecting low SNR metabolic products. A typical in vivo experiment will acquire a spectrum over 1–10 kHz sweep width using a slice selective pulse, and this acquisition is repeated until the polarization is presumed to be depleted. This type of acquisition gives data of the form $S(f,t)$, where f is the Fourier transform of the FID domain, and t is a variable proportional to the number of repetitions. The substrate and products have time-dependent signals $S(t)$ and $P(t)$, respectively. The hyperpolarized signals may be matched to functions of the form

$$\frac{\mathrm{d}S(t)}{\mathrm{d}t} = -\left(k_{\mathrm{SP}} + \frac{1}{T_{1,S}}\right)S(t) + k_{\mathrm{PS}}P(t) + u(t), \tag{8}$$

$$\frac{\mathrm{d}P(t)}{\mathrm{d}t} = -\left(k_{\mathrm{PS}} + \frac{1}{T_{1,P}}\right)P(t) + k_{\mathrm{SP}}S(\mathrm{t}) \tag{9}$$

where $T_{1,\mathrm{S}}$ and $T_{1,\mathrm{P}}$ are the spin lattice relaxation times of the substrate and product, respectively, k_{SP} and k_{PS} are the forward and reverse rate constants, and $u(t)$ is a function that models substrate delivery to the tissue. A frequently made simplification made when modeling conversion of [1-^{13}C]pyruvate to [1-^{13}C]lactate is to assume both molecules have nearly identical relaxation times ($T_{1,\mathrm{P}} = T_{1,\mathrm{S}}$) and that no significant backward flux occurs during measurement ($k_{\mathrm{PS}} = 0$). This reduces the number of unknowns to be fitted from 4 to 2 and greatly improves the noise conditioning of the problem.

Typical steps in processing 2D, slice-dynamic spectroscopy and estimating metabolic conversion metrics are summarized here:

1. Raw spectra are typically apodized in the spectral domain using a filter matched to the T_2* of the compound (on the order of 50–500 ms) to reduce noise.
2. Apodized spectra are Fourier transformed along the FID axis giving spectra of the form $S(f,t$, coils).
3. If data are displayed in magnitude, then a sum-of-squares over the coil axis may be performed giving $|S(f, t)|$ Phase sensitive detection may be used, but it requires phasing each channel individually before combination. Although phase-sensitive processing adds complexity, it simplifies detection of low-SNR metabolites, and may reduce contamination of large amplitude resonance on neighboring peaks due to apparent line-narrowing.

4. A further de-noising step may be performed on the 2D $|S(f, t)|$ data by using SVD-thresholding [21]. This step can be motivated by subsequent processing steps which can greatly enhance noise if poorly conditioned.
5. The peak amplitudes are then tracked over time to generate 1D curves of substrate $S(t)$ and product $P(t)$. This may be performed by taking the maximum value or integrating over a small frequency band.
6. A flip angle correction may be applied to account for RF-induced depolarization, but this requires accurate knowledge of the flip angle applied at each time point (*see* ref. 22 for an in-depth treatment of this topic).
7. Estimating the forward rate constant k_{SP} requires fitting the experimental data to the kinetic models such as those given in Eqs. 8 and 9. However, a frequently applied model free analysis of Hill et al. vastly simplifies the analysis of hyperpolarized metabolic kinetic data [23]. The model free approach is based on the fact that integrating $S(t)$ and $P(t)$ over time and taking their ratios gives a value proportional to this rate constant, so no deconvolution or curve fitting is required. This model free approach is simply implemented by taking the area under the curve (AUC) of the product and normalizing this value to the AUC of the substrate (*see* Fig. 4, right, for example traces of such an experiment).
8. For a more detailed treatment, the readers are referred to the open source hyperpolarized MRI toolbox scripts from UCSF.

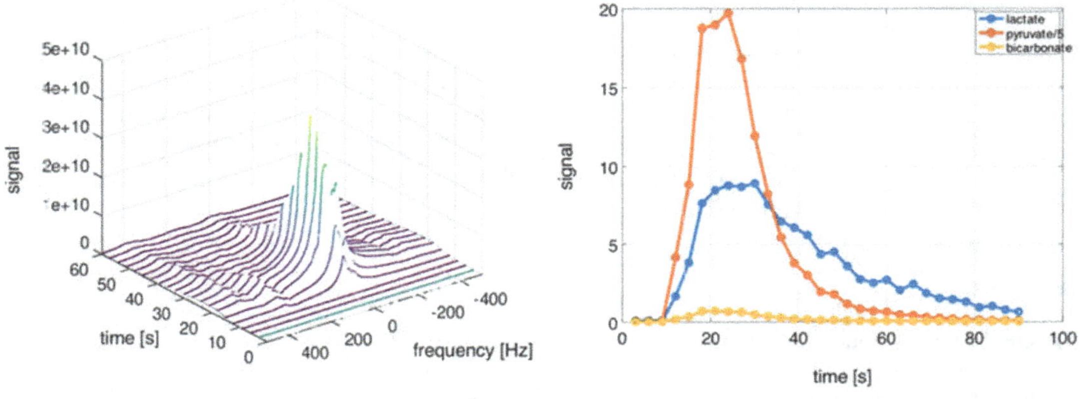

Fig. 4 Left: a typical slab-dynamic spectroscopy acquisition on a 3T scanner captures the conversion of [1-^{13}C]pyruvate (large peak on resonance) to [1-^{13}C]lactate (left, at 390 Hz) and [^{13}C]bicarbonate. Right: the traces of these three metabolites over time generated by integrating over the line width at each point. A simple measure of metabolic flux can be derived from these traces by taking the area under the curve (AUC) of a metabolic product and dividing it by the AUC of the substrate

A review paper covers the topics of kinetic modeling in great detail [22]. This toolbox can be cloned via git clone https://github.com/LarsonLab/hyperpolarized-mri-toolbox.git

9. Within this toolbox, the subfolder kinetic_modeling contains numerous scripts for fitting kinetic curves with a variety of options. See example_exchangeModel.m for a sample invocation of the main wrapper function fit_kPL() in the toolbox.

3.5 Results Validation

Most of the analysis methods outlined here will output values in physical units, so cross referencing measurements with values quoted in the literature is the chief method for validation of results. For instance, renal blood flow measurements in the range 4–10 mL/mL/min have been reported using hyperpolarized contrast agents [17]. Preliminary results show hyperpolarized-MRI-derived GFR measurements in the range of 2–3 mL/min for the rat kidney which are in close agreement with GFR measured with other modalities. A wider variation of relaxation times has been reported. For instance, [^{13}C, ^{15}N]urea T_2 values have been reported ranging from 400–800 ms to greater than 4 s [12, 13]. A further study is required to elucidate the influence of acquisition on the variance of findings in the literature.

Acknowledgments

This chapter is based upon work from COST Action PARENCH IMA, supported by European Cooperation in Science and Technology (COST). COST (www.cost.eu) is a funding agency for research and innovation networks. COST Actions help connect research initiatives across Europe and enable scientists to enrich their ideas by sharing them with their peers. This boosts their research, career, and innovation.

PARENCHIMA (renalmri.org) is a community-driven Action in the COST program of the European Union, which unites more than 200 experts in renal MRI from 30 countries with the aim to improve the reproducibility and standardization of renal MRI biomarkers.

References

1. GE MR Collaboration Community. https://collaborate.mr.gehealthcare.com
2. Reed GD accompanying source code examples for book chapter on renal MRI analysis. https://github.com/galenreed/renalC13MRIBook
3. Golman K, Ardenkjaer-Larsen JH, Petersson JS et al (2003) Molecular imaging with endogenous substances. Proc Natl Acad Sci 100:10435–10439
4. Reed GD, von Morze C, Bok R et al (2014) High resolution 13C MRI with hyperpolarized urea: in vivo T2 mapping and 15N labeling effects. IEEE Trans Med Imaging 33:362–371
5. Svensson J, Månsson S, Johansson E et al (2003) Hyperpolarized 13C MR angiography using trueFISP. Magn Reson Med 50:256–262
6. Grant AK, Vinogradov E, Wang X et al (2011) Perfusion imaging with a freely diffusible

hyperpolarized contrast agent. Magn Reson Med 66:746–755

7. von Morze C, Bok RA, Reed GD et al (2014) Simultaneous multiagent hyperpolarized 13C perfusion imaging. Magn Reson Med 72:1599–1609
8. Østergaard L, Weisskoff RM, Chesler DA et al (1996) High resolution measurement of cerebral blood flow using intravascular tracer bolus passages. Part I: mathematical approach and statistical analysis. Magn Reson Med 36:715–725
9. Johansson E, Månsson S, Wirestam R et al (2004) Cerebral perfusion assessment by bolus tracking using hyperpolarized 13C. Magn Reson Med 51:464–472
10. von Morze C, Larson PEZ, Hu S et al (2011) Imaging of blood flow using hyperpolarized [13C]Urea in preclinical cancer models. J Magn Reson Imaging 33:692–697
11. Yen Y-F, Le Roux P, Mayer D et al (2010) T2 relaxation times of 13C metabolites in a rat hepatocellular carcinoma model measured in vivo using 13C-MRS of hyperpolarized [1-13C]pyruvate. NMR Biomed 85:414–423
12. Reed GD, von Morze C, Verkman AS et al (2016) Imaging renal urea handling in rats at millimeter resolution using hyperpolarized magnetic resonance relaxometry. Tomography 2:125–137
13. Laustsen C, Stokholm Nørlinger T, Christoffer Hansen D et al (2016) Hyperpolarized 13C urea relaxation mechanism reveals renal changes in diabetic nephropathy. Magn Reson Med 75:515–518
14. Mariager CØ, Nielsen PM, Qi H et al (2017) Hyperpolarized 13C, 15N2-urea T2 relaxation changes in acute kidney injury. Magn Reson Med 80:696–702
15. Whittall KP, MacKay AL (1989) Quantitative interpretation of NMR relaxation data. J Magn Reson 84:134–152
16. Whittall KP, MacKay AL, Graeb DA et al (1997) In vivo measurement of T2 distributions and water contents in normal human brain. Magn Reson Med 37:34–43
17. Østergaard Mariager C, Nielsen PM, Qi H et al (2017) Can hyperpolarized 13C-urea be used to assess glomerular filtration rate? A retrospective study. Tomography 3:146–152
18. Baumann D, Rudin M (2000) Quantitative assessment of rat kidney function by measuring the clearance of the contrast agent Gd(DOTA) using dynamic MRI. Magn Reson Imaging 18:587–595
19. Krepkin K, Won E, Ramaswamy K et al (2014) Dynamic contrast-enhanced MR renography for renal function evaluation in ureteropelvic junction obstruction: feasibility study. Am J Roentgenol 202:778–783
20. Witney TH, Kettunen MI, Brindle KM (2011) Kinetic modeling of hyperpolarized 13C label exchange between pyruvate and lactate in tumor cells. J Biol Chem 286:24572–24580
21. Brender JR, Kishimoto S, Merkle H et al (2019) Dynamic imaging of glucose and lactate metabolism by 13C-MRS without hyperpolarization. Sci Rep 9:3410
22. Larson PEZ, Chen H, Gordon JW et al (2018) Investigation of analysis methods for hyperpolarized 13C-pyruvate metabolic MRI in prostate cancer patients. NMR Biomed 31:e3997
23. Hill DK, Orton MR, Mariotti E et al (2013) Model free approach to kinetic analysis of real-time hyperpolarized 13C magnetic resonance spectroscopy data. PLoS One 8:e71996

5

Fluorine (^{19}F) MRI to Measure Renal Oxygen Tension and Blood Volume: Experimental Protocol

Lingzhi Hu, Hua Pan, and Samuel A. Wickline

Abstract

Fluorinated compounds feature favorable toxicity profile and can be used as a contrast agent for magnetic resonance imaging and spectroscopy. Fluorine nucleus from fluorinated compounds exhibit well-known advantages of being a high signal nucleus with a natural abundance of its stable isotope, a convenient gyromagnetic ratio close to that of protons, and a unique spectral signature with no detectable background at clinical field strengths. Perfluorocarbon core nanoparticles (PFC NP) are a class of clinically approved emulsion agents recently applied in vivo for ligand-targeted molecular imaging. The objective of this chapter is to outline a multinuclear ^{1}H/^{19}F MRI protocol for functional kidney imaging in rodents for mapping of renal blood volume and oxygenation (pO_2) in renal disease models.

This chapter is based upon work from the COST Action PARENCHIMA, a community-driven network funded by the European Cooperation in Science and Technology (COST) program of the European Union, which aims to improve the reproducibility and standardization of renal MRI biomarkers. This experimental protocol chapter is complemented by a separate chapter describing the basic concept of functional imaging using fluorine (^{19}F) MR methods.

Key words Perfluorocarbon, Fluorine, Oxygenation, Perfusion, MRI, Kidney, Mice, Rats

1 Introduction

In healthy kidneys, the countercurrent design of blood vessels and tubules maintains the necessary osmolar gradient to permit efficient urinary concentration, yet the system operates under conditions of a relatively hypoxic environment in some regions that requires extensive extraction of oxygen from flowing blood [1, 2]. During acute and chronic kidney injury, ischemia challenges effective O_2 delivery to the capillary beds of the renal tubules where extraction of extra oxygen is marginal, resulting in heightened susceptibility to ischemic damage that may culminate in renal failure [3]. Besides the traditional biochemical metrics for assessing renal failure (e.g., blood urea nitrogen, creatinine), ^{1}H/^{19}F imaging offers a multi-parametric quantifiable approach to functional imaging in kidney injury that avoids the use of potentially nephrotoxic gadolinium (Gd) based contrast agents [3].

Perfluorocarbon core nanoparticles (PFC NP) are a class of emulsion agents clinically approved as blood substitutes that have been applied recently for in vivo for targeted molecular imaging and noninvasive oxygen tension (pO_2) assessment [1–3]. As compared with standard iodinated or Gd contrast agents, PFC NP are biologically inert and exhibit a good safety profile with no renal toxicity reported in both animals and human [3]. Because PFC NP (nominal size 200–250 nm) are not cleared through glomerular filtration, they do not increase kidney workload, which is a major risk factor for kidney failure with the use of other agents that undergo renal clearance [3]. For imaging purposes, the unique ^{19}F MR signal emanating from the fluorine core of PFC NP can be measured directly in vivo in quite sparse concentrations (e.g., picomolar voxel amounts) with no background signal, as contrasted with other paramagnetic or superparamagnetic moieties that exert indirect contrast effects on circulating protons [4–6]. PFC NP have been demonstrated as effective functional probes for regional blood volume as the detected ^{19}F signal intensity directly reflects the actual quantity of PFC NP within a voxel. Furthermore, for pO_2 measurements, the ^{19}F longitudinal relaxation rate (R_1) responds directly to local oxygen content in a linear manner [1, 2].

Herein we describe ^{1}H/^{19}F MRI for monitoring of renal perfusion in the kidney of rodents in a step-by-step experimental protocol. The rationale for choosing acquisition parameters is described in generic terms, together with specific parameter examples.

This experimental protocol chapter is complemented by a separate chapter describing the basic concept of functional imaging using fluorine (19F) MR methods, which is part of this book.

This chapter is part of the book Pohlmann A, Niendorf T (eds) (2020) Preclinical MRI of the Kidney—Methods and Protocols. Springer, New York.

2 Materials

2.1 Animals

This experimental protocol is applicable to mice and rats.

2.2 Lab Equipment

Enumerated below are the contrast agents and equipment components needed:

1. Perfluorocarbon Nanoparticle Preparation: PFC NP (~200–250 nm) can be formulated with a variety of PFC that are liquid at body temperature. Here we describe either perfluorooctylbromide (PFOB) or perfluoro-15-crown-5-ether (CE). The PFOB or CE emulsions are composed of 20% or 40% (v/v) of PFOB or CE, 2.0% (w/v) of a surfactant commixture, and 1.7% (w/v) glycerin in water (*see* **Note 1**).

2. Gases: O_2, N_2, and compressed air, as well as a gas-mixing system to achieve required changes in the oxygen fraction of inspired gas mixture (FiO_2). In addition to room air, the following gas mixtures are required during the experiment: 10% O_2–90% N_2 for hypoxia and 100% O_2 for hyperoxia.
3. Anesthesia: An MRI-compatible slow infusion system is needed for anesthesia with ketamine–xylazine (e.g., syringe pump). Isoflurane is not recommended for ^{19}F imaging as it could interfere with the detected ^{19}F MRI signal from PFC NP.
4. Small Animal Monitoring System: An MRI-compatible small animal physiological monitoring system (e.g., SAI Inc., USA) is needed for real time respiratory monitoring and respiratory triggering and/or gating. Respiratory gating is recommended during ^{19}F MRI acquisition because it reduces motion artifact and preserves ^{19}F signal intensity in the final images, which could otherwise be degraded by motion.
5. Small Animal Holder: a dedicated customer built small animal holder is needed to accommodate animal imaging and for maintenance of body temperature at 37 °C. A warm water blanket or warm air blower can be used for maintaining body temperature of animals (*see* **Note 2**).
6. Animal Surgery Suite: A fully equipped animal surgery suite is needed for preparing animal models of renal injury (*see* **Note 3**).

2.3 MRI Hardware

The technique described in this chapter is tailored for an 11.7 T MR system (e.g., Varian, USA) but advice for adaptation to other field strengths is given where necessary. In general, the MRI scanner should be equipped with a wide band spectrometer and a wide band RF power amplifier. The scanner needs to be functional at both ^{1}H and ^{19}F frequencies.

1. ^{1}H/^{19}F dual-tuned Coils: use actively decoupled coil pair for renal imaging applications. Such coils can be custom-built as described in our prior publications [7] or obtained from commercial coil manufacturers (*see* **Note 4**).
2. Transmit Coils: use a volume transmit coil to generate a homogeneous B_1 field that covers both kidneys. Tune and match to the ^{19}F frequency.
3. Receive Coils: Place a surface receive coil on the dorsal side of the animal to achieve high sensitivity to ^{19}F signal from the two kidneys. Tune and match to the ^{19}F frequency.

2.4 MRI Techniques

1. ^{1}H MRI: a gradient echo sequence is employed to locate two imaging slices with 2 mm thickness, positioned 1–2 mm apart, and centered respectively at the left and right kidney.

2. ^{1}H MRI: a multiecho gradient-echo blood oxygenation level dependent (BOLD) scan can be performed. For an example of parameters used for a specific setting (*see* **Note 5**).
3. ^{19}F MRI: For spin density ^{19}F MRI, TR is set to 4 s. For T_1-weighted MRI, TR is set to two respiration periods, or ~300 ms. All other imaging parameters are identical in these two sets of ^{19}F MRI (*see* **Note 6**)
4. ^{19}F MRI Oxygenation Measurement: For PFC NP dependent oxygenation measurements in fast flowing blood of major blood vessels, a Blood Flow-Enhanced-Saturation-Recovery (BESR) sequence [8] can be utilized to minimize in-flow effects on the image (*see* **Note 7**).

3 Methods

3.1 PFC Nanoparticle Formulation

1. Prepare PFC NP emulsifying 40% (v/v) of CE (Exfluor Research Corp, Round Rock, TX), 2.0% (w/v) of a surfactant commixture, and 1.7% (w/v) glycerin, in distilled water using a microfluidic apparatus (e.g., benchtop LV1 fluidizer, Microfluidics Corporation, Westwood, MA) (*see* **Note 8**).
2. Determine size and charge with a submicron particle analyzer (e.g., Zetasizer, Malvern, UK) [9, 10].

3.2 PFC NP Injection and Imaging

1. Inject PFC NP for functional perfusion imaging to quantify blood volume and oxygenation.
2. Prepare an external reference for ^{19}F signal quantification. Place the external reference close to the animal within the field of view (*see* **Note 9**).
3. Perform ^{1}H and ^{19}F imaging 10 min to 1 h after NP injection. A shorter circulation time is preferred to maximize the intravascular ^{19}F signal (*see* **Note 10**).

3.3 Coil Sensitivity Profiling for Quantification of ^{19}F Signal Intensity

1. Acquire an RF coil sensitivity map using a saline phantom positioned at the selected imaging location to correct for the signal bias created by surface coil receive profile inhomogeneity. The saline phantom is prepared to cover the entire region of imaging FOV (*see* **Note 11**).
2. Compensate for the spatial inhomogeneity of the RF coil sensitivity profile by multiplying the correction factor obtained from the phantom image (*see* **Note 12**) with the in vivo measured image signal intensity at the corresponding locations.

3.4 Calibration of ^{19}F R_1 vs. pO_2 Curve In Vitro

1. Perform an in vitro calibration of ^{19}F relaxation time (R_1) as a function of pO_2 using at least three different O_2 concentrations (e.g., 0%, 21%, 100% O_2 balanced with N_2) by bubbling gas

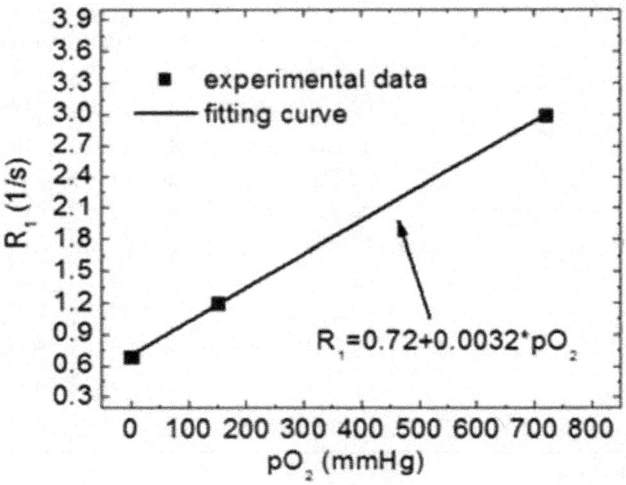

Fig. 1 In vitro calibration shows the ^{19}F R_1 ($=1/T_1$) of PFC NP as a function of pO_2. Data were collected at 11.7 T using a PFC NP phantom. Temperature of the PFC NP phantom was maintained at 37 °C. The correlation coefficient $R > 0.99$ (From Hu et al. [1])

mixtures into a PFC emulsion sample for 30 min at 37 °C (Fig. 1).

2. Perform ^{19}F T_1 measurements with inversion recovery spectroscopy at TR > 10 s, and at least ten different inversion delays (T_I) ranging from 3 ms to 5 s. Use exponential fitting to extract R_1 from T_1 measurements and linear fitting to calibrate the relationship between ^{19}F R_1 and pO_2.

3.5 Quantification of ^{19}F Based pO_2 Measurement In Vivo

1. Create two sets of images, one using a short TR and one using a long TR, for T_1 mapping (*see* **Note 13**).
2. Determine the actual TR using the external ^{19}F standard (*see* **Note 14**).
3. After determining the actual short TR, perform voxel-wise T_1 mapping of the kidney using the standard saturation recovery signal model:

$$S = S_0\left(1 - e^{\frac{TR}{T_1}}\right). \tag{1}$$

4. Translate T_1 values into corresponding pO_2 levels according to the predetermined calibration curve.

4 Notes

1. The CE signal intensity is effectively greater for narrow band reception as all fluorine atoms contribute to a single spectral peak, as compared to PFOB where chemical shifts apportion

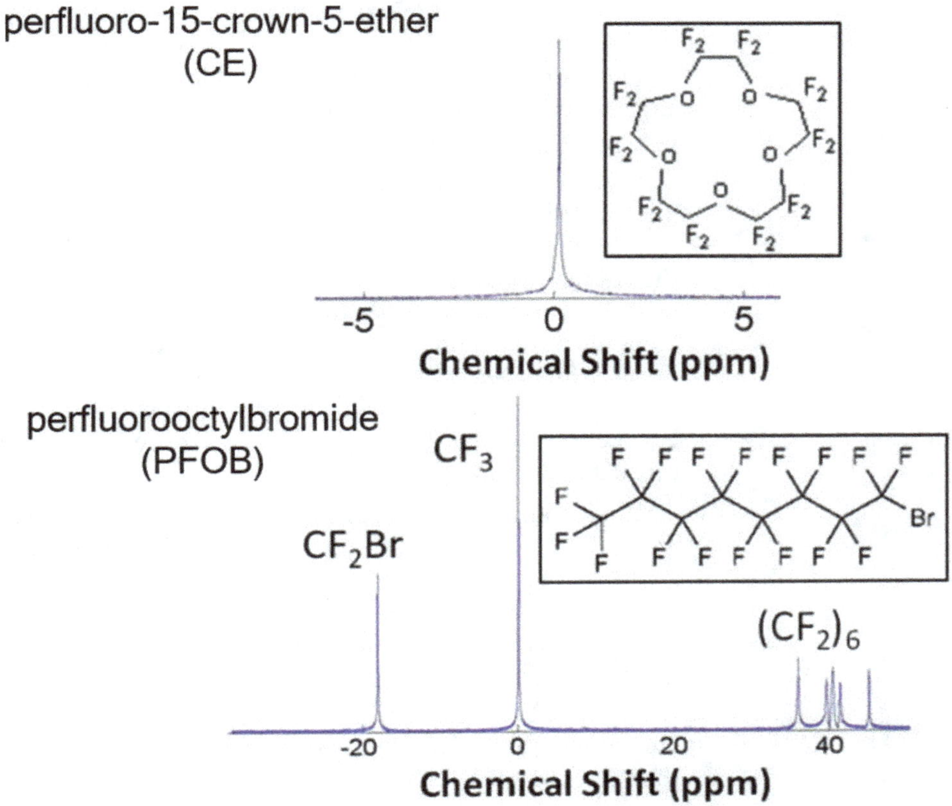

Fig. 2 Chemical structure and magnetic resonance chemical shift of perfluoro-15-crown-5-ether (CE) and perfluorooctylbromide (PFOB)

the signal into several peaks (Fig. 2). Suppliers of PFC include Exfluor Research Corporation (Round Rock, TX). The clearance half-life for PFOB is ~3–5 h depending on species and whether the PFC contrast material is molecularly targeted or not [11]. The CE materials exhibit a longer tissue residence time in bloodstream than PFOB compounds, which makes them problematic for clinical use or repeat studies. For the present protocol, no targeting ligands are attached to the surface of the PFC NP to avoid changing the pharmacokinetics of the contrast agent.

2. Potential MRI in-flow artifacts may be present on ^{1}H but not ^{19}F MR images if a warm water blanket is used. Special attention should be given when choosing the animal holder and the MRI coils as reduced animal motion during lengthy MRI acquisitions will improve image quality.
3. In general, ischemic renal injury can be produced unilaterally or bilaterally by exposing the kidneys either through the abdomen or retroperitoneally, and then clamping the renal artery for a

selected interval [1, 2]. The animal surgery suite does not need to be located in the MRI facility but should be close enough for imaging a short time after surgery and later for tissue harvest after imaging is completed if indicated.

4. Despite being slightly off-resonance for ^1H imaging, the ^{19}F coil pair should be sufficient to generate high quality anatomic images within <1 min scan time. The size of the transmit and receive coils should be designed to match the animal size, so that different coil sizes will be needed for imaging mice and rats. For imaging at field strengths lower than 11.7 T, it is recommended to use double tuned receive coils that simultaneously function at ^1H and ^{19}F frequency to assure maximal detection efficiency while avoiding potential image mismatches between ^1H and ^{19}F images that may occur as a result of manual coil retuning.
5. The imaging parameters of BOLD at 4.7 T are: TR = 100 ms, TE = 1.96 ms with 1.75 ms increment for every echo, flip angle = 10°, field of view = 26 × 26 mm^2, voxel size = 0.2 × 0.2 × 2 mm^3. Field of view and voxel size should be adjusted based on animal size to achieve optimal image quality.
6. ETL = 4, TE = 11.5 ms, receiver bandwidth = 20 kHz, voxel size = 0.4 × 0.4 × 2 mm^3, and the field of view is identical to that for ^1H BOLD imaging.
7. For an example of parameters used at 4.7 T, the imaging parameters of BESR sequence are: TR = 2.5 s; TE = 2.2 ms; number of points along recovery curve = 8; number of averages = 16; in plane resolution = 1.5 mm × 0.75 mm; slice thickness = 2 mm
8. PFC NP can be colabeled with Alexa Fluor 594 for ex vivo fluorescence microscopy examination.
9. As reference, a tube of another PFC NP formulation (e.g., perfluorodecalin) at a similar PFC concentration to that administered in vivo for the imaging studies can be used.
10. In healthy tissues, PFC NP are generally constrained to the intravascular space because of their large particle size (200–250 nm), which ensures that the measured ^{19}F signal intensity correlates linearly with intravascular blood volume. One has to also consider that during injury, PFC NP will escape from the circulation and will get trapped in tissue compartments. In this case the total fluorine signal would comprise both stationary (i.e., trapped in tissue) and flowing (i.e., in blood) PFC NP. Employ spin labeling [12] to eliminate the signal from trapped PFC NP, leaving only the signal from the flowing blood compartment. Apply diffusion gradients to suppress the signal from flowing blood [13] and acquire distinct

signal from either compartment. For O_2 measurements, a mixture of signals could occur where trapped PFC NP exist under hypoxic conditions and the flowing PFC NP under more normoxic conditions. In this case the ^{19}F relaxation times would represent an average of the two situations.

11. At 11.7 T, imaging parameters are as follows: TR = 100 ms, TE = 1.96 ms, and flip angle = 10°. For other field strengths, minimize TE and select similar TR and flip angle.
12. For each voxel location, the phantom image defines a correction factor matrix $R(x,y,z)$ that is the inverse of local signal intensity $I(x,y,z)$: $R(x,y,z) = 1/I(x,y,z)$.
13. In vivo quantification of renal T_1 and pO_2 is based on the general assumption that image signal intensity in a fast spin echo sequence follows a saturation-recovery process (Fig. 3). Because short TR or T_1-weighed ^{19}F MRI is gated with respiration, the actual short TR can vary from animal to animal.
14. Given that the ^{19}F T_1 of PFC standard is 0.9–1 s at room air oxygen tension, the signal acquired with a long TR = 4 s, that is, >3 × T_1, should approximate the ^{19}F spin-density signal of PFC NP at room temperature (Fig. 4).

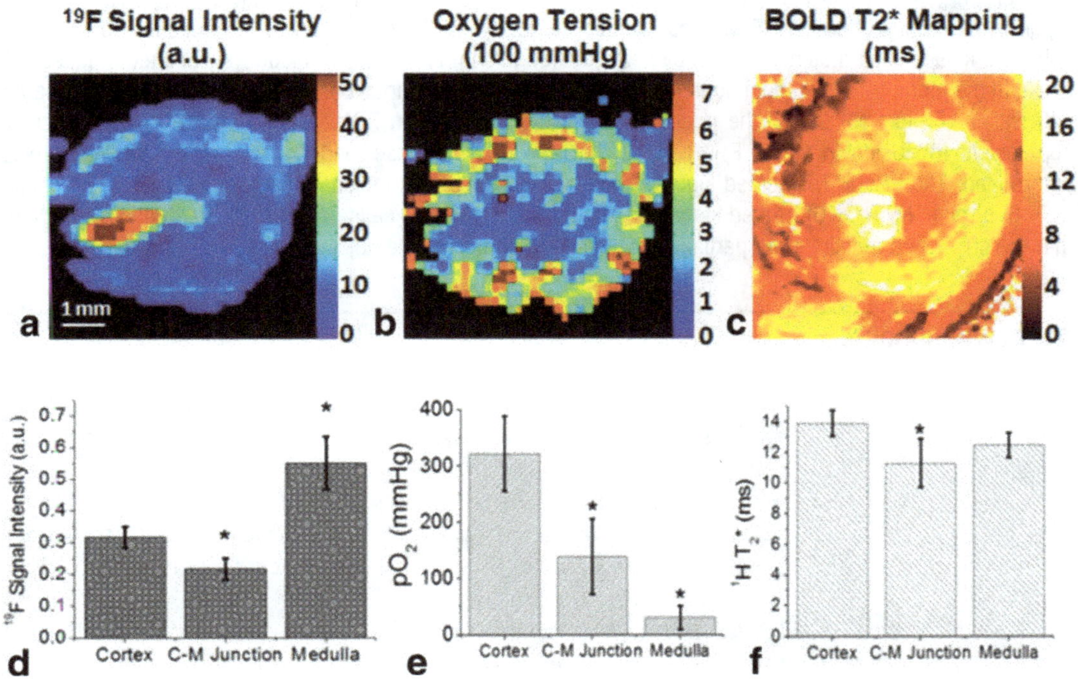

Fig. 3 (**a**, **b**) Representative renal blood volume and pO_2 mapping of healthy kidneys determined by quantitative ^{19}F MRI. (**c**) Representative ^{1}H T2* (BOLD) mapping of healthy kidneys. (**d–f**) Quantification of functional indexes in different anatomical regions. $*P < 0.05$ compared with cortex (From Hu et al. [1])

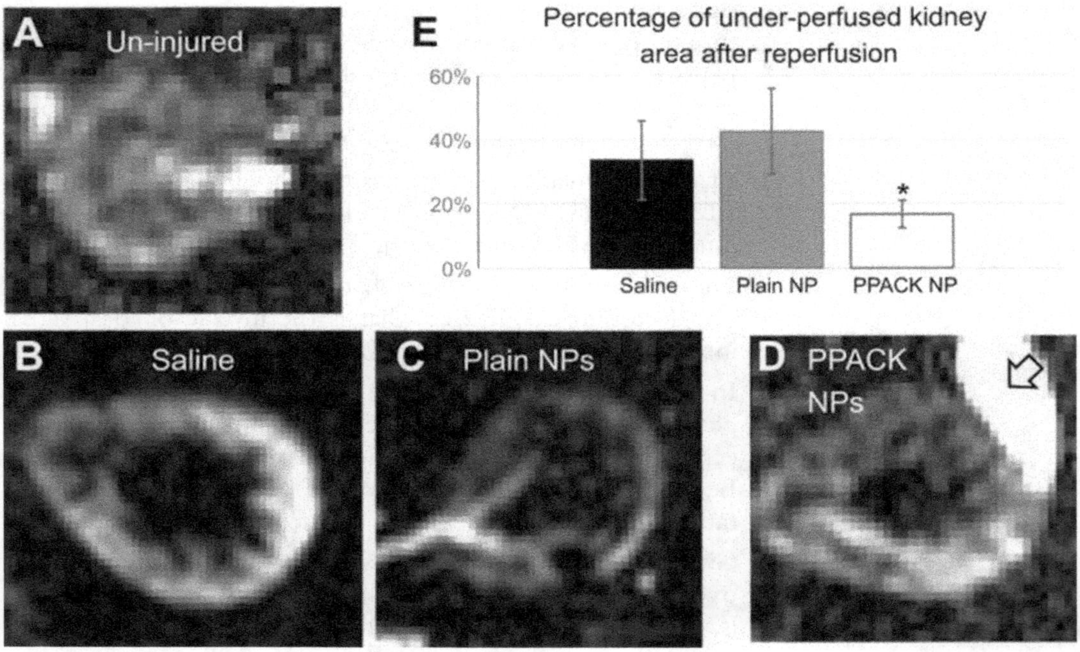

Fig. 4 Imaging of improved renal medullary perfusion after antithrombin PFC NP treatments. Here the thrombin inhibitor PPACK (phenylalanine-proline-arginine-chloromethylketone) was conjugated to the PFC NP. Mice were pretreated with PFOB PPACK NP, plain PFOB NP, or saline before ischemia induction. At 3 h after reperfusion, a single dose of CE NP was injected i.v. for ^{19}F MRI. The ^{19}F signal from circulating CE NP of uninjured kidney illustrates normal kidney perfusion (**a**). In contrast, all injured kidneys exhibited reduced ^{19}F signal in the medulla (**b–d**) reflecting the severity of regional nonreperfusion. Compared to kidneys pretreated with saline or plain NP (**b**, **c**), the improved medullary perfusion in PPACK NP treated kidneys is visually appreciable (**d**). Using in vivo ^{19}F MRI data, the ratio of nonperfused kidney area after reperfusion was determined. The PPACK NP treated kidneys ($n = 4$) developed less regional nonreperfusion than did saline ($n = 6$) or plain NP ($n = 6$) treated kidneys. $^*p < 0.05$ compared to saline or plain NP treated kidneys. Note that the arrow in d indicates the partial overlay of ^{19}F signal from the adjacent spleen (From Chen et al. [2])

Acknowledgments

This chapter is based upon work from COST Action PARENCH IMA, supported by European Cooperation in Science and Technology (COST). COST (www.cost.eu) is a funding agency for research and innovation networks. COST Actions help connect research initiatives across Europe and enable scientists to enrich their ideas by sharing them with their peers. This boosts their research, career, and innovation.

PARENCHIMA (renalmri.org) is a community-driven Action in the COST program of the European Union, which unites more than 200 experts in renal MRI from 30 countries with the aim to improve the reproducibility and standardization of renal MRI biomarkers.

References

1. Hu LZ et al (2014) Assessing intrarenal non-perfusion and vascular leakage in acute kidney injury with multinuclear H-1/F-19 MRI and perfluorocarbon nanoparticles. Magn Reson Med 71(6):2186–2196
2. Chen JJ et al (2015) Antithrombin nanoparticles improve kidney reperfusion and protect kidney function after ischemia-reperfusion injury. Am J Physiol Renal Physiol 308(7): F765–F773
3. Chen JJ et al (2013) Perfluorocarbon nanoparticles for physiological and molecular imaging and therapy. Adv Chronic Kidney Dis 20 (6):466–478
4. Goette MJ et al (2015) Balanced UTE-SSFP for 19F MR imaging of complex spectra. Magn Reson Med 74(2):537–543
5. Goette MJ et al (2015) Improved quantitative 19 F MR molecular imaging with flip angle calibration and B1-mapping compensation. J Magn Reson Imaging 42(2):488–494
6. Palekar RU et al (2015) Quantifying progression and regression of thrombotic risk in experimental atherosclerosis. FASEB J 29 (7):3100–3109
7. Hu LZ et al (2011) A generalized strategy for designing (19)F/(1)H dual-frequency MRI coil for small animal imaging at 4.7 Tesla. J Magn Reson Imaging 34(1):245–252
8. Hu LZ et al (2013) Rapid quantification of oxygen tension in blood flow with a fluorine nanoparticle reporter and a novel blood flow-enhanced-saturation-recovery sequence. Magn Reson Med 70(1):176–183
9. Winter PM et al (2003) Molecular imaging of angiogenesis in nascent Vx-2 rabbit tumors using a novel alpha(nu)beta3-targeted nanoparticle and 1.5 tesla magnetic resonance imaging. Cancer Res 63(18):5838–5843
10. Winter PM et al (2003) Molecular imaging of angiogenesis in early-stage atherosclerosis with alpha(v)beta3-integrin-targeted nanoparticles. Circulation 108(18):2270–2274
11. Kaneda MM et al (2009) Perfluorocarbon nanoemulsions for quantitative molecular imaging and targeted therapeutics. Ann Biomed Eng 37(10):1922–1933
12. Wu WC et al (2011) Renal perfusion 3-T MR imaging: a comparative study of arterial spin labeling and dynamic contrast-enhanced techniques. Radiology 261(3):845–853
13. Ichikawa S et al (2013) Intravoxel incoherent motion imaging of the kidney: alterations in diffusion and perfusion in patients with renal dysfunction. Magn Reson Imaging 31 (3):414–417

6

Analysis Protocols for MRI Mapping of the Blood Oxygenation–Sensitive Parameters T_2* and T_2 in the Kidney

João S. Periquito, Ludger Starke, Carlota M. Santos, Andreia C. Freitas, Nuno Loução, Pablo García Polo, Rita G. Nunes, Thoralf Niendorf, and Andreas Pohlmann

Abstract

Renal hypoxia is generally accepted as a key pathophysiologic event in acute kidney injury of various origins and has also been suggested to play a role in the development of chronic kidney disease. Here we describe step-by-step data analysis protocols for MRI monitoring of renal oxygenation in rodents via the deoxyhemoglobin concentration sensitive MR parameters T_2* and T_2—a contrast mechanism known as the blood oxygenation level dependent (BOLD) effect.

This chapter describes how to use the analysis tools provided by vendors of animal and clinical MR systems, as well as how to develop an analysis software. Aspects covered are: data quality checks, data exclusion, model fitting, fitting algorithm, starting values, effects of multiecho imaging, and result validation.

This chapter is based upon work from the PARENCHIMA COST Action, a community-driven network funded by the European Cooperation in Science and Technology (COST) program of the European Union, which aims to improve the reproducibility and standardization of renal MRI biomarkers. This experimental protocol chapter is complemented by two separate chapters describing the basic concept and data analysis.

Key words Magnetic resonance imaging (MRI), Kidney, Mice, Rats, T_2, T_2*, BOLD

1 Introduction

The parametric mapping of the transverse relaxation times T_2* and T_2 (or relaxation rates $R_2* = 1/T_2*$ and $R_2 = 1/T_2$) has the potential to yield inferences regarding renal oxygenation, since both parameters are sensitive to blood oxygenation [1]. The underlying mechanism rests on the inherent difference in the magnetic properties of oxygenated hemoglobin (diamagnetic) vs. deoxygenated hemoglobin (paramagnetic) [2]. The presence of deoxyhemoglobin in a voxel decreases both relaxation times, T_2* and T_2, which are the time constants governing the exponential signal decays due to spin

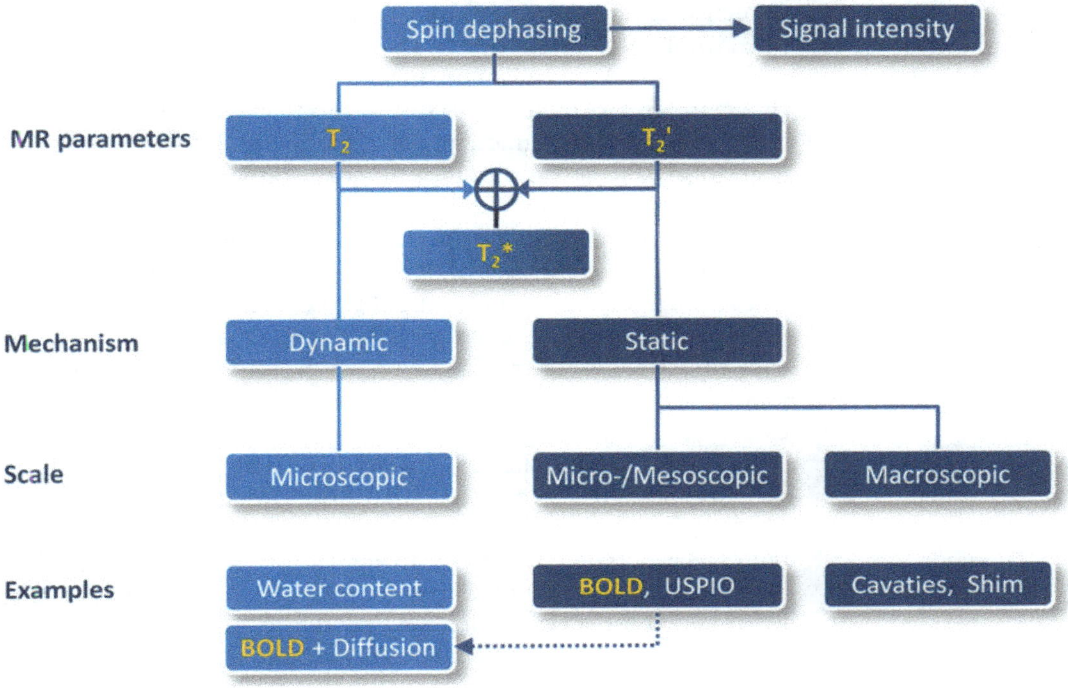

Fig. 1 Spin dephasing due to dynamic (irreversible; represented by the parameter T_2) and static (reversible; represented by the parameter T_2') sources can be quantified by calculation of T_2* and T_2 from series of MRI images with different echo times using $1/T_2^* = 1/T_2 + 1/T_2'$. The possible sources for this dephasing range from the microscopic to the macroscopic scale and their level dictates the observed attenuation in the signal intensity. Blood oxygenation affects primarily T_2* (often referred to as Blood Oxygenation Level Dependent, BOLD), but to a lesser extend also T_2 via diffusion effects in the proximity of blood vessels. USPIO: Ultra-small Superparamagnetic Particles of Iron Oxide, which can be used as intravascular contrast agents

dephasing in gradient-echo (GRE) and spin-echo (SE) MR measurements, respectively.

Possible sources for this dephasing are magnetic field inhomogeneities ranging from the microscopic to the macroscopic scale, which can be classified with respect to the echo time into microscopic dynamic spin–spin interactions—T_2, that is, typically ranging a time span between 1 and 100 ms (Fig. 1) and static mesoscopic interactions—T_2'. In fact, T_2* includes the dynamic (irreversible) dephasing effects described by T_2 plus the additional effects that are due to static (reversible) dephasing effects described by T_2'. Blood oxygenation affects primarily T_2* (often referred to as Blood Oxygenation Level Dependent, BOLD), but to a lesser extend also T_2, via water diffusion effects in the proximity of blood vessels due to local magnetic field gradients [1].

Calculation of T_2* and T_2 requires a series of MR images with different echo times. Repeated measurements with a single echo sequence using either a GRE or SE method and variable echo times (TE) would provide the most accurate T_2* and T_2 values but would require very long acquisition times [2]. In order to address this shortcoming fast multiecho MRI methods are commonly used for in vivo studies: multi-gradient-echo (MGE) for T_2* and multi-spin-echo (also called "MSME") for T_2. They provide relaxation times that slightly underestimate T_2* and overestimate T_2 (*see* **Note 1**).

The core of $T_2^{(*)}$ mapping consists of fitting the exponential model curve $S(\mathrm{TE}) = S_0 \exp.(-\mathrm{TE}/T_2^{(*)})$ to the signal intensities of each image pixel at increasing TE. For the calculation of such parameter maps from a series of $T_2^{(*)}$-weighted images software tools and plugins are provided by the MR system vendors but they may lack some features instrumental for precise $T_2^{(*)}$ mapping. For example, some important preprocessing steps may not be available, such as eliminating the first echo of T_2 data, removing echoes acquired at high TEs that may have too low signal-to-noise ratio (SNR) or applying Rician noise bias correction. Also, details about the used processing and curve fitting algorithms may not be available. It is also a limitation that the algorithms are fixed and cannot be modified for specific purposes. Therefore, depending on application, it may be advantageous to develop a dedicated analysis software program in-house. The analysis software is developed assuming 2D data was acquired, for 3D data (multiple slices) data set are separated into individual slices.

The pixel-wise signal fitting with a monoexponential model is known to introduce T_2 bias, and so for studies that require an extremely rigorous T_2 value (error $< 1\%$) a dictionary-based method has been suggested. In dictionary-matching methodologies, T_2 maps are calculated by matching the T_2 signal decay to precomputed Echo Modulation Curve (EMC), therefore accounting for all echo pathways. The use of dictionary-based methods has been suggested to improve T_2 accuracy, accounting for the stimulated echoes and effective B_1^+ field [3]. The use of dictionary-based methods is still fairly novel and its implementation and use is not covered in this chapter.

This chapter will describe both how to use the vendor's analysis tools and how to develop your own analysis software conceptually. An example of a MATLAB script described in this chapter together with a data sample (*T2analysis.m* and *data.mat*) can be downloaded from https://github.com/JoaoPeriquito/T2-s-Mapping.

This data analysis protocol is complemented by two separate chapters describing the basic concept and experimental, which are part of this book.

This chapter is part of the book Pohlmann A, Niendorf T (eds) (2020) Preclinical MRI of the Kidney—Methods and Protocols. Springer, New York.

2 Materials

2.1 Software Requirements

To calculate the parametric maps using existing tools, a software such as the following is required:

2.1.1 Essential Tools

1. MR system software *ParaVision* (version 5 or higher; Bruker Biospin, Ettlingen, Germany).
2. MR system software *Syngo* (versions MR B17 or higher; Siemens Healthineers, Erlangen, Germany). The optional toolbox *MapIt* is not necessary.
3. MR system software *Ready View* (General Electric Healthcare, Milwaukee, USA).
4. MR system software from Philips (Philips Medical Systems, Best, Netherlands).

To develop custom software for calculating the parametric maps one of the following, or other equivalent, software development environments (SDE) is required:

5. *MATLAB*® including the *Curve Fitting* toolbox (The MathWorks, Natick, Massachusetts, USA; www.mathworks.com/products/MATLAB).
6. *Python* (https://www.python.org/).
7. *Octave* (http://www.gnu.org/software/octave).
8. A MATLAB tool for Rician noise bias correction can be downloaded from https://github.com/LudgerS/MRInoiseBiasCorrection. It is also compatible with Octave and includes detailed documentation to facilitate adaptation for, for example, Python.

2.1.2 Optional Tools

An image processing software for checking data quality, such as ImageJ (free Java-based image processing program developed at the National Institutes of Health and the University of Wisconsin; https://imagej.net/). We recommend and describe here the use of Fiji (https://fiji.sc/ [4]), which is ImageJ packaged with a wide range of plugins included.

2.2 Source Data: Format Requirements and Quality Check

Before the analysis it is highly recommended to check the image quality. This check should include SNR measurements, particularly for the images with longest echo times, and the assessment of geometric image distortions, motion artifacts, or susceptibility artifacts.

The steps in this section can be performed either on the scanner console using the MR vendors system viewing software, or offline using a software such as *Fiji* (recommended as a practical tool).

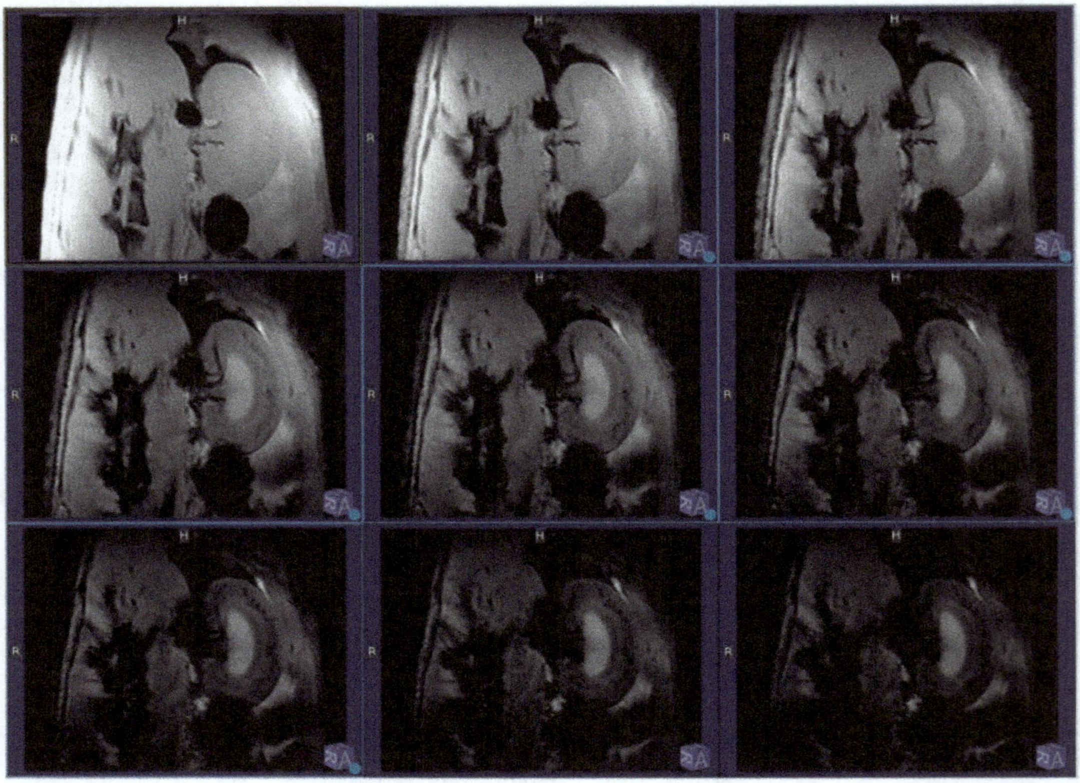

Fig. 2 Series of nine T_2*-weighted images of a healthy rat kidney acquired with a 2D MGE sequence at 9.4 T. From left to right and top to bottom, images correspond to TE = 2.14, 4.28, 6.42 ms (top row), TE = 8.56, 10.70, 12.84 ms (middle row), and TE = 14.98, 17.12, 19.26 ms (bottom row)

2.2.1 Input Requirements

As already mentioned, in order to be able to calculate $T_2^{(*)}$-maps, multiple images acquired with different echo times are needed. As an example, please refer to Fig. 2 and Fig. 3, where a series of T_2*- and T_2-weighted images suitable for mapping is presented (*see* **Note 2**). Access to specific acquisition parameters is also necessary, namely the TE of each image and in some cases the image intensity scaling parameters (offset, slope) used when storing the image data.

2.2.2 Open/Import Images

When using the scanner console:

1. Open the $T_2^{(*)}$-weighted image series in the image viewer.

   When using *Fiji* for DICOM images:

2. Import the DICOM image series using the DICOM import plugin.

   When using *Fiji* for images in Bruker format:

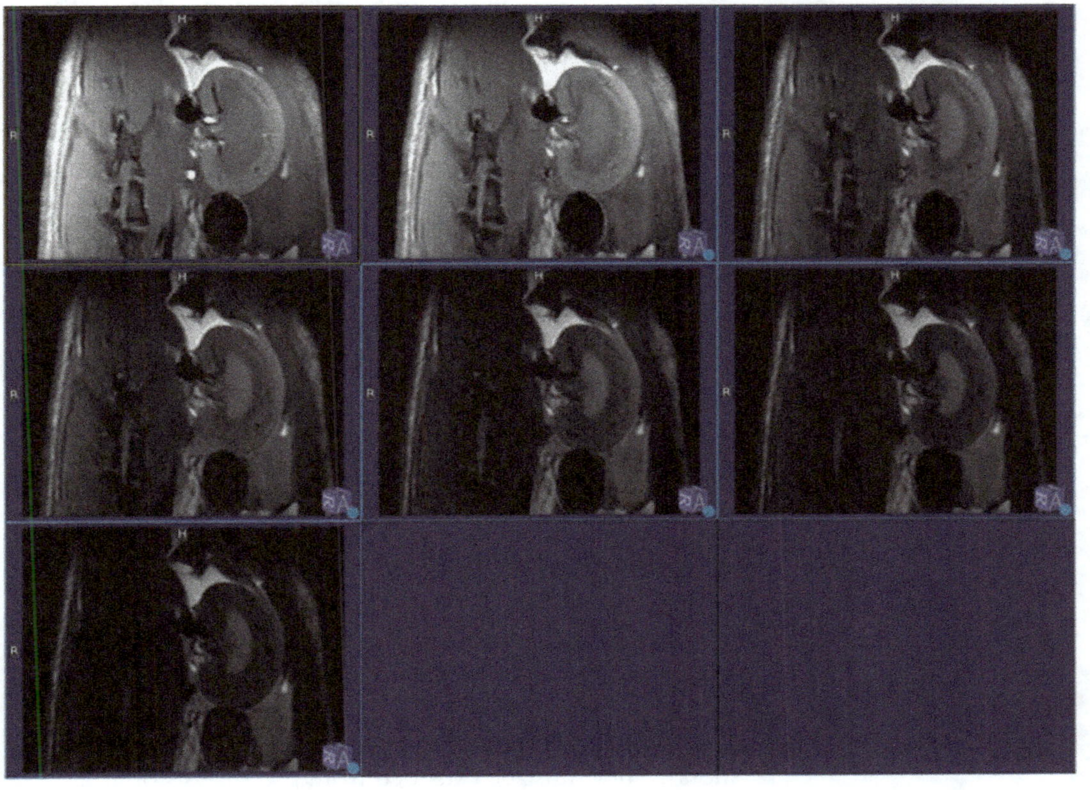

Fig. 3 Series of seven T2-weighted images of a healthy rat kidney acquired with a 2D MSME sequence at 9.4 T. Images correspond to TE = 10.0, 20.0, 30.0 ms (top row), TE = 40.0, 50.0, 60.0 ms (middle row), and TE = 70.0 ms (bottom row)

3. Browse to the data directory for the scan containing the $T_2^{(*)}$-weighted image series: /opt/PV6.0.1/data/[user_name]/[session_name]/[scan_number]/.
4. Open the "*method*" file of the scan in a text editor or by dragging it to the *Fiji* window.
5. Get the following parameters: number of slices, matrix size (e.g., 128 × 128) image type (e.g., little-endian) and byte order (e.g., 16-bit unsigned).
6. Load the image series using the RAW import function (*Import > RAW*) and providing the above parameters. The MR data file is called 2dseq and located in the subfolder "pdata/nr" (number of reconstruction) of the data directory.

2.2.3 Motion Artifacts Check

Abdominal imaging comes with complex bulk physiological motion due to the interplay of respiratory and bowel movement. If respiratory triggering of the data acquisition was used (recommended) there should only be minor motion artifacts. Check images for artifacts from motion (nontriggered acquisition) or possible residual motion (triggered acquisition).

In the image viewer or *Fiji* go to the central slice and scroll rapidly from the first to the last echo image.

1. Check for motion between the echoes. If motion is noticeable then information close to structure boundaries may not be reliable and image registration should be used for motion correction (registration is a separate topic that is not explained in this chapter).

2.2.4 Susceptibility Artifacts Check on T_2-Weighted Images*

Kidney regions adjacent to bowels or in close proximity to skin/fat/muscle boundaries or air cavities are particularly challenging to T_2* imaging and prone to loss of anatomical integrity due to geometric distortions and signal loss created by susceptibility artifacts induced by the air-filled bowels, cavities and tissue interfaces surrounding the kidneys.

1. Scroll to the images acquired at the later echoes, where susceptibility artifacts are more severe.
2. Check areas affected by susceptibility artifacts, that is, areas in the kidney with unusual and severe hypointensities (typically in the form of spherical dark "shadows"; Fig. 4).
3. Make a record of areas affected by such artifacts (notes, screenshots). They must be excluded from the analysis or at least be considered during interpretation of the result.

2.2.5 Signal-to-Noise Ratio Check

Before the analysis it is highly recommended to define an SNR acceptance threshold (*see* **Note 3**).

1. Draw a region-of-interest (ROI) over the inner medulla in the first echo image (in *Fiji* use the "Freehand Selection" tool) (*see* **Note 4**).

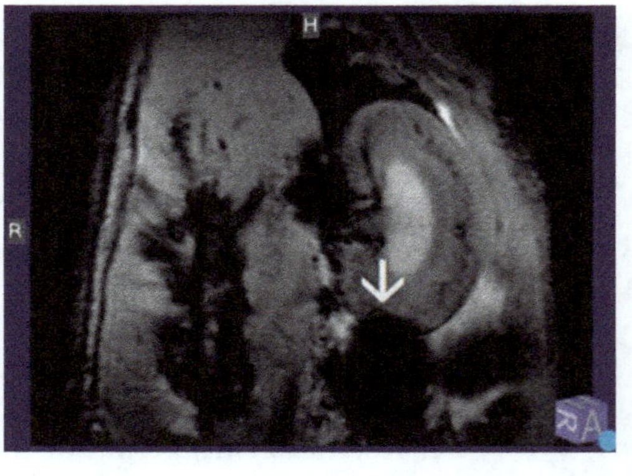

Fig. 4 T_2*-weighted image of a rat kidney that shows a susceptibility artifact at the caudal end (white arrow); image acquired with TE = 10.70 ms at B_0 = 9.4 T

2. Measure the mean signal intensity of the ROI (in *Fiji*: *Analyze > Set Measurements*; select mean and standard deviation; *Analyze > Measure*).
3. Draw an ROI over a region in the background that contains only noise without any signal or artifacts (*see* **Note 5**).
4. Measure the standard deviation of the signal within this background ROI.
5. Divide this value by 0.655 to obtain the noise standard deviation. This is necessary because the background noise in MR magnitude images differs from noise in signal regions (*see* **Note 6** if you use a multichannel RF array).
6. Calculate the SNR by dividing the mean signal of the inner medulla ROI by the noise standard deviation.
7. If the SNR is significantly below your predefined acceptance threshold, this indicates that there might be a technical problem or that the animal is not positioned correctly relative to the receiver RF coils. For more information on adequate SNR thresholds refer to **Note 7**.

3 Methods

Tools for calculating $T_2^{(*)}$-maps are provided by most MRI vendors, but, as mentioned in the introduction, we recommend creating your own analysis tool to have the maximum level of control over the processing steps and freedom to adapt them to your specific needs. Hence, this section will describe both how to use vendor's analysis tools and how to develop your own analysis software.

In both cases, mapping of T_2 and T_2^*, it may be required to exclude some data from the analysis, such as data points with insufficient SNR in the tail of the exponential decay. In the case of T_2-mapping from data acquired with a MSME method, it is also recommended to discard the first echo (*see* **Note 8**).

3.1 Data Exclusion and Model Fitting (Siemens Syngo)

When using the Siemens scanner console this is currently not possible, but one can manually select the echo images that should be included when computing the fit. Using this feature, one can exclude entire images at high TEs. We recommend using a cut-off for echo images with low SNR. Please exclude all echo images with SNR < 2.6 in the ROI of interest (*see* **Note 7**). When performing T_2-mapping, the first echo should also be excluded from the data analysis (*see* **Note 8**).

1. Load image series in the *Viewing Task Card*.
2. Using the *ROI* tool to draw an ROI on the image with the largest TE over the region of interest, and register the mean signal.

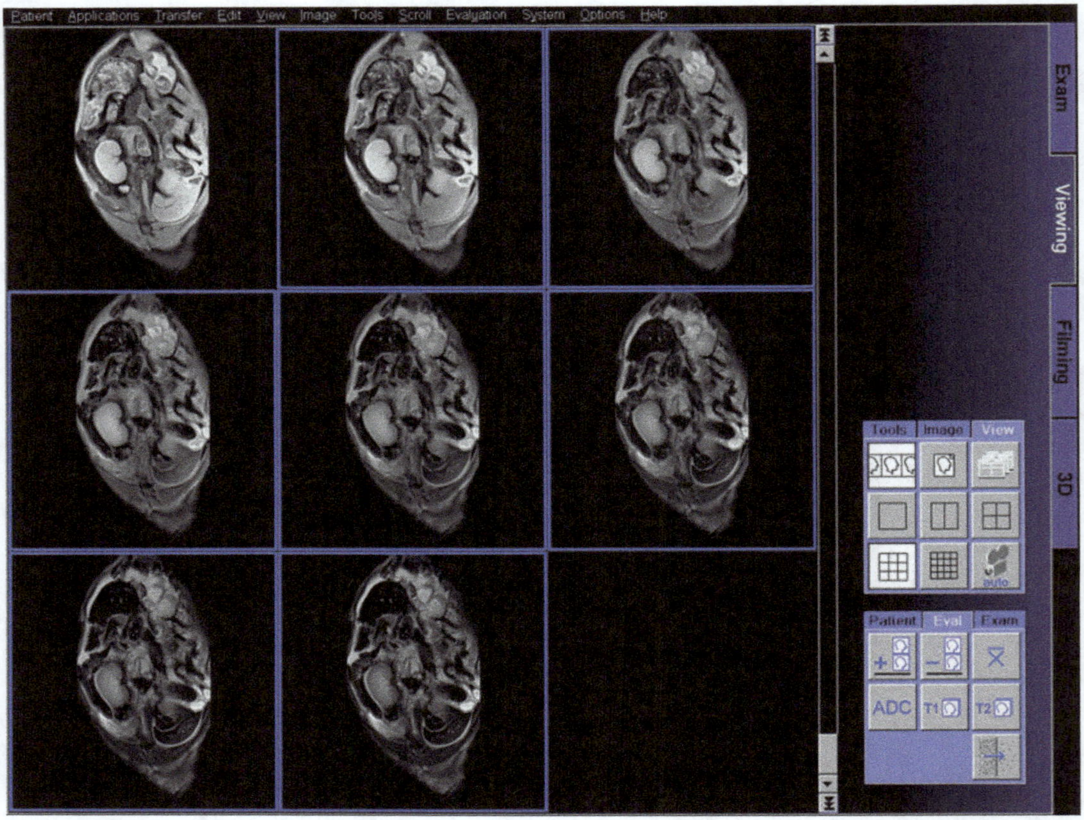

Fig. 5 Selection of echo images for $T_2^{(*)}$-mapping of a rat kidney in Siemens *Syngo*. Here T_2-mapping was performed, for which the first echo image must be excluded. Then start the $T_2^{(*)}$-map calculation with the *T2* button in the *Eval* tab in the *Control Area* panel on the bottom right

3. On the same image, use the *ROI* tool draw an ROI on the background, and register the standard deviation of the signal. Divide this value by 0.655 to obtain the noise standard deviation (*see* **Note 6** if you use a multichannel RF array).
4. Calculate the SNR by dividing the mean signal ROI by the noise standard deviation. If the SNR is below 2.6 this image should be excluded on step "8" (*see* **Note 7**).
5. Select a 3 × 3 or 4 × 4 layout in the *View* tab of the *Control Area* (right panel) in order to see all acquired echo images.
6. Select all echo images for T_2*-mapping or all echo images except the first for T_2-mapping (Fig. 5).
7. In the *Control Area* choose *Eval* > T_2 > *OK*. Two new images will appear in the viewer, the $T_2^{(*)}$-map and the S_0-map.
8. Exclude all echo images that have a SNR < 2.6 (*see* **Note 7**).

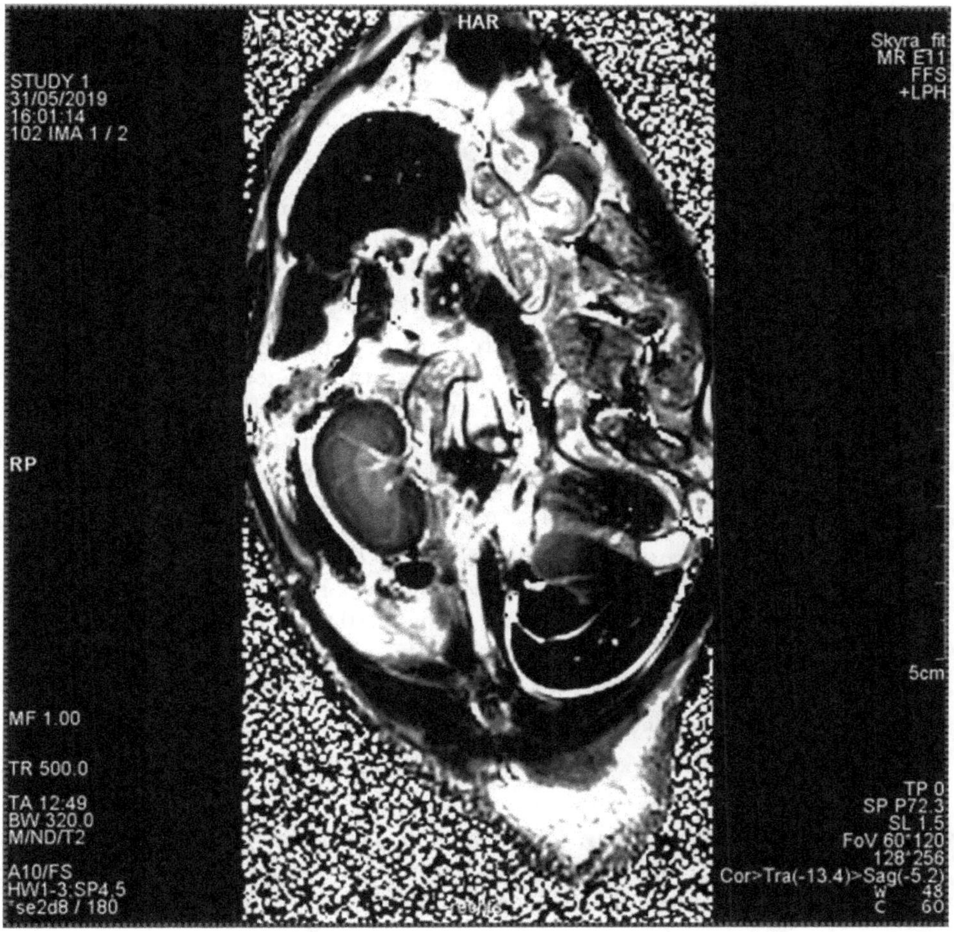

Fig. 6 T_2-map of a rat kidney calculated using the *T2-analysis* tool of Siemens *Syngo* from data acquired with a clinical 3 T scanner

9. In the *Control Area* choose *Eval* > T_2 > *OK*. A $T_2^{(*)}$-map will appear in the viewer. Use this new map for further analysis/quantification (Fig. 6).

3.2 Model Fitting (General Electric $T_2^{(*)}$ Map Ready View)

On a GE system a similar tool is used for mapping of T_2 and T_2*. The *Ready View T2 Map* protocol post processes data sets acquired using the *Cartigram* (T_2 Map) application. The *T2 Map* layout is comprised of four viewports: upper-left Map viewport: source image, upper-right viewport: curve displaying signal intensity (vertical axis) and the echo number (horizontal axis). A data point for each echo is plotted when an ROI is deposited on any of the three images. Lower left viewport: *T2 Map* Preset-1 parametric image. Lower right viewport: *T2 Map* Preset-2 parametric map.

Use these steps to post-process data sets acquired using the *Cartigram* application. The $T_2^{(*)}$ relaxation time color map is coded to capture $T_2^{(*)}$ values from the TE range of the acquired images. Blue and green reflect the longer $T_2^{(*)}$ values, yellow the intermediate $T_2^{(*)}$ values, and red and orange the shorter $T_2^{(*)}$ values. The functional $T_2^{(*)}$ map units are ms.

1. Open *ReadyView* and start the *T2map* protocol.
2. Adjust the *W/L* (window width and level) and magnification—to adjust the *W/L*, middle-click and drag over the image. To adjust the magnification factor, place the cursor over the red *DFOV* and middle-click and drag right to left.
3. Locate the desired images to view—press the Up and Down arrows to move through the images to locate the image with the area of interest. Or click and drag the red slice Location annotation. Press the Right and Left arrows to select the desired echo or click and drag the red echo annotation.
4. Open the *T2 Map* Settings screen.
5. Adjust the settings on the *T2 Map Settings* screen. Typically, the Preset Color Level sliders for both the $T_2^{(*)}$ map and parametric image are within a 10 and 90 ms range and the Threshold is 20. Typically, the Confidence Level is 0.05. A default smoothing kernel of 2 is recommended.
6. Click Compute.
7. If necessary, use the *Clip Min & Max* values. By default (25–75).
8. In the measurements panel, select the ROI icon and draw the desired region of interest. An annotation with the area, mean value and standard deviation of the ROI will appear.

3.3 Model Fitting (Philips)

1. When acquiring a $T_2^{(*)}$ (mTSE/MGE) dataset, select the *Postproc* tab and choose the option *T2*$^{(*)}$ or *R2*$^{(*)}$ ($1/T_2^{(*)}$) under the field *Calculated images* (Fig. 7).
2. Insert the maximum expected $T_2^{(*)}$ or its reciprocal ($1/T_2^{(*)}$) under the field *T2 clip value* or its reciprocal *R2*$^{(*)}$ *clip value* to specify the maximum calculated $T_2^{(*)}/R_2^{(*)}$ value for the SE sequence. Larger $T_2^{(*)}/R_2^{(*)}$ values are clipped to this value.
3. By default, $T_2/T_2{}^*$ reconstruction includes the first echo and performs a MLE fitting of the signal curve. Research customers can modify these parameters under the *Scan Control Parameters* panel select *Reconstruction* and choose the option *Include first echo for (SE) T2,R2 calc (yes/no)*, and reconstruction method (*MLE* [5, 6] or Least squares (*RLSQ*)) for $T_2^{(*)}$, $R_2^{(*)}$. If available we recommend to use *Include first echo* = *no* and the default *MLE* calculation method (*see* **Note 9**)—Warning: changing these options affects every scan until reset of the system (Fig. 8). After the acquisition, drag and drop the images in the viewer.

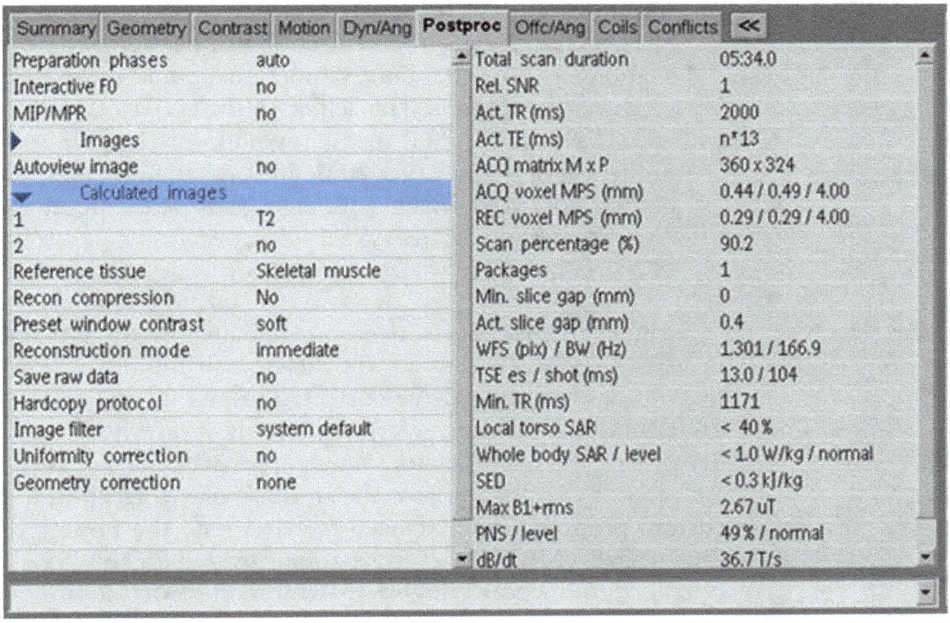

Fig. 7 Philips acquisition software *Postproc* tab. Here T_2-mapping can be performed by choosing the option *T2* or *R2* ($1/T_2$) under the field *Calculated images*

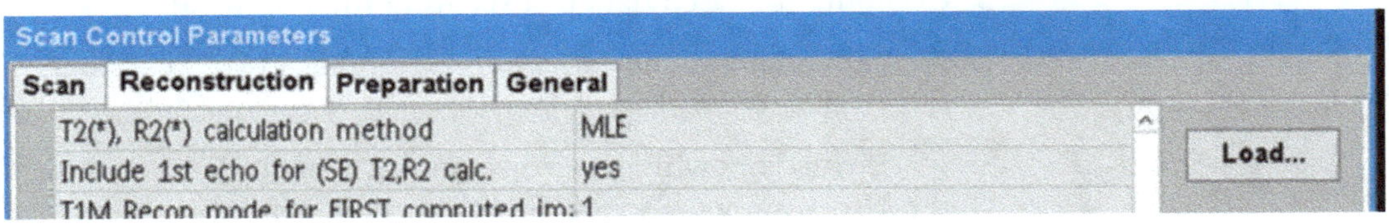

Fig. 8 Philips acquisition software *Scan Control Parameters* panel—only accessible for research customers. Here under the *Reconstruction* tab select *no* on the option *Include first echo for (SE) T2/R2 calc.* to exclude the first echo image on T_2 mapping and select *MLE* for *T2(*), R2(*) calculation method* (*see* **Note 9**)

3.4 Data Preparation and Model Fitting (Custom Program)

The following custom program for $T_2^{(*)}$ relaxometry contains code examples following MATLAB syntax. These were tested to be compatible with Octave and should be easily reproducible in Python or an equivalent SDE.

3.4.1 Data Import and Exclusion of First TE (Only for T_2)

1. Import your scan with the images obtained for different TEs.

   Bruker data: in MATLAB use the import function provided by Bruker's *pvtools*—to obtain Bruker's *pvtools* send an e-mail to Bruker mri-software-support@bruker.com.

   DICOM data: in MATLAB use the dicomread function—https://mathworks.com/help/images/ref/dicomread.html; in Python use dcmread from the pydicom package—https://pydicom.github.io/). As input you need to provide a string containing the full path of the DICOM file.

2. As previously explained, when performing T_2-mapping using a multiecho sequence, the first echo must be excluded from data analysis (*see* **Note 8**). For example, that could mean that for a series of T_2 weighted data acquired at TE = 10.0, 20.0, 30.0, 40.0, 50.0, 60.0, 70.0 ms one would only be able to fit the model curve to the TE = 20.0, 30.0, 40.0, 50.0, 60.0 ms data points: store your data in a different variable excluding the first TE (`imgData_forAnalysis = imgDataT2w(:,:,2:end); TE_forAnalysis = TE(2:end)`).

3.4.2 Rician Noise Bias Correction

MR signal intensities are overestimated in low SNR magnitude images. This bias is due to the Rician distribution of noisy MR magnitude data and can be corrected in post-processing. We can understand the processing step as multiplication with a signal-level dependent correction factor, which approaches 1 as higher SNRs are reached. To incorporate Rician noise bias correction into our custom program, we first need to determine the noise level and then utilize a MATLAB/Octave tool provided for this book under https://github.com/LudgerS/MRInoiseBiasCorrection:

1. Add the downloaded noise correction tool to the search path.

```
Addpath(genpath('...\MRInoiseBiasCOrrection)).
```

2. Compute unbiased data by executing the following:

```
imgData_corrected=correctNoiseBias(imgData_forAnalysis, sigma, 1)
```

If you work with data from a multichannel RF array, change the last argument of the function to the number of receive elements.

3.4.3 Fitting Model

The most common method is to iteratively fit the model of the $T_2^{(*)}$ decay to the signal intensity (SI) data of each pixel using the following equation:

$$S(\mathrm{TE}) = S_0 . \exp\left(-\frac{\mathrm{TE}}{T_2^{(*)}}\right) \quad (1)$$

where S_0 is a scaling factor that includes many parameters such as the proton density together with the signal gain of the system.

3.4.4 Starting Values

An important step of the curve fitting process is the choice of suitable starting values for each parameter that will be determined by the fitting algorithm (NB: different starting values may lead to different results!). Here we describe how to derive starting values from the SI of each pixel.

1. Step through all pixels in the images using for loops for the pixel coordinates *x* and *y*.

2. Store the SI of that pixel at all TEs in a vector (in MATLAB: `SI_vector = imgData_forFitting(xPix, yPix,:)`).
3. As starting value for the parameter S_0 use the first and largest SI (`startVal_S0 = SI_vector(1)`).

For estimating a starting value for $T_2^{(*)}$, one can exploit the fact that at TE = $T_2^{(*)}$ the SI has fallen to 37% of its value at TE = 0. Estimate the starting value by determining the TE whose SI is closest to 37% of the largest SI value:

4. Normalize the SI vector to a maximum value of 1 (divide by the largest SI value).
5. Subtract 0.63 from the SI vector.
6. Get the absolute values of the SI vector (resulting in only positive values).
7. Find the index of the smallest value in the vector (in MATLAB: `[min_Value,min_Index] = min(SI_norm_abs_37pct)`).
8. Get the respective echo from your echoes using the index from the last step (`startVal_T2=TE_forFitting(min_Index)`).

3.4.5 Fitting Algorithm

Least squares algorithms, such as the Levenberg–Marquardt [7] and Trust-region methods [8], are the most commonly used curve fitting algorithms for $T_2^{(*)}$-mapping. They work by minimizing a cost function, which describes the deviation of the fitted curve from the corresponding data points. With starting values near the optimal solution they quickly converge, but with starting values far away from the solution, the Levenberg–Marquardt algorithm will slow down significantly. Also, there is the risk that it may converge to a local minimum (rather than the global minimum) and hence produce an erroneous result.

In contrast, the Trust-region method (a further development of the Levenberg–Marquardt algorithm) will quickly converge, even with suboptimal starting values, and it will always find the global minimum. However, it does require the definition of lower and upper limits for the parameters to be fitted. Hence, for $T_2^{(*)}$-mapping, where such limits can easily be defined, the Trust-region method is well suited (*see* **Note 10**)

1. Create for loops for pixel coordinates *x* and *y* to step through all pixels of the image.
2. Store the SI of that pixel at all TEs in a vector (in MATLAB: `SI_vector = imgData_forFitting(xPix, yPix,:)`).
3. Define the model for the function using Equation1 (in MATLAB: `T2model = fittype('a*exp.(-x*b)', 'independent', 'x', 'dependent', 'y')`).

4. Choose the function for the fitting algorithm, that is, Trust-region or, if not available, then Levenberg–Marquardt (in MATLAB: `opts.Algorithm = 'Trust-Region'`).
5. Provide the starting values for S_0 and $T_2^{(*)}$ (in MATLAB, e.g., `opts.StartPoint = [startVal_S0 startVal_T2]`).
6. Define lower and upper limits for the fit parameters. Use for T_2* [0.1 150], for T_2 [1 1000], and for S_0 the possible range of SI in the image data (this depends on the system; for 16-bit integer it may be [1 65536]). In MATLAB, for example, `opts.Lower = [1 0.1]; opts.Upper = [65,536 150]`.
7. Execute the curve fitting for each pixel data (in MATLAB: `[fitresult, gof] = fit(TE_forFitting, SI_vector, T2model, opts);`).
8. Save the fit result for each variable in parameter maps: `mapS0(xPix, yPix) = fitresult.a; mapT2(xPix, yPix) = fitresult.b; rsquare(xPix, yPix) = gof.rsquare`.

3.4.6 Visual Display

1. Display the parameter map, which is a matrix with floating point numbers, as an image (in MATLAB: `imagesc(mapT2);`).
2. Remove axis labels and ensure that the axes are scaled such that the aspect ratio of the image is identical to that of the acquired FOV (For the case of square pixels in MATLAB: `axis off; axis equal;`).
3. Select the color map and display a color bar (in MATLAB: colormap(jet(256)); `colorbar;`) (*see* **Note 11**).
4. Set the display range for the color coding, for example, for T_2* [0 25]; and for T_2 [0 80]; (in MATLAB: `caxis([0 25]);`). An example is shown in Fig. 9.

3.5 Quantification

Quantitative values can be obtained from the parameter maps using manually drawn ROI for the different morphological regions (cortex, outer medulla, and inner medulla). Because manual ROI drawing can introduce unwanted additional variability or bias, we recommend the use of semiautomated methods, such as the concentric objects technique [9] or the morphology-based ROI placement technique [10]. For further details and step-by-step protocols for these two techniques please refer to the chapter by Riazy L et al. "Subsegmentation of the Kidney in Experimental MR Images Using Morphology-Based Regions-of-Interest or Multiple-Layer Concentric Objects."

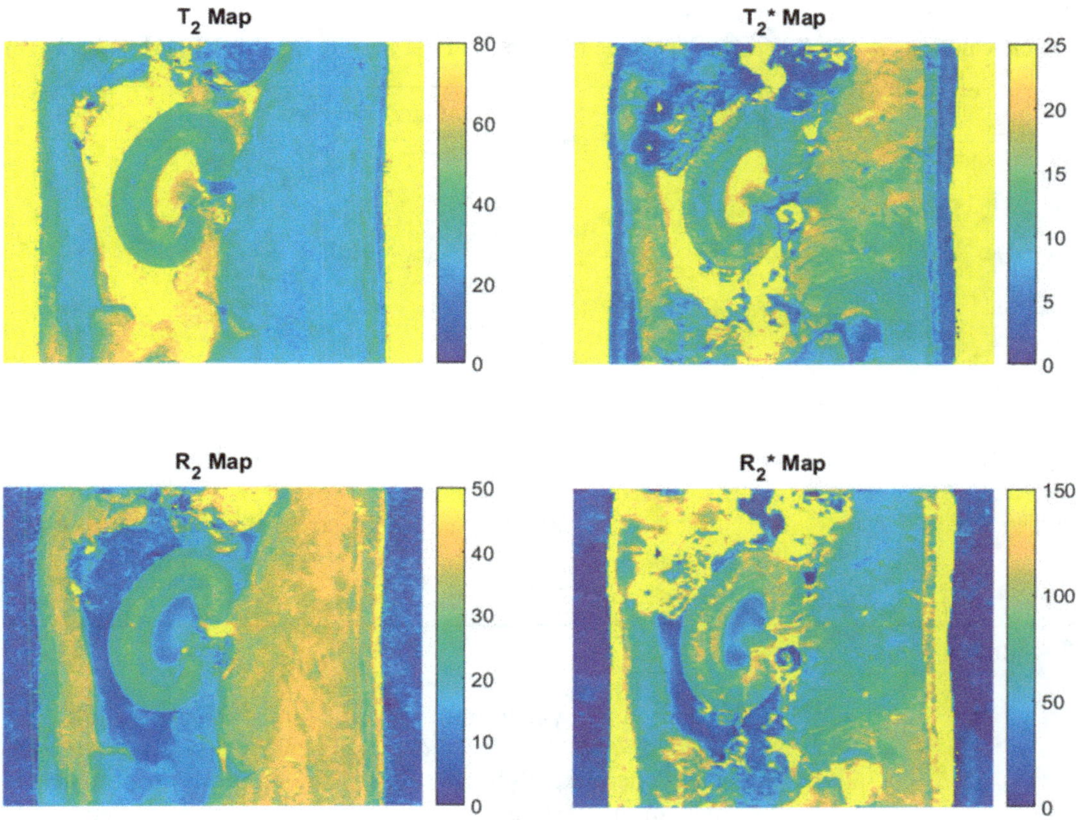

Fig. 9 $T_2^{(*)}$ in ms and $R_2^{(*)}$ in ms^{-1} maps of an healthy rat kidney calculated using a custom program developed in MATLAB (displayed using colormap *parula*) from data acquired with a preclinical 9.4 T scanner

3.6 Methods for Result Validation

3.6.1 Evaluation of Analysis Errors and Variability Using Synthetic Data

A simple approach to validate the data analysis procedure is to generate synthetic image data and then evaluate how close the results produced by the analysis are to the known true value. A series of artificial images could be created (using an in-house software program) that mimic a multiecho MR experiment. Each image could represent a chosen TE for which the signal intensity in a virtual phantom (could simply be a circle in the center of the image) has been calculated using the known exponential equation that describes the $T_2^{(*)}$ relaxation. Alternatively, more sophisticated simulation approaches as previously described in [3] could be used, accounting for the timings and characteristics of the used RF pulses so as to evaluate the effect of using the simpler monoexponential decay model. Having generated the images, Rician noise is added. This synthetic data could then be analyzed, evaluating both accuracy (how close the resulting $T_2^{(*)}$ is to the true $T_2^{(*)}$) and precision (evaluating dispersion over multiple instances with the same level of SNR).

Table 1
Typical values of T_2 and T_2* for each specific renal tissue for a healthy rat at 9.4 T [11] and 3 T [12]

Map	Inner medulla	Outer medulla	Cortex
9.4 T [8]			
R_2 [1 s^{-1}]	11.0–14.6	20.0–23.2	23.0–27.3
R_2* [1 s^{-1}]	32.1–47.2	73.9–101.1	64.8–93.6
3.0 T [9]			
R_2 [1 s^{-1}]	5.5–7.0	9.6–12.5	13.8–16.3
R_2* [1 s^{-1}]	12.8–19.8	28.3–30.3	29.5–37.5

3.6.2 Comparison with Reference Values from the Literature

The obtained values can be compared with those reported for healthy animals in the literature. Table 1 provides ranges of T_2* and T_2 for different magnetic field strengths based on current literature.

4 Notes

1. With increasing echo number additional diffusion weighting is added due to the repeated magnetic field gradients used for spatial encoding (NB: this effect is much more pronounced in small animal systems, which use much stronger gradients than clinical systems). A greater bias is introduced by the superposition of stimulated echoes in multi-spin-echo imaging, which leads to significant overestimation of T_2. It also demands the exclusion of the first echo (pure spin echo) from the analysis, because its magnitude is usually much smaller than that of the following echoes, which are combinations of spin-echoes and stimulated echoes. Although these biases depend on the acquisition parameters, they are fixed and reproducible for each protocol and hence acceptable in studies focusing on relative differences/changes, where precision is far more important than accuracy. If needed, more accurate T_2 values can be obtained from multiecho data using sophisticated post-processing, such as dictionary-matching methodologies [3].
2. Make sure your data is ordered from the lowest to the highest TE as in Figs. 2 and 3.
3. When establishing the MR technique, define an SNR acceptance threshold. The aim is to have at least three (preferably five or more) number of echoes with an SNR > 5. This threshold will depend on the expected $T_2^{(*)}$ values, which in turn depend on parameters like the magnetic field strength, shim quality, and tissue properties (pathology). Example: for a rat imaged at 9.4 T using a 4-element rat heart array receiver surface RF coil

together with a volume resonator for excitation in combination with interventions leading to strong hypoxia an SNR > 60 was needed for the image with the lowest TE. Always draw the ROI over the same region of the kidney, that is, cortex, outer medulla, or inner medulla (we use the inner medulla, which is the brightest region of the kidney). If reaching a sufficiently high SNR is a problem, consider creating ROIs and performing the $T_2^{(*)}$-fitting on the average values of these ROIs in order to boost the SNR (SNR scales with the square root of the number of pixels). Another option is to modify the acquisition protocol, reducing the attained spatial resolution to gain SNR.

4. As a good practice you should always save your ROIs for later reference. After creating an ROI click on Analyze > Tools > ROI Manager > Add. Then rename your ROI to a meaningful name (using the button "Rename on the ROI Manager).
5. When you create an ROI over a region with no signal make sure no artifacts are present. Click on Image > Adjust > Brightness and Contrast and drag the scroll bar "Minimum" to the left.
6. Sum-of-squares reconstruction of multichannel data changes the distribution of noisy MR magnitude data. Substitute the factor 0.655 by 0.682 or 0.695 for two channel and four channel data, respectively [13].
7. The Rician distribution of MR magnitude images introduces a signal level-dependent positive bias. The relative error introduced by this bias increases with decreasing SNR. For single receive element coils, an error of 10% is reached at SNR = 2.6. For two-channel or four-channel coils, the corresponding threshold is at SNR = 4.2 or 6.4, respectively, assuming sum-of-squares reconstruction. Under pathophysiological conditions $T_2^{(*)}$ can become significantly shorter and images acquired at high TEs may have a rather low SNR or may even reach noise level. This could result in a poor model curve fit and overestimate the calculated $T_2^{(*)}$. Therefore, data points at high TEs below a predefined SNR threshold should be excluded from the data analysis. Data exclusion can be done either during the acquisition (by not acquiring some echoes) or performed prior to data analysis. The latter is advantageous because the SNR cutoff to exclude data from the fitting can also be adjusted for each pixel individually.
8. When a multiecho sequence is used for T_2-mapping, the first echo must be excluded from the data analysis. The reason is that the first echo is a pure spin echo, unlike all following echoes, which are superpositions of spin-echoes and stimulated echoes. As a result, the first echo has significantly smaller amplitude than the second echo and fitting the model curve to all data points would produce a poor curve fit and an inaccurate T_2 value [10].

9. MLE option refers to "Maximum-likelihood estimator" that takes into account the Rician noise. The noise level is measured as part of the scan. This approach should be robust against noise floor estimation bias and therefore there is no need to exclude later echoes from the analysis [5, 6].
10. An approach to increase the speed of the curve fitting is using a fast mono exponential fit [14]. The MATLAB implementation of the following fit can be downloaded from https://github.com/JoaoPeriquito/T2-s-Mapping under the name *fastExpoFit.m*. The result of a simulation comparing the recommended fast mono exponential fit and the trust-region can be found at the same location under the name *fastExpoFit_Simulation.png*.
11. Pseudocolor representations can be extremely useful for analyzing $T_2^{(*)}$-maps, since they generally enhance the perception of differences within the value range of the parameter. But one needs to be careful when choosing a color map. Parameter maps displayed as images in pseudocolor can potentially be misleading. Small differences in the underlying values may be artificially emphasised by a change in color hue, or a significant parameter difference that can easily be seen in a gray-scale image may be flattened or hidden if there is little change of hue or brightness over a certain range of the color-scale. It is recommended to always use the same color map and scale to improve comparability.

Acknowledgments

The authors wish to thank Dr. Torben Schneider and Dr. Anabea Solana for the contribute of the $T_2^{(*)}$ mapping protocol for Philips and GE scanner, respectively. Portuguese Foundation for Science and Technology (FCT—UID/EEA/50009/2019), and POR Lisboa 2020 (LISBOA-01-0145-FEDER-029686).

This work was funded in part (Thoralf Niendorf, Andreas Pohlmann, Joao Periquito) by the German Research Foundation (Gefoerdert durch die Deutsche Forschungsgemeinschaft (DFG), Projektnummer 394046635, SFB 1365, RENOPROTECTION. Funded by the Deutsche Forschungsgemeinschaft (DFG, German Research Foundation), Project number 394046635, SFB 1365, R ENOPROTECTION).

This chapter is based upon work from COST Action PARENCH IMA, supported by European Cooperation in Science and Technology (COST). COST (www.cost.eu) is a funding agency for research and innovation networks. COST Actions help connect research initiatives across Europe and enable scientists to enrich their ideas by sharing them with their peers. This boosts their research, career, and innovation.

PARENCHIMA (renalmri.org) is a community-driven Action in the COST program of the European Union, which unites more than 200 experts in renal MRI from 30 countries with the aim to improve the reproducibility and standardization of renal MRI biomarkers.

References

1. Niendorf T, Pohlmann A et al (2015) How bold is blood oxygenation level-dependent (BOLD) magnetic resonance imaging of the kidney? Opportunities, challenges and future directions. Acta Physiol (Oxf) 213(1):19–38. https://doi.org/10.1111/apha.12393
2. Pohlmann A et al (2014) Detailing the relation between renal T2* and renal tissue pO2 using an integrated approach of parametric magnetic resonance imaging and invasive physiological measurements. Investig Radiol 49:547–560
3. Ben-Eliezer N, Sodickson DK, Block KT (2015) Rapid and accurate T2 mapping from multi-spin-echo data using Bloch-simulation-based reconstruction. Magn Reson Med 73:809–817
4. Schindelin J, Arganda-Carreras I, Frise E et al (2012) Fiji: an open-source platform for biological-image analysis. Nat Methods 9 (7):676–682. https://doi.org/10.1038/nmeth.2019
5. Senegas J, Knopp T, Dahnke H (2007) Dealing with spatially varying noise in T2* mapping with SENSE. Proceedings of the International Society of Magnetic Resonance in Medicine, Berlin
6. Hedström E et al (2017) Automatic T2* determination for quantification of iron load in heart and liver: a comparison between automatic inline maximum likelihood estimate and the truncation and offset methods. Clin Physiol Funct Imaging 37(3):299–304
7. Moré JJ (1978) The Levenberg-Marquardt algorithm: implementation and theory. Numerical analysis. Springer, Berlin, pp 105–116
8. Byrd RH, Schnabel RB, Shultz GA (1987) A trust region algorithm for nonlinearly constrained optimization. SIAM J Numer Anal 24(5):1152–1170
9. Piskunowicz M et al (2015) A new technique with high reproducibility to estimate renal oxygenation using BOLD-MRI in chronic kidney disease. Magn Reson Imaging 33(3):253–261
10. Pohlmann A, Cantow K, Huelnhagenm T, Grosenick D, dos Santos Periquito J et al (2017) Experimental MRI monitoring of renal blood volume fraction variations en route to renal magnetic resonance oximetry. Tomography 3(4):188–200
11. Pohlmann A et al (2013) High temporal resolution parametric MRI monitoring of the initial ischemia/reperfusion phase in experimental acute kidney injury. PLoS One 8(2):e57411
12. Thacker J, Zhang JL, Franklin T, Prasad P (2017) BOLD quantified renal pO2 is sensitive to pharmacological challenges in rats. Magn Reson Med 78(1):297–302
13. Constantinides CD, Atalar E, McVeigh ER (1997) Signal-to-noise measurements in magnitude images from NMR phased arrays. Magn Reson Imaging 38(5):852–857
14. Pei M et al (2015) Algorithm for fast monoexponential fitting based on auto-regression on linear operations (ARLO) of data. Magn Reson Med 73:843–850

7

Analysis of Renal Diffusion-Weighted Imaging (DWI) using Apparent Diffusion Coefficient (ADC) and Intravoxel Incoherent Motion (IVIM) Models

Neil Peter Jerome and João S. Periquito

Abstract

Analysis of renal diffusion-weighted imaging (DWI) data to derive markers of tissue properties requires careful consideration of the type, extent, and limitations of the acquired data. Alongside data quality and general suitability for quantitative analysis, choice of diffusion model, fitting algorithm, and processing steps can have consequences for the precision, accuracy, and reliability of derived diffusion parameters. Here we introduce and discuss important steps for diffusion-weighted image processing, and in particular give example analysis protocols and pseudo-code for analysis using the apparent diffusion coefficient (ADC) and intravoxel incoherent motion (IVIM) models. Following an overview of general principles, we provide details of optional steps, and steps for validation of results. Illustrative examples are provided, together with extensive notes discussing wider context of individual steps, and notes on potential pitfalls.

This publication is based upon work from the COST Action PARENCHIMA, a community-driven network funded by the European Cooperation in Science and Technology (COST) program of the European Union, which aims to improve the reproducibility and standardization of renal MRI biomarkers. This analysis protocol chapter is complemented by two separate chapters describing the basic concepts and experimental procedure.

Key words MRI, Kidney, Diffusion, Diffusion-weighted imaging (DWI), Apparent diffusion coefficient (ADC), Intravoxel incoherent motion (IVIM), Mouse, Rat, Analysis, Algorithm

1 Introduction

Diffusion-weighted imaging (DWI) can be implemented in many forms, and similarly analysis of DWI data is more complex than for other common quantitative modalities such as T_1, T_2, and T_2* [1, 2]. The overall goal of deriving robust biomarkers for renal function, disease identification and response, as well as monitoring of transplants and so forth [3] relies not only on the suitability of the acquisition for the question being asked, but also how that data are handled in post-processing and analysis.

The basic concepts underlying DWI, and example experimental protocols, are discussed in the chapters by Jerome NP et al. "Renal Diffusion-Weighted Imaging (DWI) for Apparent Diffusion Coefficient (ADC), Intravoxel Incoherent Motion (IVIM), and Diffusion Tensor Imaging (DTI): Basic Concepts" and by Periquito J et al. "Renal MRI Diffusion: Experimental Protocol" of this book. This chapter will cover general elements of data quality and analysis, with a view to providing example protocols for the main models employed for renal DWI. As mentioned in the chapter by Jerome NP et al. "Renal Diffusion-Weighted Imaging (DWI) for Apparent Diffusion Coefficient (ADC), Intravoxel Incoherent Motion (IVIM), and Diffusion Tensor Imaging (DTI): Basic Concepts," however, it is critical to note that analysis choices are intrinsically linked to the acquisition strategy itself, most prominently in number and direction of chosen *b*-values used, which means not only that the available choices of analysis are limited by the type of data collected but also that intended analysis should be an integral part of study planning. Analysis itself is naïve to the suitability of the choices of model and algorithm used, for example, and so this responsibility rests with the researcher.

Alternative diffusion models, as well as other mathematical signal representations without explicit physiological meaning, to the ones discussed here are numerous, and include the increasingly popular stretched exponential and kurtosis descriptions, and this field is constantly developing [4–8]. In addition to general considerations, this chapter provides explicit methods for two common diffusion models, namely, the apparent diffusion coefficient (ADC) and the intravoxel incoherent motion (IVIM) models, and describes the estimation of the corresponding diffusion parameters. While the assumption has been made that suitable data has been acquired (*see* the chapter by Periquito J et al. "Renal MRI Diffusion: Experimental Protocol"), no two datasets are alike, and these protocols are presented as guidelines that claim to be neither complete nor sufficient, and are intended only to provide a basic framework whereby a full analysis protocol can be developed. The advantages of more sophisticated algorithms than are presented here are becoming more apparent, and while the full details of these techniques are beyond the scope of this chapter, the reader is encouraged to investigate their potential when considering both analysis protocols and, where possible, study design. When retrospective analysis is performed outside the original study plan, understanding associated limitations and potential problems is crucial to delivering sound conclusions.

Once DWI data has been acquired, an appreciable portion of the available choices has already been made about how the data are presented and packaged. Analysis is thus a purely computational process that can be performed either "manually" using routines developed in-house, ideally in collaboration with specialist MR physicists or mathematicians, or by using commercially available software packages (including those available on the scanners themselves). The pros and cons of these two approaches are inversions of each other, essentially revolving around transparency of the processes and the ability to design bespoke interrogations of the data, versus using more developed and optimized analysis using tools that require less "up-front" investment of time but which can act as inscrutable "black boxes."

While many of the same issues arise for renal imaging, is it useful to remember that much of current DWI acquisition and analysis development has been in the brain and for neurological applications. While this affords a large amount of literature and advanced techniques, translating from one tissue to another requires a certain degree of circumspection regarding assumptions and reoptimization, if not protocol redesign. Finally, it should be remembered that no level of analysis can ever provide more information than is contained in the data itself, and care should be taken to avoid over-interpretation.

This analysis protocol chapter is complemented by two separate chapters describing the basic concepts and experimental procedure, which are part of this book.

This chapter is part of the book Pohlmann A, Niendorf T (eds) (2020) Preclinical MRI of the Kidney—Methods and Protocols. Springer, New York.

2 Materials

2.1 Data Format and Quality

MRI, including DWI, data are stored as either a manufacturer-specific format (e.g., Bruker) or as a medical imaging standard (e.g., DICOM, NifTI), but in essence contains a series of matrices of intensity values constituting the images, with each image indexed against the acquisition parameters including the diffusion-weighting *b*-value. The exact details of where the *b*-value is stored varies by image format, or the *b*-value may need to be explicitly added (*see* **Note 1**). Commonly, DWI schemes acquire a set of three images for nonzero *b*-value magnitudes, with the diffusion-sensitizing gradients applied in orthogonal directions; this allows for calculation of a *trace image*, where any anisotropy of diffusion is averaged out by taking the geometric mean of the intensities. If possible, the separate images should be used for analysis, since this allows for finer quality control before processing, and will retain the intrinsic weighting (i.e., more data at nonzero points) assumed by fitting algorithms.

A brief visual inspection should identify corrupted data or individual images that need to be excluded on account of severe artifacts or signal dropout, or from insufficient signal-to-noise (SNR). Images and/or cases that display gross motion or distortion may require additional processing steps before being included [9], or can be excluded (*see* Fig. 1).

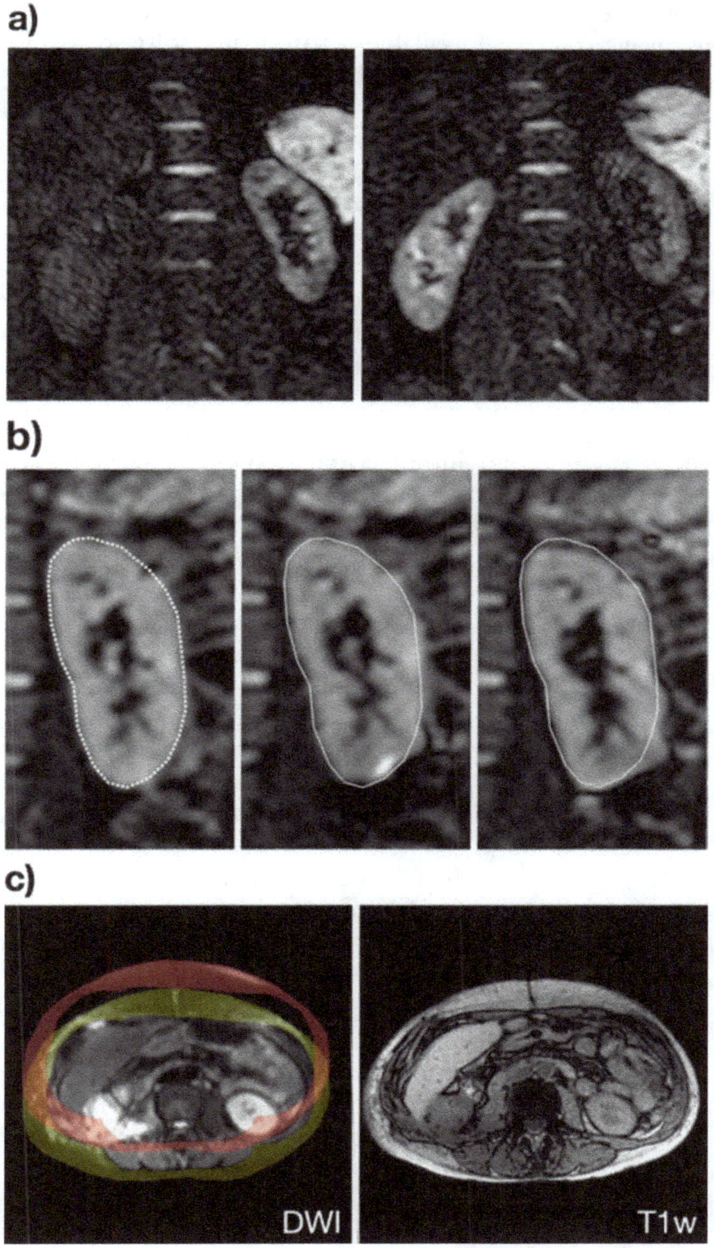

Fig. 1 Examples of images that might be considered for exclusion from analysis. (**a**) Signal drop, which can be uneven across the image, may arise from excessive movement during image readout; these images are the same *b*-value and were acquired in the same sequence, but show markedly different signal in each kidney. (**b**) Three images from the same sequence showing different degrees of distortion around the kidney edge; distortion is a dominant artifact in DWI where EPI is used, and is most prominent at magnetic susceptibility boundaries. (**c**) Imperfect fat suppression in the diffusion-weighted image across the body, combined with the chemical shift displacement of fat protons,

2.2 Software Requirements

Many common mathematical algorithms used for signal fitting are available across many software platforms with limited expertise needed to implement them, meaning analysis routines can be designed and written as needed. Commercial software such as *Matlab* include curve fitting toolboxes, whereas platforms such as *Python* and *R* contain equivalent functions and, being freely available, may present a more accessible or portable choice. In addition, these environments have the ability to handle image data (reading, sorting, displaying) and create figures, though a basic level of programming ability is required. The trade-off is more direct control versus the extra investment required to obtain proficiency with the software environment.

Several freely available software packages are able to perform both image processing and curve fitting, but attempt to give a more intuitive graphical user interface that allows out-of-the-box use, perhaps at the expense of tailored functionality. Environments such as *Fiji* (based on *ImageJ*, with additional plugins), as well as the brain-centric *FSL* and the OSX-only DICOM viewers *Horos* and *OsiriX*, provide different degrees of functionality and automation, and the option for bespoke plugins to at least some degree. The MR scanner itself and associated workstations also offer some options for processing of diffusion images, for example *ParaVision* on Bruker scanners or *SyngoVia* on Siemens, although the available choices and customizability on these systems can be limited.

In the following we present detailed instructions for implementing a custom-made analysis program.

2.3 Fitting Algorithms, Limits, and Initialization

In well-behaved systems with high quality data and appropriate models, choice of fitting algorithm is unlikely to influence the resulting parameters. In many cases, however, data are sufficiently noisy, or there may be cross-correlation between parameters in the model being used, which can mean that choice of fitting algorithm and initialization values can affect the result. These choices are subjective and are made as part of the analysis procedure, so should be reported in publications. Similarly, whether parameters are constrained to physical or anticipated physiological limits may have an effect on reported metrics. Analysis protocols should critically consider these choices as well as report them in scientific articles so that the results can be communicated within the appropriate context.

It is difficult to prescribe "best practice" in diffusion-weighted image processing, since organs and pathologies give a wide-ranging spectrum of situations. Given the highly perfused nature of the

Fig. 1 (continued) may give incorrect intensities from overlap of fat signal with target areas; here, the subcutaneous fat around the abdomen (overlay in yellow; T1w is given for comparison) is shifted up in the image (overlay in red), and will alter the observed image intensity seen for part of the kidney

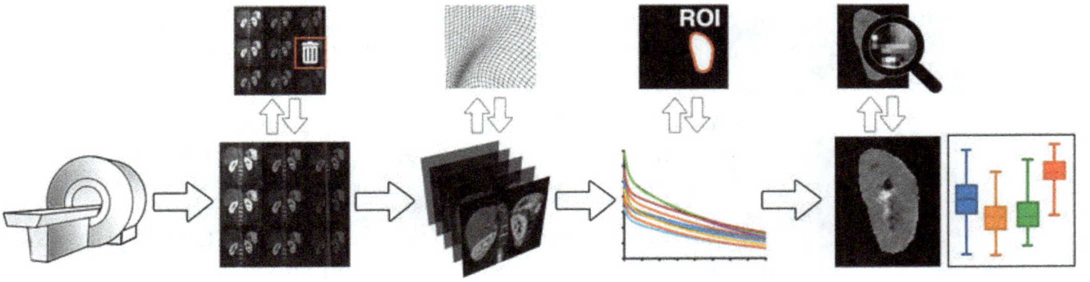

Fig. 2 General overview of the diffusion-weighted imaging pipeline, left to right: Export from the scanner gives the diffusion-weighted images, which should be reviewed for quality (SNR, artifacts, excessive motion, or distortion). The resulting data matrix can be preprocessed using registration, and corrections for eddy currents, distortion, and motion if desired. The fitting algorithm for the chosen model is run either on a region of interest, or on the whole image and the ROI drawn on the parameter maps. A further quality check on the maps and extracted results is recommended

kidney, together with the tubular structures, models such as IVIM that attempt to quantify pseudodiffusion (*see* **Note 2**) are potentially more informative than simple *ADC* measurements, although the analysis is more complex commensurate with the model, and may not give sufficient repeatability for detection of small changes [10]. Overall, standardization of protocols across studies has a value to be balanced against optimization at a local level, where translation of preclinical work into clinical use is the ultimate goal.

3 Methods

3.1 Generalized Steps for Diffusion-Weighted Image Processing

The steps listed here outline a general approach for DWI analysis (Fig. 2). The sections immediately following give more specific instructions for the ADC and IVIM models respectively, which are sufficiently different in complexity to warrant separate presentation and discussion. Notes at the end of the chapter, referenced throughout, give further detail on aspects that may need to be considered.

1. *Retrieve DWI data* to analysis platform: verify *b*-value information, and expected number of images (*see* **Note 1**).
2. *Initial quality check*: SNR threshold (*see* **Notes 3** and **4**) for exclusion of poor images, excessive signal drop-out, distortion, motion, failed fat suppression, and so on.
3. *Preprocessing*: motion correction, distortion correction, and registration if desired/applicable (*see* **Note 5**).
4. *Fitting of the model* to observed signal intensities against their acquisition parameters, normally *b*-value magnitude (*see* **Note 6**).

5. *Second quality check*: visual inspection of parameter maps, extreme values, visualization of fitted curves against the data (*see* **Note 7**).
6. *Extraction of diffusion parameters.* Summary statistics, histogram moments, and so on from a region of interest (*see* **Notes 8** and **9**).

The example protocols below are the constituent parts of a custom-made analysis program, designed to illustrate each step clearly and explicitly (and are thus not optimized for speed), and are presented in pseudo-code using functions and syntax in Matlab (Mathworks, Natick, USA). The wide number of equivalent choices and flexibility of some steps involved in DWI analysis are ignored in favor of presenting the main thread of a workflow that is easy to recreate, and so the reader is encouraged to appreciate the purpose of each step, which can usually be performed in a number of ways with different functions, rather than the specific implementation.

3.2 Diffusion Weighted Imaging: Apparent Diffusion Coefficient (ADC)

3.2.1 Preparation of Image Data for Fitting

1. Retrieve the data to the required folder structure and verify contents.
2. Load image data to matrix structure, aiming to create a 3D matrix of stacked images for each slice (a single slice is presented for simplicity here), with *b*-value in the 3rd dimension (*see* **Note 10**).

```
DICOM: matrix(:,:,i) = dicomread(<i_th_DICOM_filename>);
Bruker: [img,hdr] = read_2dseq(<series/pdata/1>);
```

3. Create a 'bVals' vector variable with the corresponding *b*-values, checking for the correct number of repetitions and the correct order (*see* **Notes 11** and **12**).
4. Review the images for quality: sufficient SNR, artifacts, and so on. Identify and remove any nonqualifying images from the img matrix, and correct bVals to match.

```
exclude = [0 0 0 1 0 0 0 1 1 0 0];
img = img(:,:,~logical(exclude));
bVals = bVals(~logical(exclude));
```

Optional steps at this stage include distortion, eddy current, and motion correction, and image registration (*see* **Notes 5** and **13**).

3.2.2 Least Squares Fitting for Apparent Diffusion Coefficient ADC

1. Define the model for fitting, where the two variables in *X* are *S0* and *ADC* (*see* **Note 14**):

```
curveADC = @(X,bVals) (X(1)*exp(-bVals*X(2)));
```

2. Assign empty matrices for the two resulting maps, using the dimensions of the images (*see* **Note 15**):

```
S0map = NaN(nRows,nCols);
ADCmap = NaN(nRows,nCols);
```

3. For each voxel, loop through each row (*i*) and column (*j*) and extract the signal data

```
for i = 1:nRows; for j = 1:nCols;
Sb = img(i,j,:);
```

4. Estimate initial values for the variables to be fitted; use the $b = 0\ \mathrm{s/mm^2}$ value for *S0*, and approximate *ADC* by taking the gradient of the log signal between two points (*see* **Notes 16** and **17**). *See* also Subheading 3.2.4 for discussion of linearization of *ADC* estimation and fitting.

```
S0_est = Sb(1);
ADC_est = (log(max(Sb))-log(min(Sb)))/
(max(bVals)-min(bVals));
X_est = [S0_est ADC_est];
```

5. Run the least-squares curve fitting routine, using the initial estimates and providing lower and upper boundaries for the estimates if desired (*see* **Note 18**). Assign the results to the allocated results maps:

```
limL = [0 0]; limU = [Inf Inf];
res = lsqcurvefit(curveADC,X_est,bVals,Sb,LimL,LimU);
S0map(i,j) = res(1);
ADCmap(i,j) = res(2);
end; end; % close the row/column loops
```

Some of the options available for least-squares curve fitting include the choice of algorithm, boundary conditions, stopping criteria, number of iterations, and so forth. In general, for well-behaved data the initial estimates will be good and the fitting should converge quickly.

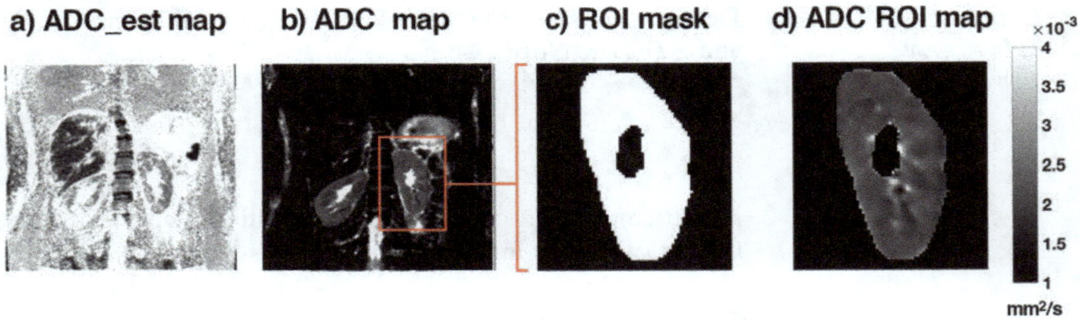

Fig. 3 Example maps from a healthy volunteer illustrating the steps for *ADC* analysis. (**a**) Initial linear estimate of *ADC* gives initial values for least-squares fitting. (**b**) Resulting *ADC* map. (**c**) A binary mask for the region-of-interest drawn on the *ADC* image. (**d**) *ADC* values ready for extraction

3.2.3 Extraction of Parameter Results

1. Review the results maps to visually inspect the results. Data plotted against a signal curve generated from the fitted values for any voxel in the image (*i,j*) should alert to any issues with either the fitting process or the data itself.

```
Sb = img(i,j,:);
S0 = S0map(i,j);
ADC = ADCmap(i,j);
figure; hold on;
plot(bVals, Sb, 'o'); % show the data
% show the fitted curve
plot(0:max(bVals), S0*exp(-ADC*(0:max(bVals))), 'r-');
```

2. Define the region of interest on the *ADC* map and use this to create a list of voxel coordinates within the ROI. For display, creating a binary mask is also useful (Fig. 3).

```
imagesc(ADCmap);
roi = impoly(); % draw ROI on image
mask = createMask(roi);
ADCmask = ADCmap .* mask;
```

3. Extract the *ADC* values from the ROI to a single matrix for summarizing (mean, median, percentiles, etc.).

```
ADClist = ADCmask(find(ADCmask));
ADC_mean = mean(ADClist);
```

3.2.4 Linear Regression and Matrix Inversion for ADC

Fitting of DWI to the monoexponential ADC model can be achieved with either nonlinear fitting of the signal directly, as above, but can also be treated as a linear regression fitting problem (which is computationally faster) if the natural log of the signal intensities is used (*see* **Note 17**). For the minimal acquisition of only two *b*-values, there is no ambiguity and the initial estimate calculation shown in Subheading 3.2.2 gives the result.

Taking the signal logarithm also allows for the use of matrix manipulations to perform the linear fitting, which again is computationally faster and handles the whole image simultaneously (*see* **Note 19**).

3.2.5 Computed Diffusion Images

Following calculation of *S0* and *ADC* maps, it becomes possible to create synthetic images at any desired *b*-value based on these values, which may increase conspicuity of lesions at higher *b*-values where noise would dominate in experimentally acquired images. Extension of this technique using an additional echo time *TE* allows similar control for computed T_2 weighting, which may assist with T_2 shine-through from fluid [11, 12].

3.3 Intravoxel Incoherent Motion (IVIM)

Fitting of the more complex IVIM model introduces associated complexity on the analysis, in particular the initialization and algorithm used for fitting [13]. Notably, the fitting for IVIM is inherently nonlinear, and cannot be easily linearized for speed. While more advanced fitting routines become popular (*see* Subheading 3.3.6), the major obstacle to successful IVIM fitting is ultimately the appropriateness of the model to the quality of data available.

In the protocol below, which shares much with the *ADC* protocol in Subheading 3.2, we present the segmented method as a method of initializing a full least-squares fit. The segmented method benefits from speed and stability, and can be used as an estimator in its own right, although it relies on prior assumptions. Parameters from segmented fitting may be fixed for the subsequent least-squares fitting if desired [14–16]. In all cases, the user is strongly encouraged to critically examine the results from IVIM fitting.

3.3.1 Preparation of Image Data for Fitting

This is identical to the preparation steps for *ADC* in Subheading 3.2.1.

1. Retrieve the data to the required folder structure and verify contents.
2. Load image data to matrix structure, aiming to create a 3D matrix of stacked images for each slice (a single slice is presented for simplicity here), with *b*-value in the third dimension (*see* **Note 10**).

```
DICOM: matrix(:,:,i) = dicomread(<ith_DICOM_filename>);
Bruker: [img,hdr] = read_2dseq(<series/pdata/1>);
```

3. Create a bVals vector variable with the corresponding *b*-values, checking for the correct number of repetitions and the correct order (*see* **Notes 11** and **12**).

4. Review the images for quality: sufficient SNR, artifacts, and so on. Identify and remove any nonqualifying images from the img matrix, and correct bVals to match.

```
exclude = [0 0 0 1 0 0 0 1 1 0 0];
img = img(:,:,~logical(exclude));
bVals = bVals(~logical(exclude));
```

Optional steps at this stage include distortion, eddy current, and motion correction, and image registration (*see* **Notes 5** and **13**).

3.3.2 Segmented Fitting for Diffusion Coefficient D

This section is largely the same as fitting for *ADC* in Subheading 3.2.2, with the exception that it is on a subset of the data in order to derive *D*. The parameter *SD* is the equivalent of *S0* but for the *D* compartment only, and is used to estimate *f* in the next section.

1. Choose a threshold *b*-value beyond which it is assumed that the pseudodiffusion signal contribution is negligible; this is commonly around 200 s/mm^2. Create a new (not overwritten) data matrix containing only these images, and matching bVals vector.

```
Bcut = 200;
imgD = img(:,:,[find(bVals >= Bcut)]);
bValsD = bVals(find(bVals >= Bcut));
```

2. Define the model for fitting, directly analogous to *ADC*, where the two variables in X are *SD* and *D*:

```
curveD = @(X,bVals) (X(1)*exp(-bVals*X(2)));
```

3. Assign empty matrices for the two resulting maps, using the dimensions of the images (*see* **Note 15**):

```
SDmap = NaN(nRows,nCols);
Dmap = NaN(nRows,nCols);
```

4. For each voxel, loop through each row (*i*) and column (*j*) and extract the signal data:

```
for i = 1:nRows; for j = 1:nCols;
Sb = imgD(i,j,:);
```

5. Estimate initial values for SD and D by taking the gradient of the log signal between two points (*see* **Note 16**).

```
SD_est = Sb(1);
D_est = (log(max(Sb))-log(min(Sb)))...
/(max(bValsD)-min(bValsD));
X_est = [SD_est D_est];
```

6. Run the least-squares curve fitting routine, using the initial estimates and providing boundaries for the estimates if desired (*see* **Note 18**). Assign the results to the allocated results maps:

```
limL = [0 0]; limU = [Inf Inf];
res = lsqcurvefit(curveD,X_est,bValsD,Sb,limL,limU);
SDmap(i,j) = res(1);
Dmap(i,j) = res(2);
end; end; % close the row/column loops
```

3.3.3 Segmented Fitting for Pseudodiffusion Fraction f

The calculation (not strictly a fitting) of f, similar to fitting for D^* that follows, can also be performed on a voxelwise basis within the loops used for the fitting of D. The presentation here is to emphasize the stepwise nature of this procedure.

1. Derive estimate of f by calculating the fraction of $S0$ (the signal at $b = 0$ s/mm^2) that does not arise from the D component. Use the mean $b = 0$ s/mm^2 image if there are more than one.

```
b0img = mean(img(:,:,find(bVals == 0)),3);
fmap = (b0img - SDmap) ./ b0img;
```

3.3.4 Fitting for Pseudodiffusion Coefficient D*

Having estimated D and f using the segmented method above, D^* can be estimated by a second fitting process of the residuals after subtracting the calculated signal from the D component. Though not exactly equivalent, it is common to fix the D and f values and perform a least-squares fit only for D^* using all the data (*see* **Note 20**). These estimates can be sufficient on their own to provide a result, or they can be used as initial estimates for subsequent nonlinear fitting of all the parameters in the IVIM model (*see* Subheading 3.3.5).

The dependency of IVIM parameters on the specific details of the fitting process is not simple [17], and pseudodiffusion parameters in particular are known to be less repeatable [18]. It is worth reiterating here that DWI acquisition and analysis are closely interwoven, and the utility of derived parameters is ultimately reliant on the acquisition of suitable data.

1. Allocate a matrix for the D^* values (*see* **Note 21**) and the pseudodiffusion fraction signal intensity.

```
Dsmap = NaN(nRows,nCols); SDsmap = NaN(nRows,nCols);
```

2. Define the IVIM model for fitting of D^* (*see* **Note 20**). Note that this uses the fixed values for SD and D so is placed inside the voxel loops.

```
for i = 1:nRows; for j = 1:nCols;
SD = SDmap(i,j); D = Dmap(i,j); F = fmap(i,j);
curveDs = @(X,bVals) ( X(1)*exp(-bVals*X(2)) +...
SD*exp(-bVals*D) );
```

3. Extract the voxel data for the fitting.

```
Sb = img(i,j,:);
```

4. Estimate initial values for the fitted parameters; in this case D^* can be initialized as $10 \times D$, and *SDs* is derived from *f* from the $b = 0$ s/mm^2 image.

```
SDs_est = F*b0img(i,j); Ds_est = 10*D;
X_est = [SDs_est Ds_est];
```

5. Run the fitting routine, assign the results to maps, and close the loops.

```
limL = [0 0]; limU = [Inf Inf];
res = lsqcurvefit(curveDs,X_est,bVals,Sb,limL,limU);
SDsmap(i,j) = res(1); Dsmap(i,j) = res(2);
end; end;
```

3.3.5 Least-Squares Fitting for Full IVIM Model

The segmented fitting described above should provide good initial values for a full least-squares fitting, using the same framework. Approximation of *f* and D^* is more challenging than for D (Fig. 4).

1. Define model.

```
curveIVIM = @(X,bVals) ( X(1)*(X(2)*exp(-bVals*X(3)) +...
(1-X(2))*exp(-bVals*X(4)) ));
```

2. Assign matrices for maps.

```
S0full = NaN(nRows,nCols);
ffull = NaN(nRows,nCols);
```

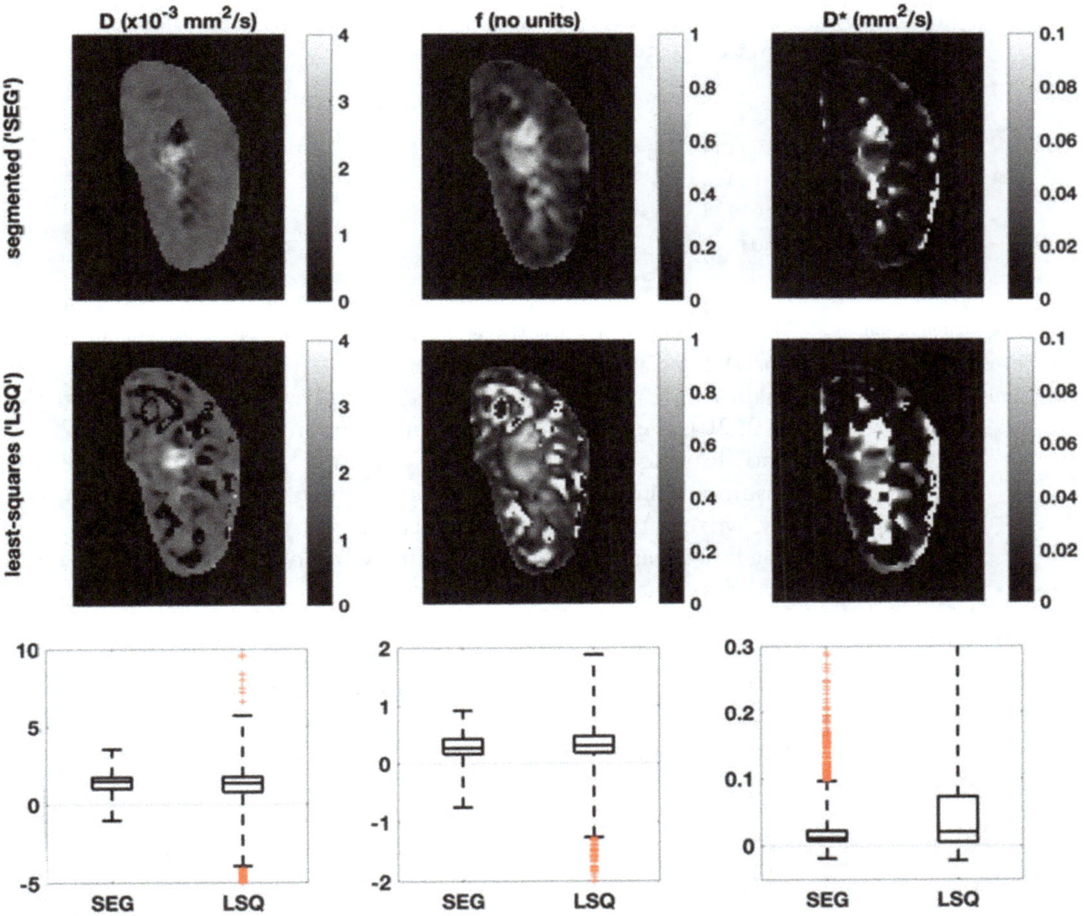

Fig. 4 IVIM parameter maps derived from (top row) segmented approach and (middle row) least-squares using segmented values for initialization. Box plots of the parameter values for the ROI (bottom row, outliers indicated in red) show the voxel spread in more detail and illustrate the relationship between returned parameters and the specifics of the analysis protocol, although the summary parameters are largely similar

```
Dsfull = NaN(nRows,nCols);
Dfull = NaN(nRows,nCols);
```

3. Begin voxel loop and assign initial values.

```
for i = 1:nRows; for j = 1:nCols;
X_est = [b0img(i,j) fmap(i,j) Dsmap(i,j) Dmap(i,j)];
```

4. Run fitting routine.

```
Sb = img(i,j,:);
limL = [0 0 0 0]; limU = [Inf Inf Inf Inf];
res = lsqcurvefit(curveIVIM,X_est,bVals,Sb,limL,limU);
```

5. Assign results to maps and close loops.

```
S0full(i,j) = res(1);
ffull(i,j) = res(2);
Dsfull(i,j) = res(3);
Dfull(i,j) = res(4);
end; end;
```

3.3.6 Spatial Information and Bayesian Fitting Algorithms

Another class of algorithms that have found promising applications for IVIM data are Bayesian methods that utilize additional information not normally considered in conventional fitting strategies [19, 20]. If each voxel is fitted independently, as for the segmented and least-squares approaches outlined above, it is implicitly assumed there is no interrelation between different voxels; in reality, voxels that are either adjacent or within the same tissue (or lesion) are likely to share diffusion and pseudodiffusion characteristics, at least to some degree.

The assumption of spatial similarity can be leveraged against the IVIM model with the view to improving the performance of the fitting, by allowing cross-talk between voxels throughout a series of iterations. These algorithms, by their nature, require many more calculations and so take substantially longer to run; nevertheless, they require no extra data to be acquired and so can be performed retrospectively, and have been shown to produce not only more visually appealing parameter maps but also more meaningful results [17, 21].

4 Methods for Results Validation

4.1 Validation of Fitting Algorithm

One simple way to validate the fitting procedure is to run (and initially develop) the code on synthetic data, generated using known parameters, and to compare the results [21, 22]. A more rigorous validation of the entire pipeline, including data acquisition and transfer, can be performed by scanning a test object with known diffusion parameters [23] using the study protocol.

Curve fitting routines should be able to supply additional output, such as stopping condition and number of iterations used, and these may be useful for troubleshooting, for example identifying where results have hit boundaries or found local minima.

4.2 Visualization of Fitted Curves

Generating signal curves using the derived parameters, and comparing against the original data, is a straightforward way of validating results, and allows examination of areas of interest or apparently spurious results (extreme or suspect values commonly arise from

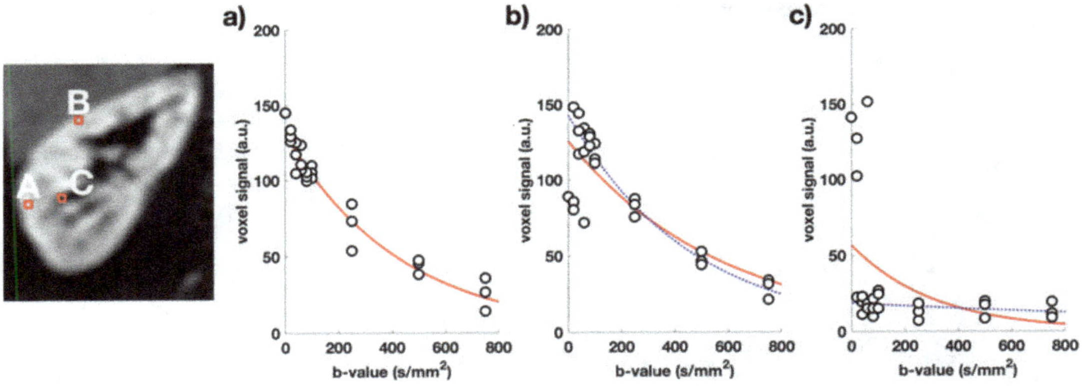

Fig. 5 Typical fitted curves overlaid on the experimental data from voxels in the healthy kidney, with locations indicated in the calculated S0 map shown. (**a**) Good fitting within the kidney parenchyma. (**b**) A voxel near the boundary is susceptible to respiratory motion, with some samples coming from within the liver tissue; the ADC from all the data (red curve) is an underestimation compared to excluding images with substantial motion (blue curve). (**c**) A similar effect is responsible for returning an incorrect curve for a voxel in the renal hilum. Note that exclusion of the same four images would avoid both of these problems, or alternatively registration may ameliorate it to some degree

partial volume or motion in voxels at tissue boundaries, *see* Fig. 5). Identification of particular issues may suggest changes to the analysis routine or, in more severe cases, amendments to the analysis or acquisition protocols. In particular for IVIM results, if the underlying pseudodiffusion fraction is limitingly small (or very large, though this is not expected), the parameter D^* can take essentially any value without affecting the associated signal curve and thus the quality of the fit. This is an intrinsic problem with the model performance in this region of the parameter space, and cannot be solved by acquiring better data.

4.3 Residuals and Systematic Bias

Examining the residuals from the fitting, which are expected to be normally distributed if the model correctly describes the underlying signal, may also highlight bias in the model. Systematic deviation of the residuals over *b*-values is an indication that the selected signal representation is not optimal, though this does not necessarily preclude it from providing useful parameters (Fig. 6).

4.4 Information Criteria and Model Selection

It may become apparent, from examination of the data, that original assumptions made about the applicability of different models may not be valid. Comparisons of different models must take account of the complexity of the model (number of variable parameters) as well as the number of samples, since additional parameters will always provide a better fit if only residual signal is considered.

There are several forms of such measures, the dominant one being the Akaike information criteria (*AIC*), formulated using the

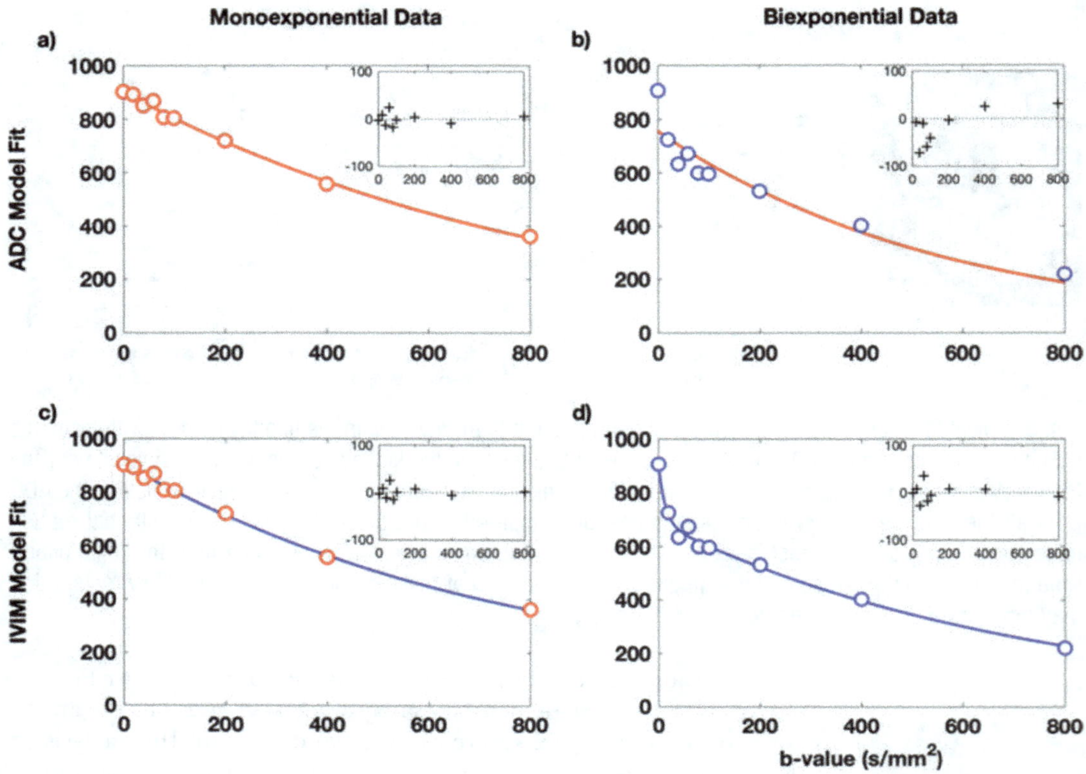

Fig. 6 Example sample fits for synthetic monoexponential (left column, data in red) and biexponential (right column, data in blue) data, fitted with the ADC (top row, curve in red) and IVIM (bottom row, curve in blue) models. Residual signal from each fitting are inset. Where the model matches the underlying signal curve, in (**a**) and (**d**), the residuals are normally distributed. Underfitting the model in (**b**) shows bias in the residuals. Overfitting the data in (**c**) gives a visually acceptable curve and comparable residuals to ADC, but returns $f = 0.98$, $D^* = 0.0012$ mm^2/s, and $D = -0.005$ mm^2/s, which should be flagged as problematic; critical assessment of results should highlight such issues

residual sum-of-squares differences between the observed data and the fitted values at those points (*RSS*) and the number of data points *k*:

$$\text{AIC} = -2 \cdot \ln(\text{RSS}) + 2k \tag{1}$$

The AIC thus gives a numerical value that can be compared across models, with lower (or more negative) values being preferred, although the relationship of the AIC to model validation is not straightforward and is sometimes criticised for being too liberal in favoring overly complex models. Nevertheless, it can often provide evidence for questioning assumptions about suitability. Note that an assessment by AIC indicates only which model is best supported by the data, and is not a validation of the model (Fig. 7).

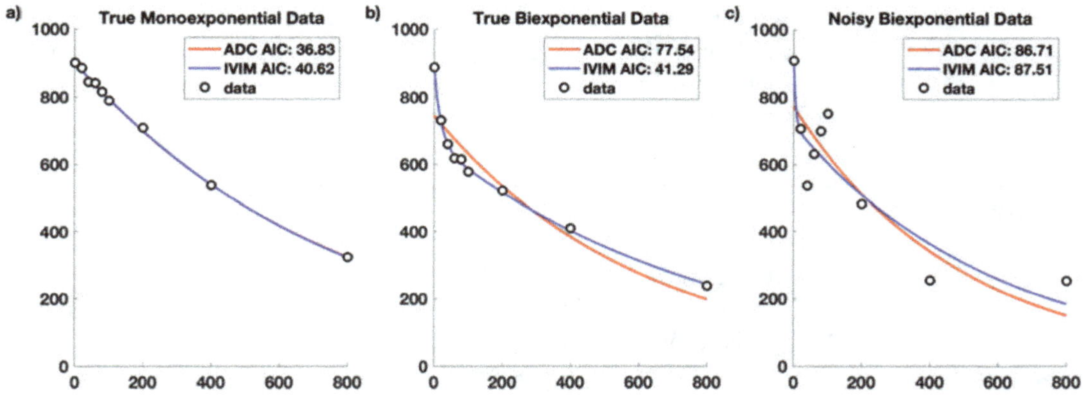

Fig. 7 Comparison of models using the Akaike information criterion (AIC) illustrates what complexity of model is supported by the data but does not necessarily indicate the underlying truth if the data are not of high quality. For (**a**) monoexponential and (**b**) biexponential synthetic data with low noise, the appropriate model fit gives the favorable (lower) AIC value for ADC and IVIM models, respectively, indicated by the lower AIC values in the legend. In (**a**), ADC and IVIM curves are identical, but the simpler ADC model (fewer variables) is favoured. (**c**) With enough noise added, however, the underlying biexponential nature is obscured, and the monoexponential fit with fewer parameters is favored. Axes shown are x: b-value (mm^2s^{-1}) and y: signal (a.u.)

4.5 Covariance and Repeatability

It is critical in quantitative studies to assess the robustness of the derived metrics, and the gold standard for this is to include repeatability studies where the same objects are measured (at least, but commonly only) twice in the same way, and the resulting metrics compared [24]. This is more achievable in preclinical studies, and helps to establish the scale of changes in metrics that can be reliably interpreted as arising from underlying physiological changes. Previous work on the *ADC* in extracranial cancer has shown it to be generally robust [25], whereas there is less certainty about the repeatability of parameters arising from more complex models [10, 18].

Without the benefit of repeated measurements, analyzing the covariance matrix of fitted parameters—that is to say, the extent to which combinations of parameters have the same effect on the fitted curve, can be illuminating. The covariance matrix is a standard output from many fitting routines; high values indicate redundancy between parameters, which in itself is not disqualifying but may indicate a mis-match between the chosen model and the available information in the data.

4.6 Final Analysis Quality Check

Critical assessment of DWI results, no less than the principles of good study design, is essential to avoid wasted time and effort, not to mention the animals used for study, in generating meaningless results. Diffusion-weighted imaging is extremely sensitive to spin motion, which is not simple, and the complexity of the diffusion signal curve is compounded by the additional subtleties of modeling and analysis. In general, mistakes arise as a result of incorrect assumptions; a review of such assumptions—including attempting to identify those made unconsciously, for example the role of parameters automatically set by the scanner (*see* **Note 22**)—is therefore a vital part of any diffusion analysis protocol.

5 Notes

1. *Location of b-values.* For Bruker data, the method file in the experiment directory contains the full acquisition parameter list; this file is human-readable but is best treated as a reference list where *b*-values can be found by searching for the text "Bval." Export of Bruker data to DICOM varies by software version but may not include the *b*-value in the export. For DICOM files extracted from clinical scanners, the *b*-value is normally located in a private field—for example (0019,100c) in Siemens data—and can be accessed using functions such as dicominfo(<DICOM_filename>) with an appropriate dictionary file. NIfTI files do not contain *b*-value information as standard in their header.
2. *Pseudodiffusion*, rather than perfusion, is a more accurate name for the volume fraction and coefficient associated with the second compartment of the IVIM model, given that it describes only the phenomenon and avoids physiological inference. Particularly in the kidney, the pseudodiffusion observed may arise from both vascular and tubular structures. Even in tissues without the complication of tubular or ductal structures, the term pseudodiffusion should be used, since the apparent pseudodiffusion fraction is known to be dependent on acquisition parameters [26].
3. *A review of images* prior to processing should be performed to ensure that assumptions made about the format and packaging of the data are valid. This includes any naming and/or export order conventions; incorrect assumptions about data presentation and provenance may also introduce errors into results or interfere with smooth processing.
4. *Signal-to-noise* (SNR) for the relevant region is calculated as the mean of the signal divided by the standard deviation of the background noise signal, found from a comparable region containing only noise (i.e., outside the object). This should be tested at the highest *b*-values in particular; it is common to require SNR above a suitable threshold (e.g., 5) for inclusion in the calculation, unless a noise contribution is explicitly included in the model.
5. *Image registration* to account for motion and distortion is a large topic in its own right and there are many strategies available, essentially divided into rigid and non-rigid

techniques. It is useful to avoid averaging within the scanner, for example of separate diffusion directions to form trace images, which can lock in motion errors. Prospective motion correction acquisitions (e.g., gating to respiration) may still require motion correction; more efficient sampling with increased averaging alleviates this problem overall, and allows a wider range of processing options [27, 28].

6. Conventionally, all parameters except *b*-value remain constant through the acquisition, and so *b*-value is the only independent variable. For more complex acquisitions, fitting across several parameters such at *TE* or Δ are needed [26, 29]. For DTI, direction of diffusion-weighting is fitted as well as *b*-value.
7. An *additional quality or "sanity" check* is advised after the fitting procedure; invalid assumptions about model applicability or data quality should become apparent either in the resulting values, or from visual inspection of the parameter maps or fitted curves. Resulting values should always be critically assessed and not just accepted.
8. *Region of interest definition.* Depending on the research question, it may be appropriate to define a region of interest (ROI) based on a calculated parameter map (e.g., *ADC*) or a representative high-*b*-value image, or to transfer an ROI from another modality (e.g., DCE). In the latter cases, it is not necessary to perform diffusion modeling over the whole image, which can save considerable computation where more complex models and algorithms are used. In general, calculation of the parameter map across the whole image gives a better visual overview and may reveal features otherwise missed.
9. The *definition of regions of interest* (ROIs) can be done before or after the model fitting. If done before, the signal through the ROI can be summed (or averaged) and fitted to give a single parameter set to reflect the entire ROI. This approach minimizes the influence of noise, but is predicated on all ROI voxels being the same class of tissue and discards spatial information. Conversely, calculation of entire-image parameter maps can highlight spatial features and help guide to ROI definition. Summary statistics drawn from voxel-wise maps after fitting also discards spatial information, and each voxel fit will be subject to more noise but allows for reporting and analysis of ROI histogram moments.
10. *Reading Bruker format* data into Matlab is not a standard function; the read_2dseq suggested here is available for download from Mathworks [30]. Another alternative, with more direct equivalents in other programming languages, is to read the file directly:

```
file = fopen('<2dseqFile>', 'r');
data = fread(file, 'int16');
img = reshape(data,imageDim1,imageDim2,nSlices,nBVals);
thisSlice = squeeze(img(:,:,sliceNumber,:));
fclose(file);
Other platforms are able to read Bruker format directly, or
convert to a more accessible format (e.g., NIfTI).
```

11. *The order of b-values* is irrelevant for the fitting, but it is convention to handle them in a consistent (usually ascending) order. If the *b*-values are known but without assignation to specific images, the correct assignment can be inferred from the overall image signal intensity if there is sufficient change in contrast between successive images. *b*-value magnitude cannot be inferred from the images if the values are not recorded.
12. *b-values* are usually specified as nominal values entered on the console (e.g., 100 s/mm^2) but, in reality, are modified by the use of the imaging readout gradients themselves (which, like the diffusion-encoding gradients pulses, have both magnitude and direction). It is more correct to use the full *b*-value matrix in the fitting [31], although the imaging gradient contributions are often considered small (e.g., "100" = 105 s/mm^2).
13. *Registration* and/or motion correction can be applied within the diffusion series, or to a separate reference image (e.g., T2w). Distortion correction from eddy currents in EPI images can also be ameliorated by registration to T2w images, or by using phase reversed image pairs if acquired [32].
14. *The S0 maps* from ADC and IVIM fitting are expected to be qualitatively similar to the $b = 0$ s/mm^2 images (for DWI acquisitions with two *b*-values they are equivalent) and are often not considered to be interesting. Nevertheless, the *S0* map is generated using all data and thus may have less influence from confounding factors (noise, distortion, etc.) and may highlight issues arising from the fitting process.
15. When using *custom fitting routines*, certain programming practices such as memory preallocation can save substantial computation time and are worth the extra investment of effort. Full optimization of code is a much larger task, and will give diminishing returns beyond a certain level.
16. *Division by zero*, for example in voxels outside the object (and which are not of interest), may result in infinities or errors that halt the routine. These can be excluded from the fitting loop, assigned an arbitrary default value, or values in Sb can be incremented to an arbitrary small value (e.g., 1) that will not appreciably affect the outcome.

```
Sb = 1 + img(i,j,:);
```

17. *Normalization of signal data* to the $b = 0$ s/mm^2 value is not necessary, and may introduce inaccuracy if the observed signal value at $b = 0$ s/mm^2 is not representative of the underlying *S0* (e.g., in the presence of appreciable perfusion).
18. *Imposing limits* on fitted variables, perhaps to physiological or physical, is possible in many fitting algorithms. One potential pitfall with this approach is if limit values returned from a failed fitting are treated as legitimate (i.e., converged) values, they may bias summary measures. This is an easy oversight if summary statistics are taken and parameter maps/histograms are not examined.
19. *Matrix inversion* is an efficient implementation of linear regression (using the log signal). The whole image can be used at once, although since the 3D data matrix is reshaped for the calculation, care must be taken to reconstruct the resulting maps with the correct dimensions.

```
si = size(img);
dataVect = reshape(img+1,(si(1)*si(2)),si(3));
dataVectLog = log(dataVect');
A = [ones(length(bVals),1) -bVals'];
res = inv(A'*A)*A'*dataVectLog;
res(1,:) = exp(res(1,:));
ADCmap_MI = reshape(res(2,:),si(1),si(2));
```

20. *Segmented fitting for* D^* can take many flavors, essentially revolving around which parameters are allowed to be free and which are fixed. For example in this implementation, f is already fixed but could be recalculated following fitting for *SDs*. The use of the segmented method as initialization for a full least-squares fitting is an iterative process and can minimize the influence of noise in the $b = 0$ s/mm^2 image, and uncertainty in choosing a suitable Bcut threshold [33].
21. One major need in the IVIM community is the standardization of terminology, including the exact formulation of the model, and even the parameter symbols. This article uses D^* to denote pseudodiffusion coefficient, but owing to the use of the asterisk in Matlab to denote the product, D^* is written Ds in the code.
22. The effect of *diffusion time* (delay between the gradient-encoding pulses, Δ) is yet to be fully described, although it is known to influence IVIM parameters in a similar way to echo time, *TE* [26, 29]. It is thus important to fix, record, and report this during acquisition, similar to *TE*.

Acknowledgments

N.P.J. wishes to acknowledge support from the liaison Committee between the Central Norway Regional Health Authority and the Norwegian University of Science and Technology (Project nr. 90065000).

This work was funded in part (Joao Periquito) by the German Research Foundation (Gefoerdert durch die Deutsche Forschungsgemeinschaft (DFG), Projektnummer 394046635, SFB 1365, RE NOPROTECTION . Funded by the Deutsche Forschungsgemeinschaft (DFG, German Research Foundation), Project number 394046635, SFB 1365, RENOPROTECTION).

This publication is based upon work from COST Action PAR ENCHIMA, supported by European Cooperation in Science and Technology (COST). COST (www.cost.eu) is a funding agency for research and innovation networks. COST Actions help connect research initiatives across Europe and enable scientists to enrich their ideas by sharing them with their peers. This boosts their research, career, and innovation.

PARENCHIMA (renalmri.org) is a community-driven Action in the COST program of the European Union, which unites more than 200 experts in renal MRI from 30 countries with the aim to improve the reproducibility and standardization of renal MRI biomarkers.

References

1. Wolf M, de Boer A, Sharma K et al (2018) Magnetic resonance imaging T1- and T2-mapping to assess renal structure and function: a systematic review and statement paper. Nephrol Dial Transplant 33:ii41–ii50
2. Pruijm M, Mendichovszky IA, Liss P et al (2018) Renal blood oxygenation level-dependent magnetic resonance imaging to measure renal tissue oxygenation: a statement paper and systematic review. Nephrol Dial Transplant 33:ii22–ii28
3. Caroli A, Schneider M, Friedli I et al (2018) Diffusion-weighted magnetic resonance imaging to assess diffuse renal pathology: a systematic review and statement paper. Nephrol Dial Transplant 33:ii29–ii40
4. Taouli B, Beer AJ, Chenevert T et al (2016) Diffusion-weighted imaging outside the brain: consensus statement from an ISMRM-sponsored workshop. J Magn Reson Imaging 44:521–540
5. Notohamiprodjo M, Chandarana H, Mikheev A et al (2014) Combined intravoxel incoherent motion and diffusion tensor imaging of renal diffusion and flow anisotropy. Magn Reson Med 1532:1526–1532
6. Rosenkrantz AB, Padhani AR, Chenevert TL et al (2015) Body diffusion kurtosis imaging: basic principles, applications, and considerations for clinical practice. J Magn Reson Imaging 42:1190–1202
7. Jensen JH, Helpern J, Ramani A et al (2005) Diffusional kurtosis imaging: the quantification of non-Gaussian water diffusion by means of magnetic resonance imaging. Magn Reson Med 53:1432–1440
8. Bennett KM, Schmainda KM, Bennett RT et al (2003) Characterization of continuously distributed cortical water diffusion rates with a stretched-exponential model. Magn Reson Med 50:727–734
9. Le Bihan D, Poupon C, Amadon A, Lethimonnier F (2006) Artifacts and pitfalls in diffusion MRI. J Magn Reson Imaging 24:478–488
10. Orton MR, Jerome NP, Rata M, Koh D-M (2018) IVIM in the body: a general overview. In: Le Bihan D, Iima M, Federau C, Sigmund EE (eds) Intravoxel incoherent Motion MRI. Pan Stanford Publishing Pte. Ltd., Singapore, pp 145–174
11. Cheng L, Blackledge MD, Collins DJ et al (2016) T2-adjusted computed diffusion-

weighted imaging: a novel method to enhance tumour visualisation. Comput Biol Med 79:92–98

12. Blackledge MD, Leach MO, Collins DJ, Koh D-M (2011) Computed diffusion-weighted MR imaging may improve tumor detection. Radiology 261:573–581
13. Gurney-Champion OJ, Klaassen R, Froeling M et al (2018) Comparison of six fit algorithms for the intravoxel incoherent motion model of diffusionweighted magnetic resonance imaging data of pancreatic cancer patients. PLoS One 13:1–18
14. Meeus EM, Novak J, Withey SB et al (2017) Evaluation of intravoxel incoherent motion fitting methods in low-perfused tissue. J Magn Reson Imaging 45:1325–1334
15. Barbieri S, Donati OF, Froehlich JM, Thoeny HC (2016) Impact of the calculation algorithm on biexponential fitting of diffusion-weighted MRI in upper abdominal organs. Magn Reson Med 75:2175–2184
16. Park HJ, Sung YS, Lee SS et al (2017) Intravoxel incoherent motion diffusion-weighted MRI of the abdomen: the effect of fitting algorithms on the accuracy and reliability of the parameters. J Magn Reson Imaging 45:1637–1647
17. Vidić I, Jerome NP, Bathen TF et al (2019) Accuracy of breast cancer lesion classification using intravoxel incoherent motion diffusion-weighted imaging is improved by the inclusion of global or local prior knowledge with bayesian methods. J Magn Reson Imaging 50 (5):1478–1488
18. Jerome NP, Miyazaki K, Collins DJ et al (2016) Repeatability of derived parameters from histograms following non-Gaussian diffusion modelling of diffusion-weighted imaging in a paediatric oncological cohort. Eur Radiol 27:345–353
19. Orton MR, Collins DJ, Koh DM, Leach MO (2014) Improved intravoxel incoherent motion analysis of diffusion weighted imaging by data driven Bayesian modeling. Magn Reson Med 71:411–420
20. Freiman M, Perez-Rossello JM, Callahan MJ et al (2013) Reliable estimation of incoherent motion parametric maps from diffusion-weighted MRI using fusion bootstrap moves. Med Image Anal 17:325–336
21. While PT (2017) A comparative simulation study of bayesian fitting approaches to intravoxel incoherent motion modeling in diffusion-weighted MRI. Magn Reson Med 78:2373–2387
22. Meeus EM, Novak J, Dehghani H, Peet AC (2018) Rapid measurement of intravoxel incoherent motion (IVIM) derived perfusion fraction for clinical magnetic resonance imaging. Magn Reson Mater Phys Biol Med 31:269–283
23. Jerome NP, Papoutsaki M-V, Orton MR et al (2016) Development of a temperature-controlled phantom for magnetic resonance quality assurance of diffusion, dynamic, and relaxometry measurements. Med Phys 43:2998–3007
24. Shukla-Dave A, Obuchowski NA, Chenevert TL et al (2018) Quantitative imaging biomarkers alliance (QIBA) recommendations for improved precision of DWI and DCE-MRI derived biomarkers in multicenter oncology trials. J Magn Reson Imaging. https://doi.org/10.1002/jmri.26518
25. Winfield JM, Tunariu N, Rata M et al (2017) Extracranial soft-tissue tumors: repeatability of apparent diffusion coefficient estimates from diffusion-weighted MR imaging. Radiology 284:88–99
26. Jerome NP, D'Arcy JA, Feiweier T et al (2016) Extended T2-IVIM model for correction of TE dependence of pseudo-diffusion volume fraction in clinical diffusion-weighted magnetic resonance imaging. Phys Med Biol 61: N667–N680
27. Jerome NP, Orton MR, D'Arcy JA et al (2014) Comparison of free-breathing with navigator-controlled acquisition regimes in abdominal diffusion-weighted magnetic resonance images: effect on ADC and IVIM statistics. J Magn Reson Imaging 39:235–240
28. Jerome NP, Orton MR, D'Arcy JA et al (2015) Use of the temporal median and trimmed mean mitigates effects of respiratory motion in multiple-acquisition abdominal diffusion imaging. Phys Med Biol 60:N9–N20
29. Clark C, Hedehus M, Moseley ME (2001) Diffusion time dependence of the apparent diffusion tensor in healthy human brain and white matter disease. Magn Reson Med 45:1126–1129
30. Yen C. read_2dseq :quickly reads Bruker's 2dseq MRI images. In: MATLAB Cent File Exch. https://www.mathworks.com/matlabcentral/fileexchange/69177-read_2dseq-quickly-reads-bruker-s-2dseq-mri-images
31. Zubkov M, Stait-Gardner T, Price WS (2014) Efficient and precise calculation of the b-matrix elements in diffusion-weighted imaging pulse sequences. J Magn Reson 243:65–73
32. Holland D, Kuperman JM, Dale AM (2010) Efficient correction of inhomogeneous static

magnetic field-induced distortion in echo planar imaging. Neuroimage 50:175–183
33. Wurnig MC, Kenkel D, Filli L, Boss A (2016) A standardized parameter-free algorithm for combined intravoxel incoherent motion and diffusion kurtosis analysis of diffusion imaging data. Invest Radiol 51:203–210

8

Renal MRI Diffusion: Experimental Protocol

João S. Periquito, Martin Meier, Thoralf Niendorf, Andreas Pohlmann, and Neil Peter Jerome

Abstract

Renal diffusion-weighted imaging (DWI) can be used to obtain information on the microstructure of kidney tissue, and has the potential to provide MR-biomarkers for functional renal imaging. Here we describe in a step-by-step experimental protocol the MRI method for measuring renal diffusion coefficients in rodents using ADC or IVIM models. Both methods provide quantification of renal diffusion coefficients; however, IVIM, a more complex model, allows for the calculation of the pseudodiffusion and fraction introduced by tissue vascular and tubular components. DWI provides information of renal microstructure contributing to the understanding of the physiology and the underlying processes that precede the beginning of pathologies.

This chapter is based upon work from the COST Action PARENCHIMA, a community-driven network funded by the European Cooperation in Science and Technology (COST) program of the European Union, which aims to improve the reproducibility and standardization of renal MRI biomarkers. This experimental protocol chapter is complemented by two separate chapters describing the basic concept and data analysis.

Key words Magnetic resonance imaging (MRI), Kidney, Mice, Rats, Diffusion, ADC, IVIM

1 Introduction

Diffusion weighting imaging (DWI) is an MR imaging technique sensitive to the motion of water molecules within a voxel of tissue. The random movement, also known as Brownian motion, of fluid molecules makes them spread out until a boundary stops them. In general, extracellular water molecules will have a larger net displacement over time than intracellular molecules. Intracellular molecules have more chances to collide with cell walls, organelles, and macromolecules. Diseases and pathologies that influence tissue properties and structure may either increase or decrease the diffusion behavior of water in tissues, which can be quantified using DWI [1, 2].

In DWI, the image contrast is based on the displacement of water molecules. Voxels where molecules present a larger displacement during the diffusion-sensitization preparation will appear darker on the resulting image.

Sensitization to diffusion can be achieved by using an extra pair of magnetic field gradients during the pulse sequence, generating images with diffusion-weighting determined by the magnitude, duration, and separation of the gradients, which can be quantified by the acquisition parameter *b*-value [3].

The DWI signal decay across a series of images with different diffusion-weightings can then be analyzed, using more or less complex mathematical models, to quantify the diffusion parameters. Ideally, the acquisition should be designed considering the signal model one wishes to use. The simplest model considers only the apparent diffusion coefficient (ADC), an empirical parameter reflecting the overall water molecule motion in the tissue averaged over one or more directions using a small number of *b*-values. ADC can be estimated by fitting a monoexponential curve to the DWI signal as a function of b-value, and fitting signal curves on a pixel-by-pixel basis allows construction of diffusion parameter maps [4].

Perfusion in tissue introduces a pseudodiffusion component to the DWI signal, which cannot be quantified using the ADC model (but it will influence the calculated ADC if low b-values are included). A more complex model is needed to take separate out this effect. Intravoxel incoherent motion (IVIM) intends to model flow processes, which manifest as pseudodiffusion with a larger coefficient, by assuming the DWI signal as a function of the *b*-value is not monoexponential but biexponential. This method requires the acquisition of several *b*-values before the pseudodiffusion decays away, especially between *b*-values of 0 and 200 s/mm^2 [5].

This experimental protocol chapter is complemented by two separate chapters describing the basic concept and data analysis, which are part of this book.

This chapter is part of the book Pohlmann A, Niendorf T (eds) (2020) Preclinical MRI of the Kidney—Methods and Protocols. Springer, New York.

2 Materials

2.1 Animals

This experimental protocol is tailored for mice (variants of C57BL/6) with a body mass of 15–35 g. Advice for adaptation to rats is given as *Notes* where necessary.

2.2 Lab Equipment and Chemicals

1. Anesthesia: typically, 0.5–1.5% isoflurane is used for anesthesia administered to the mice using an anesthetic gas vaporizer (Leica Biosystems, Maryland, USA). For nonrecovery experiments, urethane solution (Sigma-Aldrich, Steinheim,

Germany; 20% in distilled water) can provide anesthesia for several hours with comparatively fewer side effects on renal physiology, which is an important issue. For nonrecovery experiments urethane solution (Sigma-Aldrich, Steinheim, Germany; 20% in distilled water) can provide anesthesia for several hours with comparatively fewer side effects on renal physiology, which is an important issue. For an in-depth description and discussion of the anesthesia please refer to the chapter by Kaucsar T et al. "Preparation and Monitoring of Small Animals in Renal MRI."

2. Gases: O_2, N_2, and compressed air, as well as a gas-mixing system (FMI Föhr Medical Instruments GmbH, Seeheim-Ober Beerbach, Germany) or general inhalation anesthesia equipment, including an anesthetic vaporizer, a flow meter, and an induction chamber.

2.3 MRI Hardware

The general hardware requirements for renal ^{1}H MRI on mice and rats are described in the chapter by Ramos Delgado P et al. "Hardware Considerations for Preclinical Magnetic Resonance of the Kidney." The technique described in this chapter has been tailored for MR preclinical systems at magnetic fields higher than 3 T but advice for adaptation to other field strengths is given where necessary. No special or additional hardware is required, except for the following:

A physiological monitoring system that can track the respiration and which is connected to the MR system such that it can be used to trigger the MRI scanner with respiration. Typically, we use the MR-compatible rodent monitoring and gating system (Small Animal Instruments, New York, USA) equipped with an air-pillow to monitor breathing rate.

2.4 MRI Techniques

The diffusion MRI pulse sequence includes a diffusion preparation responsible for the diffusion sensitization. Specifically, sensitisation to diffusion and/or other motion of water molecules is achieved by inclusion of an extra pair of magnetic field gradients during the acquisition, generating images with varying degrees of diffusion-weighting. The degree of diffusion weighting depends on the area of each of the diffusion gradients (amplitude G and duration δ) as well as the time spacing between the pair (Δ); the resulting weighting is commonly specified by the compound parameter *b*-value (Fig. 1). The diffusion module is followed by fast image readout such as echo planar imaging (EPI). Other readouts are available for DWI (*see* **Note 1**), but DW-EPI is the standard since it provides the higher SNR in acceptable acquisition times, and so will be used in this chapter.

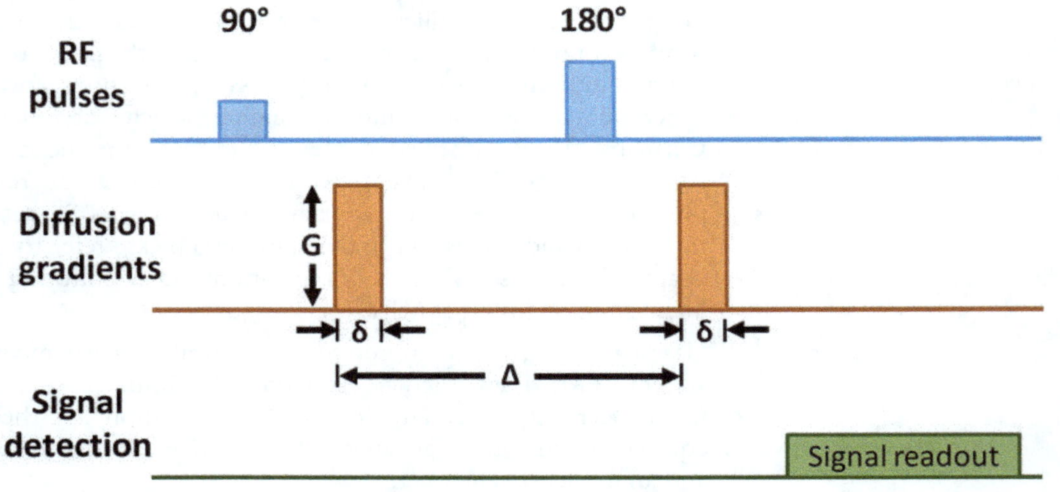

Fig. 1 Diffusion preparation ("Diffusion gradients"). The degree of diffusion weighting (measured by the "*b*-value" [mm/s^2]) depends on the area of the extra pair of gradients (amplitude G and duration δ) as well as the time spacing between them (Δ): $b = \gamma^2 G^2 \delta^2 \left(\Delta - \frac{\delta}{3}\right)$

3 Methods

3.1 MR Protocol Setup

All the mentioned MR parameters are adjustable; the provided suggestions are based on experience, but the end protocol is likely to be adjusted from these values. For more details on what goes toward making these decisions please refer to the chapter by Jerome NP et al. "Renal Diffusion-Weighted Imaging (DWI) for Apparent Diffusion Coefficient (ADC), Intravoxel Incoherent Motion (IVIM), and Diffusion Tensor Imaging (DTI): Basic Concepts"of this book.

3.1.1 DW-EPI for ADC

1. Load the DW-EPI sequence.
2. Sequence type: 2D Echo Planar Imaging sequence with diffusion preparation module that has a defined Δ and δ and a G which can be incremented within a single scan. This is a standard sequence on Bruker MRI systems, called "DW-EPI."
3. The diffusion parameters are then adjusted to allow detection of incoherent movement of molecules. The range of displacements measured with DWI is typically in the order of 1–20 μm, allowing for quantitative measurements that reflect micromorphological and physiological changes in tissues. As a recommendation a $\delta = 3.5$ ms and a $\Delta = 8.5$ ms should be used (*see* **Note 2**).
4. Set up your *b*-values to the following values: 0, 200, 600 s/mm^2 over three orthogonal directions *x*: (1,0,0), *y*: (0,1,0) and *z*: (0,0,1).

5. Repetition time (TR): choose ~500 ms for good signal stability and signal-to-noise per time (SNR/t) efficiency. TR will be limited by the length of the excitation pulse, length of echo train and the number of slices you acquire.
6. Echo time (TE): use the shortest TE. Acquisition bandwidth should be considered to shorten the inter-echo-time.
7. Segments: as low as possible to reduce scan time, however 1 segment (single-shot) might create unacceptable distortions on phase encoding. A high number of segments will increase scan time and makes the acquisition more prone to motion artifacts. As a recommendation two segments should be used (multishot DW-EPI) with a matrix size of 172 × 172 with an FOV of 30 × 30 mm.
8. Acquisition bandwidth (BW): ~ 350.000 Hz, one wants to acquire as many lines of k-space as possible to minimize motion distortions of the images. For that reason, it is advantageous to have a low inter-echo-time. Larger inter-echo-times are not advisable because the SNR in the kidney will be so low that these images must be excluded.
9. Enable fat saturation. On ultrahigh field systems this works well to avoid fat signal overlaying the kidney due to chemical shift. At lower field strengths it might work less efficient.
10. Enable the respiration trigger (per slice). This is essential to reduce motion artefacts, reduce motion blurring and unwanted intensities variations among the images acquired with different *b*-values (*see* **Note 3**).
11. Choose as phase-encoding direction the L-R direction and adapt the geometry so that the FOV in this direction includes the entire animal.
12. Use frequency encoding in head-feet (rostral-caudal) direction to avoid severe aliasing. Adjust the FOV to your needs keeping in mind that in this direction the FOV can be smaller than the animal and a smaller FOV permits a smaller acquisition matrix, and in turn a shorter echo-spacing.
13. Increase the number of averages to improve signal-to-noise ratio by a factor of $\sqrt{\text{averages}}$, especially important for higher *b*-values (use nine averages as a recommendation).
14. To reach a steady-state magnetization is advisable to use dummy scans, two as a recommendation.
15. For an example of a specific parameter set please *see* **Notes 4** and **5**.
16. For adaptation of the geometry to rats (*see* **Note 6**).

3.1.2 DW-EPI for IVIM

1. Load the DW-EPI sequence.
2. Use the same parameters as DWI-EPI for ADC (TE, TR, matrix size, dummy scans, averages, bandwidth, segments).
3. Keep the same diffusion parameters as for the ADC but increase the number of *b*-values from 3 to at least 7 (e.g., 0, 50, 100, 200, 400, 600, and 740 s/mm^2) to probe fast diffusion from blood perfusion.

3.2 In Vivo DWI

3.2.1 Animal Preparation

1. Anesthetize the animal and transfer it to scanner. For an in-depth description and discussion of the anesthesia please refer to the chapter by Kaucsar T et al. "Preparation and Monitoring of Small Animals in Renal MRI."
2. Start the temperature monitoring system, apply some surgical lubricant to the temperature probe and place it in the rectum of the animal.
3. Attach the respiration sensor (e.g., balloon) to the chest of the animal using adhesive tape. Start and set up the respiratory monitoring system. If necessary, adjust the position of the respiration sensor until the amplitude of the respiration trace is sufficiently large for the system to reliably detect the trigger points at the beginning of expiration (*see* **Note 3**).

3.2.2 Scanner Adjustments and Anatomical Imaging

1. Acquire a fast pilot scan to obtain images in three orthogonal planes *x*, *y*, and *z*.
2. Acquire anatomical images in several oblique orientations to facilitate planning a coronal slice orientation with regard to the long axis of the kidney, as described in the chapter by Pohlmann A et al. "Essential Practical Steps for MRI of the Kidney in Experimental Research" (open-access).
3. Perform localized shimming on the kidney as described in the chapter by Pohlmann A et al. "Essential Practical Steps for MRI of the Kidney in Experimental Research" (open-access). NB: shimming is crucial for DW-EPI (*see* **Note 7**), because a poor shim can lead to large distortions and add errors in the measured diffusion coefficients.
4. Acquire a 3D B_0 field-map without adaptation of the geometry (optional; *see* **Notes 8** and **9**).

3.2.3 Baseline Condition

1. Load the 2D multishot EPI sequence, adapt the slice orientation to provide a coronal or axial view with respect to the kidney (in scanner coordinates this is double-oblique).
2. In the monitoring unit set the trigger delay so that the trigger starts at the beginning of the expiratory plateau (no chest or diaphragm motion) and the duration such that it covers the

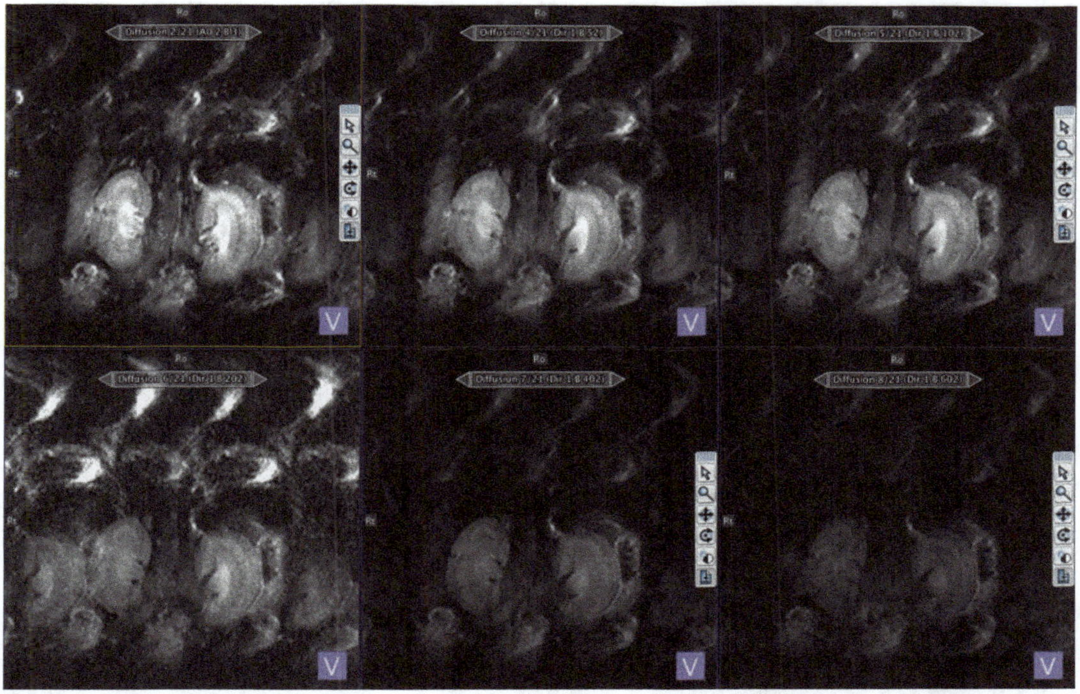

Fig. 2 Series of six diffusion-weighted images of a healthy mouse kidney acquired with DW-EPI sequence at 7.0 T. Images correspond to *b*-values: 0, 50, 100, 200, 400, and 600 mm/s^2. EPI readouts are prone to magnetic susceptibility artifacts, low-phase encoding bandwidth leads to ΔB_0 induced frequency dispersions which causes image distortion. When using a segmented EPI readout a phase deviation occurs between the different segments in k-space leading to ghosting artefacts visible in the above images [7]

entire expiratory phase, that is, until just before inhalation starts (1/2–2/3 of breath-to-breath interval) (*see* **Note 3**).

3. In the monitoring unit set the trigger delay so that the trigger starts at the beginning of the expiratory plateau (no chest or diaphragm motion) and the duration to a short value, such as 10 ms (*see* **Note 3**).
4. Run the EPI scan. Example images are shown in Fig. 2.

4 Notes

1. Other readouts apart from EPI can be use in DWI such as rapid acquisition with relaxation enhancement (RARE) (Fig. 3) which is less prone to suffering from geometric distortion specially at ultrahigh magnetic fields [6].
2. Gradients systems might differ from MR scanner to MR scanner even for the same magnetic field. If the gradient system cannot reach *b*-value of 600, consider to adjust $\delta = 3.5$ ms and

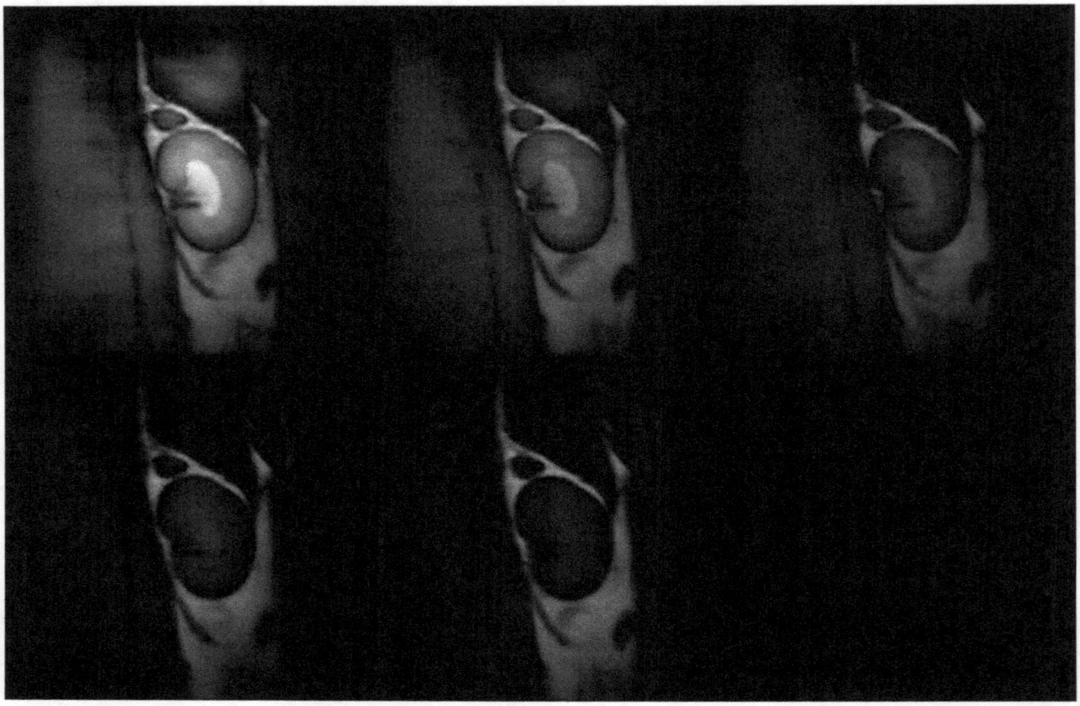

Fig. 3 Series of five diffusion-weighted images of a healthy mouse kidney acquired with single-shot DW-RARE sequence at 9.4 T. Images correspond to *b*-values: 0, 200, 300, 400, and 600 mm/s^2. A RARE readout can be used to minimize the magnetic susceptibility artifacts which cause geometric distortions on DW-EPI. DW-RARE is not commercially available, pulse programming skills are needed to implement it [6]

a $\Delta = 8.5$ to higher values. Record and report all diffusion parameters used.

3. You must monitor the respiration continuously throughout the entire experiment.
4. *Example for ADC of a 30 g mouse at 7 T (Bruker small animal system)*: TR = 500 ms; 3 *b*-values: 0, 200, 600 s/mm^2, diffusion directions: 3 (orthogonal), effective TE = 56.87 ms; Segments = 2; averages = 9; slice thickness = 1.2 mm; slice orientation = axial; frequency encoding = head-feet; FOV = 30 × 30 mm; matrix size = 172 × 172; Bandwidth = 350.000 Hz; fat suppression = on; scan time ≈ 80 s.
5. *Example for ADC of a 270 g rat at 9.4 T (Bruker small animal system)*: TR = 500 ms; 3 *b*-values: 0, 200, 600 s/mm^2, diffusion directions: 3 (orthogonal), effective TE = 56.87 ms; Segments = 2; averages = 9; slice thickness = 1.2 mm; slice orientation = axial; frequency encoding = head-feet; FOV = 45 × 45 mm; matrix size = 172 × 172; Bandwidth = 350.000 Hz; fat suppression = on;, scan time ≈ 80 s.

6. For rats increase the FOV to the body width and keep the matrix size the same or similar. The relative resolution is then identical and the SNR should also be similar, because the larger rat RF coil provides worse SNR (e.g., eight-channel rat body phase array receive coil vs eight-channel mouse body phase array receive coil).
7. Shimming is particularly important, since macroscopic magnetic field inhomogeneities affect EPI readout and might create severe geometric distortions. Shimming should be performed on a voxel enclosing the kidney using either the default iterative shimming method or the Mapshim technique (recommended).
8. *Example parameters for field mapping of a 30 g mice at 9.4 T (Bruker small animal system)*: use the vendors default protocol *AnyObject* > *AnyRegion* > *Adjustments* > *ADJ_B0MAP.* TR = 20 ms; flip angle = 30°; first echo = 1.60 ms; echo spacing = 3.57 ms; fat/water in-phase = on; slice orientation = main orientations (no angles) and offset = 0; FOC = (58 × 58 × 58) mm; matrix size =64 × 64 × 64; resolution = (0.904 × 0.904 × 0.904) mm; respiration trigger = off; acquisition time = 1–2 min.
9. This serves to keep a record of the B_0 influence on the measured DW-EPI images. It allows explanation of unusually distortions due to an imperfect shim.

Acknowledgments

This work was funded, in part (Thoralf Niendorf, Andreas Pohlmann, and Joao Periquito), by the German Research Foundation (Gefoerdert durch die Deutsche Forschungsgemeinschaft (DFG), Projektnummer 394046635, SFB 1365, RENOPROTECTION. Funded by the Deutsche Forschungsgemeinschaft (DFG, German Research Foundation), Project number 394046635, SFB 1365, RENOPROTECTION).

This chapter is based upon work from COST Action PARENCHIMA, supported by European Cooperation in Science and Technology (COST). COST (www.cost.eu) is a funding agency for research and innovation networks. COST Actions help connect research initiatives across Europe and enable scientists to enrich their ideas by sharing them with their peers. This boosts their research, career, and innovation.

PARENCHIMA (renalmri.org) is a community-driven Action in the COST program of the European Union, which unites more than 200 experts in renal MRI from 30 countries with the aim to improve the reproducibility and standardization of renal MRI biomarkers.

References

1. Hahn EL (1950) Spin echoes. Phys Rev 80:580–594
2. Carr HY, Purcell EM (1954) Effects of diffusion on free precessions in nuclear magnetic resonance experiments. Phys Rev 94:630–635
3. Stejskal EO, Tanner JE (1965) Spin diffusion measurements: spin echoes in the presence of a time-dependent field gradient. J Chem Phys 42:288–292. https://doi.org/10.1063/1.1695690
4. Le Bihan D et al (1950) Imagerie de diffusion in-vivo par resonance magnetique. CR Acad Sci 15:1109–1112
5. Le Bihan D et al (1988) Separation of diffusion and perfusion in intravoxel incoherent motion MR imaging. Radiology 168(2):497–505
6. Periquito J et al (2020) Diffusion-weighted renal MRI at 9.4 Tesla using RARE to improve anatomical integrity. *Scientific Reports* 9(1):1–12
7. Paul K et al (2015) Diffusion-sensitized ophthalmic magnetic resonance imaging free of geometric distortion at 3.0 and 7.0 T: a feasibility study in healthy subjects and patients with intraocular masses. Investig Radiol 50:309–321

9

Hardware Considerations for Preclinical Magnetic Resonance of the Kidney

Paula Ramos Delgado, Ekkehard Küstermann, André Kühne, Jason M. Millward, Thoralf Niendorf, Andreas Pohlmann, and Martin Meier

Abstract

Magnetic resonance imaging (MRI) is a noninvasive imaging technology that offers unparalleled anatomical and functional detail, along with diagnostic sensitivity. MRI is suitable for longitudinal studies due to the lack of exposure to ionizing radiation. Before undertaking preclinical MRI investigations of the kidney, the appropriate MRI hardware should be carefully chosen to balance the competing demands of image quality, spatial resolution, and imaging speed, tailored to the specific scientific objectives of the investigation. Here we describe the equipment needed to perform renal MRI in rodents, with the aim to guide the appropriate hardware selection to meet the needs of renal MRI applications.

This publication is based upon work from the COST Action PARENCHIMA, a community-driven network funded by the European Cooperation in Science and Technology (COST) program of the European Union, which aims to improve the reproducibility and standardization of renal MRI biomarkers. This chapter on hardware considerations for renal MRI in small animals is complemented by two separate publications describing the experimental procedure and data analysis.

Key words Magnetic Resonance Imaging (MRI), Kidney, Mice, Rats, Hardware, RF coils, Renal MRI

1 Introduction

The detection, staging, and monitoring of kidney diseases (KD) using measurements of renal function and structure is critical in clinical nephrology. The use of animal models in kidney research promotes the understanding of disease and therapy mechanisms. While current imaging modalities such as computed tomography or ultrasound can provide some information on structural changes in the kidney, these approaches offer limited insights into functional changes.

Magnetic resonance imaging (MRI) is a noninvasive imaging technology that offers an unparalleled level of anatomical and functional detail, along with diagnostic sensitivity. MRI is suitable for longitudinal studies due to the lack of exposure to ionizing radiation. Together with established imaging techniques, novel approaches such as dynamic contrast-enhanced MRI (DCE-MRI), arterial spin labeling (ASL), blood oxygen level dependent MRI (BOLD), and diffusion-weighted imaging (DWI) can provide a broad characterization of the kidney, including renal vascular perfusion, oxygenation, and glomerular filtration rate.

For performing dedicated MR measurements of the kidney, the appropriate MRI hardware should be carefully chosen to balance the competing demands of image quality, spatial resolution and imaging speed, tailored to the specific scientific objectives of the investigation. This chapter is intended to outline the key hardware components of an MRI scanner and to provide an overview of currently established technologies, with the goal to guide the appropriate hardware selection that meets the needs of preclinical MRI of the kidney.

This chapter on hardware considerations for renal MRI in small animals is part of the book Pohlmann A, Niendorf T (eds) (2020) Preclinical MRI of the Kidney–Methods and Protocols. Springer, New York.

2 Static Magnetic Field Strength (B_0)

A superconducting magnet that generates a constant homogeneous magnetic field is the core hardware component of an MRI scanner. This strength of this static magnetic field (B_0) is proportional to the net polarization produced within the sample. The detected MR signal on a receive RF coil depends on ${B_0}^2$, whereas the noise increases linearly with B_0 [1]. B_0 governs the signal-to-noise ratio (SNR), which is the currency for MR image quality. This provides strong motivation and momentum to move to increasingly higher magnetic field strengths for preclinical and clinical renal MRI applications [2–4]. The proportionality of SNR with B_0 is linear in the quasi-static regime, as demonstrated theoretically [5, 6] and experimentally [7]. For higher magnetic field strengths, wave propagation and the increasing resonance frequencies must be considered [2]. Additionally, an experimental study on intrinsic SNR behaviour with increasing B_0 field strengths (3.0, 7.0, and 9.4 T) in the human brain reported a superlinear increase in SNR (SNR $\propto B_0^{1.65}$) [7]. This observation was also confirmed in a simulation study [8].

Relaxation time constants of biological tissues also change with the magnetic field strength, thus influencing the SNR as well as the contrast-to-noise ratio (CNR), which ultimately has an impact on the image quality. The longitudinal relaxation time (T_1) increases nonlinearly with increasing B_0 [1, 9–11]. The transversal relaxation (T_2) and T_2* decrease at different slopes linearly [1, 9, 12–14]. These dependencies on B_0 are responsible for the reduced

T_1-weighted contrast and increased BOLD effect at higher magnetic field strengths (*see* **Note 1**). MRI methods based on T_2*-weighting (e.g., susceptibility weighted imaging, BOLD) will benefit from the T_2* shortening, and thus increase in sensitivity at high magnetic field strengths, which underlies their broad application in renal MRI. An example of renal T_2*-mapping ($R_2^* = 1/T_2^*$) is the study of oxygenation and haemodynamics in renal disorders (for a review *see* [15]). MR spectroscopy also benefits from the enhanced signal dispersion achieved at higher magnetic field strengths, which results in better resolved spectra, and permits improved accuracy of metabolite identification and quantification [1, 16].

However, MRI at high magnetic field strengths is susceptible to more severe B_0 and B_1 inhomogeneities, compared to lower field strengths. These inhomogeneities are primarily due to differences in the magnetic susceptibility at tissue interfaces. Susceptibility artifacts present themselves as T_2*-induced signal losses (or even signal voids) in areas with very high B_0 gradients, low phase-encoding bandwidth-related image distortion and off-resonance effects caused by ΔB_0-induced frequency dispersions. MRI of the kidney poses additional challenges due to the anatomical context. The kidneys are adjacent to bowels, in close proximity to skin/fat/muscle boundaries (e.g., perirenal fat) or in areas containing cavities might be particularly prone to susceptibility artifacts.

Artifacts are visible as signal losses at interfaces between fat and tissue or air and tissue (susceptibility artifacts), image blurring, image distortion, and broadening of spectral lines in MRS, which interferes with the reliable differentiation of metabolites. B_0 inhomogeneities can be mitigated using B_0 shimming (*see* Subheading 3).

B_1 inhomogeneities lead to variations in the flip angle driven by the RF pulse excitation. B_1 inhomogeneities affect tissue contrast and SNR, appearing as signal intensity variations or losses across the field of view. Nonuniformities in B_1 are caused by the RF coil (e.g., surface RF coil, *see* Subheading 4) or by the creation of standing waves and constructive/destructive interferences within the object under investigation, due to the reduction of the effective wavelength which at higher field strengths becomes shorter, and can approach the dimensions of the specific anatomical structures under study [17]. While the RF wavelength inside tissue at 3.0 T (~128 MHz) is about 30 cm, at 7.0 T (~300 MHz) it is reduced to about 13 cm [18] and to 6.5 cm at 14.0 T (~600 MHz). In preclinical renal MRI, this is not a major concern, as the size of the abdomen in small animals is typically much smaller than the RF wavelength.

RF power requirements for spin excitation increase quadratically with B_0. This imposes major concerns, especially for human applications, since the RF power deposition can easily reach the regulatory limits specified by IEC guidelines for the specific absorption rate (SAR) [16]. This constraint can be adressed by modification and adaptation of MR pulse sequences, acquisition strategies, and RF coils [18, 19]. In the case of preclinical studies, these issues have received less attention since there are no enforced SAR guidelines for small animals. Nevertheless, the physiological effects of tissue heating due to heavy RF deposition in experimental animals could be a serious confounding factor in preclinical studies that should not be ignored.

2.1 SNR Comparison for Magnetic Field Strength

The SNR gains resulting from increasing B_0, field have been computationally estimated for brain MRI to range from $B_0^{1.2}$ (close to the brain surface) up to $B_0^{2.1}$ (at the center of the head) [8]. Pohmann et al. [7] investigated the field dependence of SNR for magnetic field strengths ranging between 3.0 T and 9.4 T using gradient echo techniques, and reported that SNR increases superlinearly ($B_0^{1.65}$). Using this relationship, the calculated relative SNR (normalized for the typical case of a 3.0 T scanner) and resolution gains (in μm, in-plane resolution 1 mm) corresponding to all static magnetic field strengths from 1.5 T to 21.1 T are shown in Table 1.

The increase in SNR provided by higher magnetic field strengths can be invested in enhanced spatial resolution or improvements in imaging speed. The triad of B_0, spatial resolution, and imaging speed form the so-called SNR conundrum in which the competing constraints of SNR, CNR, spatial resolution, and imaging speed govern the image quality. For example, increasing the matrix size for a certain field of view will increase the spatial resolution—which will permit the visualization of more subtle anatomical structures in the kidney—but at a cost of reducing the SNR, or signal intensity per pixel/voxel. Although resolution in the frequency-encoding direction can be conveniently enhanced by increasing the matrix size without major scan time penalty, increasing spatial resolution along the phase-encoding direction substantially prolongs the scan time. Boosting the SNR is also possible by modifying the size of the field of view or the slice thickness: the larger these parameters are, the more signal is acquired. Another way to further increase SNR is signal averaging, which reduces the noise but comes at the cost longer scan times. Depending on the individual experimental context, longer scan times may be a reasonable price to pay (especially for ex vivo studies). For in vivo studies, animal welfare considerations call for the minimum scan time possible to achieve the scientific objective, and shorter scans promote higher throughput of individual animals to improve the experimental sample size.

Additional strategies to gain SNR include the use of SNR-promoting rapid imaging techniques such as RARE imaging, and dedicated RF coil technology, including cryogenically cooled RF coils (*see* Subheading 4).

Table 1
Relative SNR and resolution gain with increasing static magnetic field strength

Magnetic field, B_0 (T)	Relative SNR gain	Resolution gain (in-plane 1 mm) (μm^2)
1.5	0.3	(1550 × 1550)
3.0	1.0	(495 × 495)
4.7	2.1	(235 × 235)
7.0	4.0	(122 × 122)
9.4	6.6	(75 × 75)
11.7	9.4	(52 × 52)
14.0	12.7	(39 × 39)
16.4	16.5	(30 × 30)
17.6	18.5	(27 × 27)
21.1	25.0	(20 × 20)

SNR values were computed as proportional to $B^{1.65}$. The relative SNR gain was calculated relative to that of 3.0 T

2.2 Magnetic Field Strengths Used in Recently Published Studies

To provide guidance as to which B_0 is necessary or sufficient for preclinical MRI of the kidney, a total of 121 publications published over the past 10 years were reviewed. Of these, 66 publications reported on renal MRI in rats, and 55 in mice. Figure 1 shows the number of publications found per magnetic field strength for renal MRI in rats and mice. In rats, a total of 25 publications (38%) were performed at 3.0 T, closely followed by 9.4 T with 20 papers (30%). In mice the preferred magnetic field strength was 7.0 T (25 publications, 46%). The magnetic field strengths of 9.4 T (8 papers, 15%), 3.0 T (7 papers, 13%), and 11.7 T (6 publications, 11%) were also used for MRI studies of mouse kidney.

Figure 2 illustrates the number of publications per magnetic field strength, listed by year for rats and mice. In rats, the number of studies performed at 3.0 and 9.4 T was quite stable for the last 7 years. Studies at 4.7 T (7 papers, 11%) were also widely reported, as shown in the trends displayed since 2009. The use of field strengths of 1.5 and 7.0 T (7 and 6 publications, respectively) varied during the period under investigation. In contrast, 7.0 T was established as the typical magnetic field strength for preclinical MRI of the kidney in mice during this period. In the last few years, 11.7 T and 16.4 T have also emerged as MR systems suitable for the study of the mouse kidney.

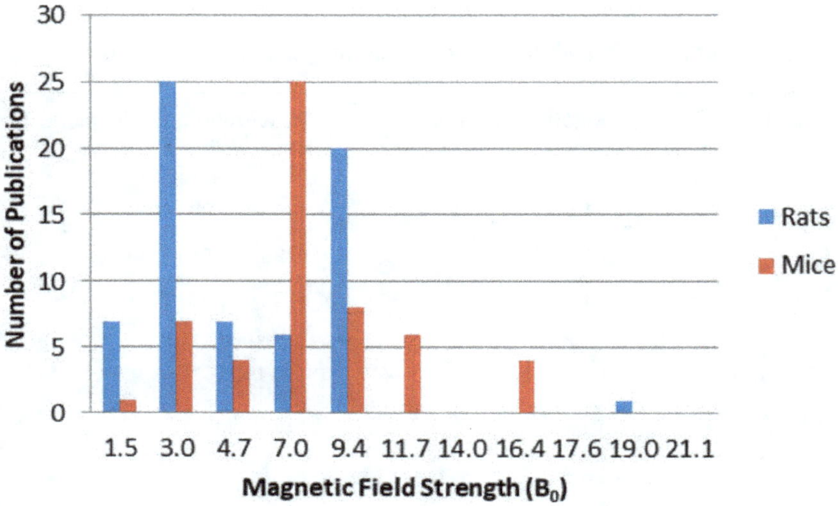

Fig. 1 Number of publications per magnetic field strength for renal MRI in rats and mice, within a total of 121 reports on preclinical renal MRI published in the past 10 years

3 Gradient Systems

To enable the spatial localisation of the MR signal, magnetic field gradients are used, which are provided by gradient coils. Gradient coils produce a linear variation of the magnetic field as a function of the spatial position (X-, Y-, and Z-direction) modifying the resonance frequency for spatial encoding of the MR signal.

Typical parameters governing the performance of the gradient system are the peak gradient strength, the rise time, and the slew rate. The peak gradient strength is the maximum achievable gradient strength (in mT/m). Typical peak gradient amplitudes in preclinical scanners are in the range of 200–1000 mT/m. Clinical scanners used for preclinical MRI of the kidney provide maximum gradient amplitudes ranging between 45 mT/m and 82 mT/m. The gradient rise time is the time needed to change the gradient field from zero to the peak amplitude (in ms). The gradient slew rate is the most important parameter, and refers to the speed at which a gradient can be switched. It is defined as the peak gradient strength divided by the gradient rise time (in T/m/s). This defines the maximum scanning speed, since it influences the minimum achievable repetition time (TR) and echo time (TE), as well as the echo spacing in fast imaging techniques such as RARE or EPI (*see* **Note 2**). Typical slew rates in preclinical scanners are in the range of 640–9000 T/m/s. Clinical scanners used for preclinical MRI of the kidney offer slew rates ranging between 150 T/m/s and 200 T/m/s. Gradient coils can be driven in two modes: (a) constant rise time, in which the slew rate is adapted for each gradient amplitude and (b) maximum slew rate, where the rise is adjusted for each gradient amplitude.

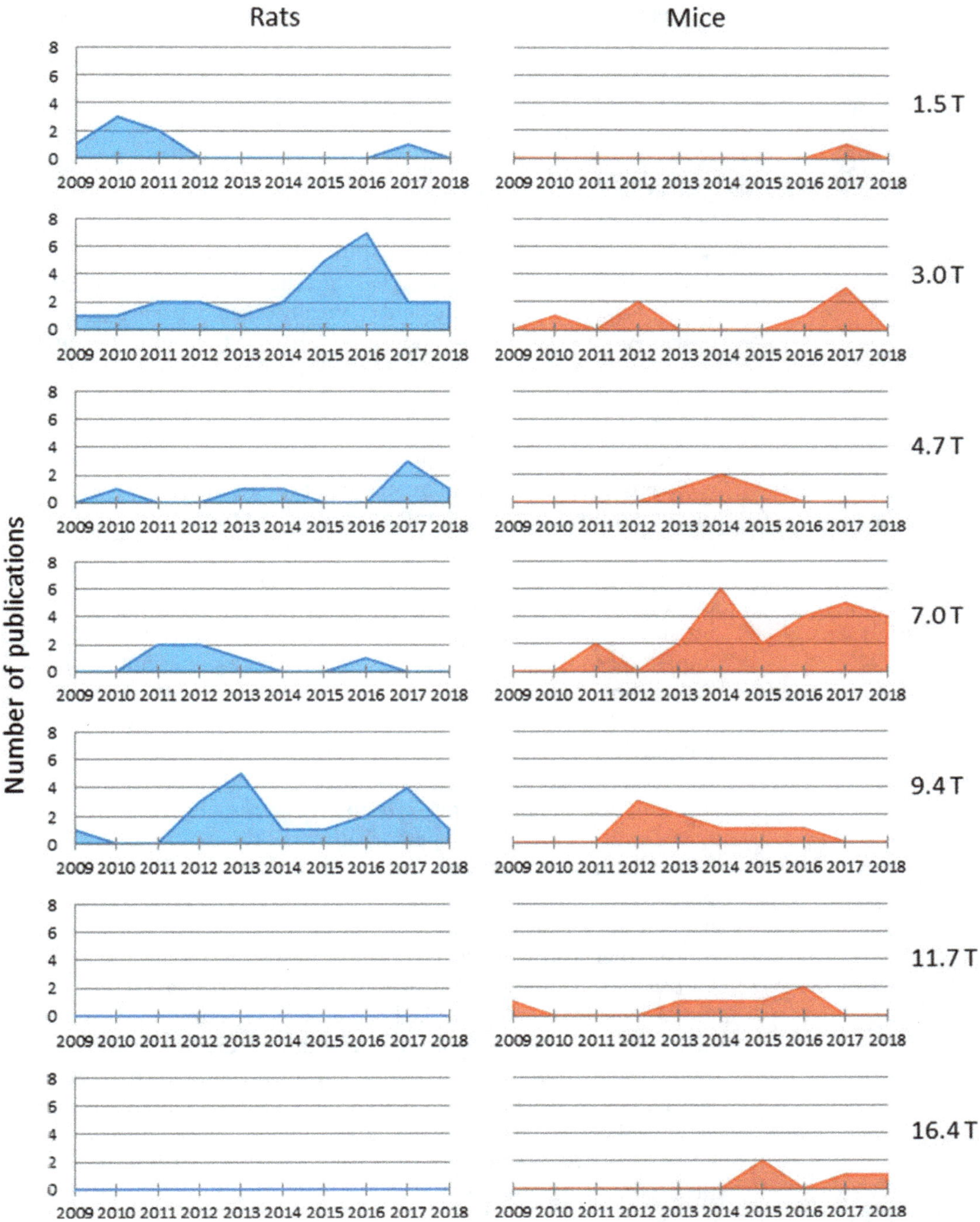

Fig. 2 Number of selected publications ordered by magnetic field strength and year, within a total of 121 reports published in the past 10 years (2009–2018) for preclinical renal MRI in rats and mice

The duty cycle defines the amount of time during which the gradient system can be run at maximum power amplitude (in % time). This parameter depends not only on the gradient system specifications mentioned above but also on the specific MR imaging technique used. Typical duty cycles in existing preclinical scanners can reach almost 100%. For this purpose, gradient coils are water-cooled to ensure proper heat dissipation and temperature management.

The accuracy of the spatial representation depends on the quality of the linear magnetic field gradients and on the homogeneity of the static magnetic field (typically given in parts per million, ppm). Any deviation will appear as object distortion in the image, and thus a correction procedure called "shimming" is typically performed. During system installation, the manufacturer places small metal plates inside the scanner bore to improve the uniformity of the main magnetic field in a static and permanent manner—this is "passive" shimming. The distribution of these ferromagnetic pieces is adjusted over several iterations until the achieved magnetic field uniformity meets the vendor's specification. In addition to passive shimming, resistive shim coils are used for B_0 homogenization. These adjustments are performed with a shim calibration tool on an empty magnet, and therefore the B_0 homogeneity becomes impaired as soon as a sample or subject (human or animal) is placed inside the magnet bore.

An "active" shimming procedure can be conducted during measurement adjustments with every MR scan. This is crucial for techniques such as fat suppression or MR spectroscopy, since the introduction of any matter—an object or animal—inevitably introduces local magnetic field perturbations of the main static magnetic field, which then must be actively compensated for. Especially at the boundaries between tissue and air-filled areas, where magnetic field distortions are pronounced due to the different magnetic susceptibility which can cause severe signal losses and image distortions. Corrective magnetic fields produced by electrical RF coils, designated as shim gradients [20] which are superimposed upon the main magnetic field. Typically, the shim gradient system contains a set of first-order gradients which impose linear field changes in the X-, Y-, and Z-directions, and some second order gradients, which create spherical harmonics in the Z^2, ZX, ZY X^2-Y^2, and XY directions [21]. Some MR systems are also equipped with more sophisticated shim gradients which provide third and fourth order correction terms [22].

Depending on the specific pulse sequence and imaging technique used, the scientist has to adjust these magnetic field corrections to meet certain quality prequisites. Especially with T_2*-weighted sequences (e.g., gradient-echo or EPI sequences) the image quality improves with improved B_0 homogeneity. MR spectroscopic methods are even more demanding [23]. Usually, state-of-the-art MR systems provide automated methods to perform the B_0 shimming task, but the user still needs to check the performance and correct the shim settings manually if necessary.

For B_0 shimming a global approach covering the entire FOV, or a localized shim covering a target area can be used. In general, the smaller the region of interest the better the achievable B_0 homogeneity. In the case of renal MRI, the B_0 homogeneity achieved after shimming across one kidney will be better than that for the whole abdomen, with air-filled lungs and gut. In the case of tissues that are moving due to respiration, cardiac activity or peristaltic motion, the magnetic field distortions change over time, which require different strategies. The time-averaged global shim would be the fastest and easiest solution, if this is sufficient. Alternatively, shimming—and also data acquisition—would be performed in synchrony with the breathing by using a trigger signal from a physiological monitor [24].

4 Radio Frequency (RF) Coils

Besides the static magnetic field and the spatial encoding with the gradient system, MRI requires transmission of RF pulses and reception of the MR signal from the sample or subject.

For signal excitation, the RF transmit resonator, or RF coil, sends RF pulses with a particular frequency, bandwidth, shape, duration, amplitude, and phase modulation to tilt the net magnetization vector oriented in parallel with the main magnetic field during equilibrium. B_0 (typically assigned as the Z-direction), is tilted into the perpendicular transverse (X-Y) plane by a given flip angle α. After excitation, the magnetization precesses back to equilibrium and induces a signal in the RF receive coil (for a comprehensive review *see* [25]).

Depending on the transmission and reception capabilities, three general types of RF coils are commonly used: (1) transmit-receive (Tx/Rx) or transceiver RF coils, (2) transmit-only (Tx) RF coils, and (3) receive-only (Rx) RF coils. These generally have two types of geometry: (1) volume RF coils and (2) surface RF coils. Both RF coil types and geometries determine the amount of tissue or organ coverage and sensitivity to the MR signal.

Volume RF resonators are designed to produce a uniform RF field over a large field-of-view (FOV), and are typically used as transmit-receive RF coils or transmit RF coils (using a surface RF coil for reception). The most widely used type of volume RF coils in both human and preclinical MRI are birdcage resonators [26, 27] driven in quadrature mode. This means that two spatially orthogonal RF channels are used for RF transmission as well as signal reception. This RF coil configuration provides a 41.4% SNR gain over simple single channel or "linear" RF coils, due to the coherent signal increases which scale linearly with the number of channels, while the incoherent noise increases with the square root of the number of channels. For example, Chang et al. [28] used this RF coil setup in a renal hypoxia study in a mouse model after myocardial infarction of different sizes using BOLD MRI. Other types of volume resonators include saddle RF coils, Helmholtz RF coils, and the transverse electromagnetic (TEM) resonators, among others.

Smaller anatomical coverage and FOVs, but enhanced SNR, are provided by surface RF coils. Due to the principle of reciprocity, the closer the position of the RF coil is to the tissue of interest, the higher is the attainable SNR. However, the sensitivity drops with increasing distance to the RF coil surface, which thus results in a reduced FOV, and an inhomogeneous sensitivity profile [29]. Within a short distance of typically up to ~1 cm, a surface RF coil outperforms a volume RF coil in terms of sensitivity. Since the kidneys are located beneath the skin, surface RF coils positioned directly above are used for optimal signal reception in renal MRI. This is advantageous not only for X-nuclei MR imaging (*see* Subheading 5) but also for other applications with low SNR, such as perfusion or diffusion-weighted imaging.

Surface RF coils may be used as transmit/receive devices or as receive-only RF coils in conjunction with a volume RF coil used for homogeneous RF transmission. The first option is technically very simple since only one RF coil is necessary, which occupies less space. In the case of small animal imaging, it is most likely a simple single-turn loop with at least two tunable capacitances for tuning and matching. Images will show a strong spatially varying SNR decay, due to the addition of the inhomogeneous excitation and reception profiles [30]. This effect may be mitigated, for example, by using adiabatic excitation RF pulses [31].

The second option involves the use of two RF coils (Tx: volume RF coil, Rx: surface RF coil) which are tuned to the same resonant frequency. To avoid RF coupling between both coils, the surface RF coil must be detuned during transmission while the volume RF coil must be detuned during reception. Thus, both RF coils must include an option, using active and passive diodes, to allow for tuning and detuning during the MR experiment. This is the most common setup, since it improves the SNR in comparison with a Tx/Rx volume RF coil, while still maintaining a homogeneous B_1. For example, Hüper et al. [32] used a four-element quadrature surface receive RF coil in combination with a transmit volume RF coil to investigate renal perfusion in acute and chronic renal allograft rejection in translational mouse models. The use of the surface RF coil improved the SNR from 15 (with a standard transceive volume RF coil) to 35.

Further SNR gains in small animal MRI are achieved with arrays of surface RF coils for signal reception [33], which are typically used together with a volume RF coil for signal excitation (*see* **Notes 3** and **4**). The use of RF coil arrays for brain imaging is especially widespread, and these are routinely offered by manufacturers. State-of-the-art small-animal MRI systems are usually equipped with 4–16 Rx channels, to which custom-tailored RF coils may be connected. Less popular are metamaterial-inspired RF coils, which have been developed for superficial tissue imaging in order to provide the best compromise of high SNR over a large FOV, while using only one receive channel [34].

Depending on the size of the sample and the RF coil, and their corresponding temperatures and resistances, their noise electronic contribution varies [35–37]. This factor is even more crucial in preclinical applications where the noise contribution of the RF coil, capacitors, sample, shield, receive electronics, and transmission lines are important [26]. This fact is exploited in small-animal imaging by the use of cryogenically cooled (cryo-cooled) RF coils. By lowering the temperature of the receiver chain, the noise contributions corresponding to temperatures and resistances can be reduced [38–40], thus achieving a significant increase in SNR, which has been reported in the literature (for a review *see* [15]). Unfortunately, only negligible effects are achieved in human MR [15, 41]. With increasing size of the sample, the relative contribution to the noise increases, and eventually becomes the dominating noise source—this is the default situation for human MR. Thus, only small animal MR applications will benefit from this cooling approach, since the noise contributions from the sample and RF coil are in the same order of magnitude. The SNR gain achieved with such cryo-cooled RF coils is higher at lower static magnetic fields [15, 26, 42]. A recognized limitation of cryo-cooled surface RF coils is that only transceive capabilities are supported, resulting in nonuniform excitation and reception profiles, which might hamper quantitative measurements.

Another option for the small-animal MR imaging of the kidney is the use of clinical scanners together with RF coils tailored for the human hand/wrist or knee. These are typically 8- to 16-element RF coil arrays which provide quasi-homogeneous excitation and reception profiles. Although these RF coils have a small size, they are not optimized for small-animal imaging and are not designed with matching/tuning capabilities. Moreover, RF coils tailored for rodent imaging are designed for a broad range of loadings (i.e., from almost empty to full loading, with a typical frequency-diameter product in the range 2–30 MHz · m [26]), in comparison to the clinical setups. Therefore, these clinical RF coils will achieve a lower efficiency than that of dedicated RF coils designed for preclinical MR systems. Alternatively, RF coils tailored for renal MRI of small rodents provided by RF coil manufactures can be connected with clinical MR scanners to enhance the fill factor and SNR.

In the following subsections, examples of possible RF coil setups are shown from different vendors. A list of the available MR system and RF coil vendors can be found in Table 2.

4.1 Commercially Available RF Coils Suitable for Kidney MRI in Rats

Due to the considerable anatomical homology with humans, rats have become one of the most commonly use rodents in animal research, particularly, in preclinical MRI. With a weight of 150–450 g, both clinical and preclinical MR systems and RF coils can be used to perform renal MR experiments:

Clinical MR System

- Tx/Rx wrist RF coil (e.g., Siemens eight-channel wrist RF coil, Fig. 3A).
- Tx/Rx knee RF coil (e.g., Siemens 15-channel knee RF coil, Fig. 3B).

Preclinical MR System

- Tx/Rx volume resonator (e.g., Bruker Biospin, Ettlingen, Germany, quadrature rat body RF coil with inner diameter (ID) = 72 mm (Fig. 3C), 82 mm or 86 mm; RAPID Biomed, Rimpar, Germany 2 × 4-channel volumetric rat array with ID = 72 mm).
- Tx/Rx quadrature volume resonator (e.g., MRI.TOOLS GmbH, Berlin, Germany, supporting an ID ranging from 54 mm to 86 mm and magnetic field strengths of 3.0 T, 4.7 T, 7.0 T, 9.4 T, and 11.T (Fig. 3D).
- Rx surface RF coil (e.g., 2 × 2 RAPID Biomed, Rimpar, Germany) rat cardiac surface array RF coil; 4 × 1 element (e.g., Bruker Biospin, Ettlingen, Germany) rat cardiac surface array RF coil, Fig. 3E) in combination with Tx volume resonator (e.g., Bruker rat body RF coils with ID 72 mm (Fig. 3F), 82 mm or 86 mm).

4.2 Commercially Available RF Coils Suitable for Kidney MRI in Mice

Mice are the most commonly used rodent in biomedical research. Their genetic similarity to humans has made them extremely useful, allowing the development of mouse models of many human diseases. Mice have an average weight of 15–40 g, making them too small for standard human RF coils:

Clinical System

- There are no standard human RF coils that are small enough to be suitable for mice MRI. Alternatively, a Tx/Rx quadrature volume resonator (MRI.TOOLS GmbH, Berlin, Germany), supporting an ID ranging from 30 mm to 45 mm and magnetic field strengths of 3.0 and 7.0 T can be used for renal MRI with clinical MR scanners (Fig. 4A).

Table 2
List of vendors of MR equipment and RF coils

	Vendor	Website
Clinical MRI	Canon Medical Systems	us.medical.canon
	General Electric Medical Systems Inc.	www.gehealthcare.com
	MRI Devices Corp.	www.allmri.com
	MR Instruments Inc.	www.mrinstruments.com
	MRI.TOOLS GmbH	www.mritools.de
	NOVA Medical Inc.	www.novamedical.com
	RAPID Biomedical GmbH	www.rapidbiomed.de
	Philips Medical Systems	www.medical.philips.com
	ScanMed	www.scanmed.com
	Siemens Medical Systems	www.siemens-healthineers.com
	Tesla Engineering Limited	www.tesla.co.uk
Preclinical MRI	Bruker BioSpin MRI GmbH	www.bruker.com
	Doty Scientific, Inc.	www.dotynmr.com
	MR Solutions	www.mrsolutions.com
	MRI.TOOLS GmbH	www.mritools.de
	RAPID Biomedical GmbH	www.rapidbiomed.de

Preclinical System

- Tx/Rx volume resonator (Bruker Biospin, Ettlingen, Germany) quadrature mouse body RF coil with ID = 35 mm, Fig. 4B); 2 × 4 -channel volumetric mouse array (RAPID Biomed, Rimpar, Germany) with 35 mm ID.
- Tx/Rx quadrature volume resonator (MRI.TOOLS GmbH, Berlin, Germany, supporting an ID ranging from 30 mm to 45 mm and magnetic field strengths of 3.0 T, 4.7 T, 7.0 T, 9.4 T, and 11.T (Fig. 4A).
- Rx surface RF coil (e.g., RAPID Biomed, Rimpar, Germany) 2 × 2 mouse cardiac surface array RF coil; 2 × 2 element mouse cardiac surface array RF coil (e.g., Bruker Biospin, Ettlingen, Germany, Fig. 4B) in combination with Tx volume resonator (e.g., Bruker Biospin, Ettlingen, Germany) quadrature mouse body RF coils with ID 72 mm (as shown in Fig. 4E), 82 mm or 86 mm).
- Tx/Rx 2 × 2 element array rat/mouse CryoProbe (e.g., Bruker Biospin, Ettlingen, Germany, Fig. 4C).

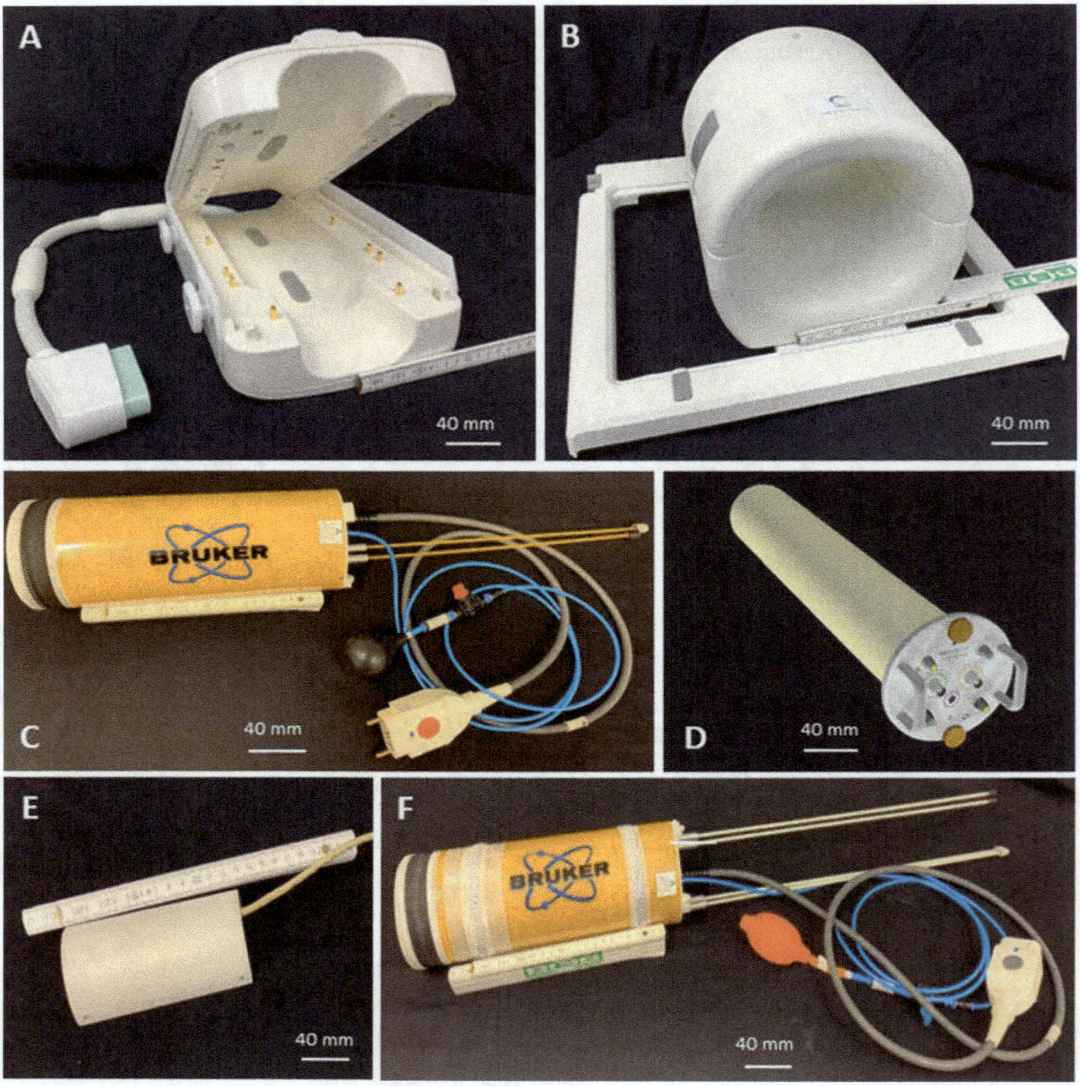

Fig. 3 Example RF coils suitable for kidney MRI of the rat. (**a**) Siemens 8-channel wrist RF coil, (**b**) Siemens 15-channel knee RF coil, (**c**) Bruker quadrature rat body RF coil with inner diameter (ID) 72 mm, (**d**) MRI.TOOLS GmbH quadrature rat body RF coil with ID of 72 mm, (**e**) 4×1 element Bruker rat cardiac Rx surface array RF coil, (**f**) Bruker rat body Tx volume resonator with ID 72 mm.

5 Multinuclear Imaging

The most frequent MRI method in biomedical research is proton (^{1}H) imaging. Hydrogen is the most abundant nucleus in living organisms. It also is the nucleus which is the most sensitive to interactions with an external magnetic field, due to its high gyromagnetic ratio ($\gamma = 42.576$ MHz/T).

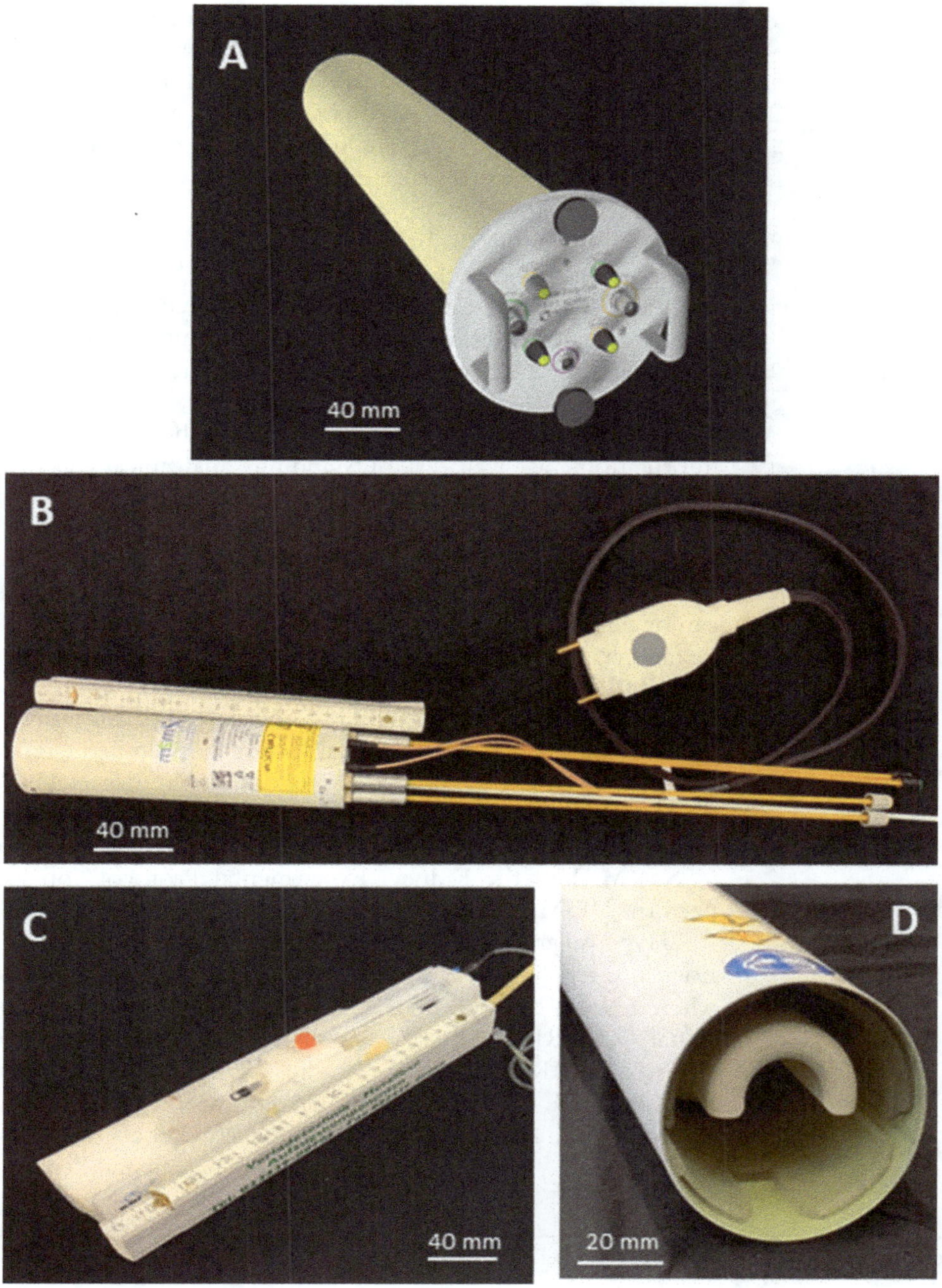

Fig. 4 Example RF coils suitable for kidney MRI of the mouse. (**a**) MRI.TOOLS GmbH quadrature mouse body RF coil with an ID = 42 mm, (**b**) Bruker quadrature mouse body RF coil with 35 mm ID, (**c**) Bruker 2 × 2 element mouse cardiac surface array RF coil, (**d**) Tx/Rx quadrature surface RF coil with cryo-cooling technology (CryoProbe)

In preclinical renal MRI, structural and functional information is typically investigated using in vivo ^{1}H MR imaging of the kidney. Techniques such as T_2/T_2* mapping, arterial spin labeling (ASL), dynamic contrast-enhanced imaging (DCE-MRI) or diffusion-weighted imaging (DWI) are performed in order to study the oxygenation, perfusion, clearance rate, and water and metabolite motion within the kidneys.

Physiometabolic probing is supported by imaging and spectroscopic applications of other nuclei such as ^{13}C, ^{17}O, ^{23}Na, ^{35}Cl, ^{39}K, ^{31}P, and ^{19}F [43]. The detection of X-nuclei is challenging because of the low intrinsic SNR due to the smaller γ, compared to ^{1}H, and by the lower abundance of these nuclei in biological tissues.

Increasing B_0 is the most effective way to increase sensitivity—the benefits of higher B_0 are unique metabolic and functional information, as well as outstanding anatomical detail [44–47]. X-nuclei MR also benefits from the increase in SNR achieved with cryo-cooled transceive surface RF coils, which are currently available for ^{13}C, ^{31}P, ^{19}F, and ^{1}H [48, 49].

Changes in the biodistribution of endogenous metabolites that can be detected with ^{23}Na- or ^{31}P-MR have been demonstrated to be markers of renal disease [50–53]. For more details on preclinical ^{23}Na-MRI protocols, see the chapters by Grist JT et al. "Sodium (^{23}Na) MRI of the Kidney: Basic Concept" and "Sodium (^{23}Na) MRI of the Kidney: Experimental Protocol." Similarly, renal perfusion, oxygenation, and inflammatory cell infiltration can be investigated using ^{19}F-MRI [54–57]. *See* the chapters by Grist JT et al. "Sodium (^{23}Na) MRI of the Kidney: Basic Concept" and "Sodium (^{23}Na) MRI of the Kidney: Experimental Protocol" on how to perform ^{19}F-MRI renal studies in rodents.

Hyperpolarization techniques have great potential for explorations into renal metabolic diseases (e.g., hyperpolarized ^{13}C-MRI), where SNR is boosted up to a 20,000-fold compared to conventional ^{13}C-MRI [58]. Experimental protocols to perform hyperpolarized ^{13}C-MRI in preclinical studies are provided in the chapters by von Morze C et al. "Hyperpolarized Carbon (^{13}C) MRI of the Kidneys: Basic Concept" and by Laustsen C et al. "Hyperpolarized Carbon (^{13}C) MRI of the Kidney: Experimental Protocol."

6 Physiological Monitoring

A major difference between clinical and preclinical MRI is the need to anesthetize the animals prior to imaging. Since most anaesthetic drugs produce physiological changes (temperature decrease, depression of cardiorespiratory function, etc.), monitoring the anaesthetized animals is a very crucial aspect in preclinical MRI studies. Even in the most simple case, that is, the scanning of spontaneously breathing animals without any further intervention or treatment, respiration and temperature of the animal has to be monitored continuously during the scan in order to guarantee the appropriate anaesthetic status and to avoid hypothermia. In particular, hypothermia is a critical issues in rodent imaging, since mice have a low mass vs. a large surface which promotes heat loss [59, 60]. This problem is less severe in rats due to their larger weight, but it is not negligible [61]. Heating systems must be therefore used to maintain temperature homeostasis.

Physiological monitoring of the animal is even more essential in functional MR imaging, since changes may produce confounding effects on the outcome of the MR experiment [62]. Careful monitoring and recording of physiological data should be performed at all times during the experiment to ensure the validity of the results and their reproducibility. The frequency of physiological monitoring depends on the invasiveness of the experimental procedure as well as the time after induction of anaesthesia. As a rule of thumb, the more invasive the procedure and the longer the time under anaesthesia, the more frequent the physiological monitoring of the animal should be performed. Additionally, the correct positioning of the animals on the animal bed systems, along with careful intubation (if needed) are essential to ensure respiratory and circulatory comfort during imaging, and to promote recovery of the animal after the experiment.

Typical physiological parameters monitored during MR experiments include temperature, heart rate, and respiration rate. Many manufacturers already offer these three monitoring channels, and are ready to use these signals for the purpose of gating or triggering the MR imaging techniques. Additionally, information on blood pressure, blood oxygen saturation, transcutaneous pCO_2, or pH can also be collected. In some cases, invasive withdrawal of blood samples is necessary—this is a very difficult task since the sampling has to be executed using long tubes with considerable dead volumes and very limited visual control.

Finally, all equipment must allow for remote physiological monitoring, and strictly comply with MR safety requirements. Several integrated animal handling solutions for physiological monitoring and anaesthesia are commercially available. Examples are given in Table 3.

7 Practical Points to Consider When Planning a Study

The aim of this chapter is to outline the main hardware components required for preclinical MRI of the kidney and to guide the appropriate hardware selection to meet the individual needs.

This section is intended to provide a summary of the prequisites needed and to help prepare for preclinical renal MR applications:

Table 3
Examples of commercially available equipment for physiological monitoring in preclinical MRI

Physiological parameter (s)	Examples of vendor equipment
Temperature	Omniflex (Neoptix, Inc., Canada) Fiber optic temperature probes (SA Instruments, Inc. Stony Brook, NY, USA) RightTemp (Kent Scientific Corp., Torrington, CT, USA) MultiSens (Opsens Solutions, Canada)
Respiration rate/ECG and gating	BioVet (m2m imaging, Cleveland, OH, USA) Model 1030 Monitoring & Gating system (Small Animall Instruments, Inc. Stony Brook, NY, USA)
Blood pressure	CODA monitor (Kent Scientific Corp., Torrington, CT, USA)
Blood oxygen saturation, heart rate	Pulse oximeter (SA Instruments, Inc. Stony Brook, NY, USA) MouseOx (STARR Life Sciences Corp., USA)
Transcutateous pCO_2	Capnograph (SA Instruments, Inc. Stony Brook, NY, USA) CapnoScan (Kent Scientific Corp., Torrington, CT, USA)
Several	PhysioSuite (Kent Scientific Corp., Torrington, CT, USA) PLUGSYS (Harvard Apparatus, Holliston, MA, USA)

7.1 MRI System

7.1.1 Clinical or Preclinical?

With a 3.0 T clinical MR system, renal MRI of rats is feasible with acceptable image quality and spatial resolution. However, if possible, we recommend to use a dedicated ultrahigh field MR system tailored for small-animal imaging with a magnetic field strength of 7.0 or 9.4 T. The reason is that the SNR gain achieved with preclinical MR scanners compared to that at lower B_0 is instrumental for achieving good spatial and temporal resolution, as well as for reducing the scan times needed to perform MR examinations.

7.1.2 Should I Consider Moving to a High Magnetic Field Strength?

As discussed above (*see* Subheading 2), the use of a higher magnetic field strength results in an increase in SNR proportional to B_0 ($SNR \propto B_0^{1.65}$). This means that renal MR images will achieve greater SNR that can be traded off for to achieve higher spatial resolution or reduced scan time as needed (*see* Table 1). Also, higher B_0 increases the BOLD effect. In general, all methods based on T_2*-weighting will benefit from an increase in the magnetic field strength. MR spectroscopy applications also profit from the increased B_0. Therefore, we strongly recommend the use of a high B_0 for these MR applications. However, not all facilities have such high field MR scanners readily available, in which case it might be advisable to perform the experiments using a lower magnetic field system, as opposed to moving animals, equipment, and personnel to another facility.

7.1.3 Higher Magnetic Fields Are All Rainbows and Unicorns, and Should Always Be Used, Right?

Not necessarily! Be aware that higher magnetic field strengths suffer from greater B_0 and B_1 inhomogeneities than lower field strengths, which must be corrected in order to fully benefit from the boost in SNR. Also, due to the B_0-dependent changes of the relaxation properties, the method-specific and protocol-specific imaging parameters have to be adopted in order to generate similar image contrasts that are comparable to those achieved at lower B_0. If the focus is the transfer of MR methods from preclinical models to clinical applications, use of the same static magnetic field strength is advisable. The "loss" of SNR may be partially compensated for by the use of cryo-cooled RF coils, which would be more cost-effective than the procurement of a high field small animal MR scanner.

7.1.4 OK, But ... Which B_0 Is Everyone Else Using?

The move to higher magnetic field strengths is supported by a large body of literature (see Figs. 1 and 2) which reports the most typical magnetic field strengths for rats to be 3.0 and 9.4 T and for mice to be 7.0 and 9.4 T. The continued use of 3.0 T scanners for rats is mainly due to the use of readily available clinical MR systems, which are then adapted for rat MR experiments. However, these are typically performed using hand/wrist or knee RF coils tailored for clinical applications in humans, and are not optimized for animal imaging, with the main disadvantages being a loss of signal due to incorrect loading, and the inability to match and tune the RF coil.

7.1.5 What About the Gradient System?

Depending on the MR application of your choice, a high gradient slew rate might be needed. Fast imaging techniques need fast gradient switching speeds, since this parameter influences the minimum achievable repetition time (TR), echo time (TE), and the echo spacing. However, a higher slew rate means a greater monetary investment will be needed at the acquisition of a new MR scanner. Equally, the duty cycle is a crucial parameter in hardware-demanding sequences, which generally includes all fast imaging techniques. We recommend the procurement of a gradient system tailored according to the individual experimental needs.

7.2 RF Coil Setup

7.2.1 Which Kind of RF Coil Should I Use to Get the Most Juice from My Clinical MR Scanner?

The best option is to use a hand/wrist RF coil; a knee RF coil is a second-best option. Both of these are RF coil arrays which provide high SNR and full FOV coverage. However, these RF coils are tailored for clinical applications in humans and are not optimized for animal imaging, with the main disadvantages being a loss of signal due to incorrect loading and the inability to match and tune the RF coil. Also, the clinical MR system must be adapted for rat MR experiments (mice are too small and do not provide enough loading in clinical systems). Alternatively, dedicated RF coils provided by RF coil vendors which are customized for renal MRI of rats can be connected to the clinical MR scanner.

7.2.2 Which RF Coil Setups Are the Most Suitable for Renal Applications in My Preclinical MR Scanner?

The anatomical position of the kidneys suggests placement of the RF coil in close proximity to the dorsal skin of the animal. We recommend the use of a surface RF coil for signal reception together with a volume RF coil for excitation. This is the most common setup since it improves the SNR in comparison with a Tx/Rx volume RF coil, while still maintaining a homogeneous B_1. Also, be aware that this setup needs the synchronized detuning of the RF coils in turns in order to avoid RF coupling between the two coils (the surface RF coil must be detuned during transmission while the volume RF coil must be detuned during reception).

7.3 X-Nuclei

7.3.1 What If I Want to Perform X-Nuclei MRI/MRS?

Broadband RF chains, including the transmission path and the receive path, together with RF coils specifically tailored for X-nuclei are needed. Due to the typically low SNR inherent to X-nuclei MR applications, a good option would be the use of a cryo-cooled RF coil. Imaging of a single kidney can be performed in mice using a mouse cryo-cooled RF coil. To image both kidneys simultaneously in mice, a rat cryo-cooled RF coil could be used. However, bear in mind that cryo-cooled RF coils are designed as transceive surface RF antennae, and provide inhomogeneous transmit and sensitivity profiles. Therefore, if your MR application needs exact T_1 contrasts or quantification based on absolute signal intensities, a B_1 correction must be performed.

7.4 Animal Handling and Physiological Monitoring

Please also *see* the chapter by Kaucsar T et al. "Preparation and Monitoring of Small Animals in Renal MRI."

7.4.1 How Should I Position the Rodent in the Animal Bed Prior to the Experiment?

This depends on the kind of RF coil being used. Typically, the kidneys are measured from the dorsal side using a combination of a volume RF coil for RF pulse transmission and a surface RF coil to receive the MR signal. The volume RF coil will be placed inside the bore and fixed, while the surface RF coil is typically displaceable or is fixed on the animal bed. The position of the animal will then be adapted according to this setup.

7.4.2 What Is the Essential Physiological Monitoring that Should Be Performed During Small-Animal Renal MR Experiments?

The essential physiological monitoring includes respiration, which is also used for triggering, and body temperature, which should be maintained at a normal level.

7.4.3 What Other Physiological Parameters Can I Measure, and Which Equipment Should I Use?

A wide variety of MR compatible equipment exists in the market that allows for measurement of temperature, respiration rate, blood pressure, blood oxygen saturation and respiration rate, and transcutaneous pCO_2, among others. *See* Table 3 for exemples of commercially available equipment for physiological monitoring in preclinical MRI.

7.5 Image Acquisition

7.5.1 Should I Perform B_0 Shimming in Every MR Study?

Preferably, yes. Active shimming protocols homogenize the B_0 field in a small region of interest, and help to improve the performance of T_2*-weighted MR protocols such as EPI. For performing MRS of the kidney (or any other organ), shimming should always be completed during the MR study adjustments. In general, we recommend to always perform shimming in every renal MR study.

7.5.2 Should I Always Do Triggering of the Signal? What Are my Options?

Renal MR imaging should be synchronized with animal respiration, preferably triggered to the exhalation phase [32, 63]. If possible, the animals should be allowed to breathe spontaneously under anaesthesia.

8 Notes

1. After the decade of the brain and the (re)discovery of the brain–heart–kidney network, a new era of kidney imaging is expected. The most important brain research tool is fMRI, and it has served as strong motivation for continued technological improvements in hardware development. Similar techniques are valuable for renal imaging. BOLD-based and BV/BF-based techniques greatly benefit from higher magnetic fields, providing a higher SNR, a higher CNR, and better spatial resolution. Nevertheless, the use of higher magnetic fields brings new problems that call for new hardware solutions.
2. Although there is an increased demand on gradient performance, this will exacerbate the problems associated with acoustic noise. New gradient designs should take into account the acoustic noise pressure level as a parameter. Gradient systems that are targeted to the region of interest only may be a solution. The higher gradient performance with increased bandwidth, as well as the increased physiological noise, reduce the gain in the SNR. A limit of the tissue contribution to thermal noise may be found by new RF coil designs.
3. Modern MRI systems come equipped with multiple receiver units allowing parallel acquisition. A combination of small, multielement receive-only RF coils with parallel imaging is a game changer in the way MRI data are acquired. Reducing the RF coil size will allow for the acquisition of data from a small region of interest with higher sensitivity, because of the close proximity of the RF coil to the region, and thus limited noise contribution from tissue. The use of multiple elements, which are decoupled from each other, will help to achieve extended tissue coverage.
4. A problem associated with parallel imaging arises in the storage and processing of large amounts of data. Therefore, considerable effort must be invested into the handling of "Big Data." Boosting the data transfer rate, the use of array processors and the application of renal MRI will push the limits of data science.

Acknowledgments

This work was funded in part (Thoralf Niendorf, Andreas Pohlmann) by the German Research Foundation (Gefoerdert durch die Deutsche Forschungsgemeinschaft (DFG), Projektnummer 394046635, SFB 1365, RENOPROTECTION. Funded by the Deutsche Forschungsgemeinschaft (DFG, German Research Foundation), Project number 394046635, SFB 1365, RENOPROTECTION).

This publication is based upon work from COST Action PARENCHIMA, supported by European Cooperation in Science and Technology (COST). COST (www.cost.eu) is a funding agency for research and innovation networks. COST Actions help connect research initiatives across Europe and enable scientists to enrich their ideas by sharing them with their peers. This boosts their research, career, and innovation.

PARENCHIMA (renalmri.org) is a community-driven Action in the COST program of the European Union, which unites more than 200 experts in renal MRI from 30 countries with the aim to improve the reproducibility and standardization of renal MRI biomarkers.

References

1. de Graaf RA, Brown PB, McIntyre S, Nixon TW, Behar KL, Rothman DL (2006) High magnetic field water and metabolite proton T_1 and T_2 relaxation in rat brain in vivo. Magn Reson Med 56(2):386–394. https://doi.org/10.1002/mrm.20946
2. Ladd ME (2018) The quest for higher sensitivity in MRI through higher magnetic fields. Z Med Phys 28(1):1–3. https://doi.org/10.1016/j.zemedi.2017.12.001
3. Moser E, Laistler E, Schmitt F, Kontaxis G (2017) Ultra-high field NMR and MRI—the role ofmagnet technology to iIncrease sensitivity and specificity. Front Phys 5:33. https://doi.org/10.3389/fphy.2017.00033
4. Niendorf T, Barth M, Kober F, Trattnig S (2016) From ultrahigh to extreme field magnetic resonance: where physics, biology and medicine meet. MAGMA 29(3):309–311. https://doi.org/10.1007/s10334-016-0564-1
5. Hoult DI (2000) Sensitivity and power deposition in a high-field imaging experiment. J Magn Reson Imaging 12:46–67. https://doi.org/10.1002/1522-2586(200007)12:1<46::AID-JMRI6>3.0.CO;2-D
6. Hoult DI, Richards RE (1976) The signal-to-noise ratio of the nuclear magnetic resonance experiment. J Magn Reson 24(1):71–85. https://doi.org/10.1016/0022-2364(76)90233-X
7. Pohmann R, Speck O, Scheffler K (2016) Signal-to-noise ratio and MR tissue parameters in human brain imaging at 3, 7, and 9.4 Tesla using current receive coil array. Magn Reson Med 75:801–809. https://doi.org/10.1002/mrm.25677
8. Guérin B, Villena JF, Polimeridis AG, Adalsteinsson E, Daniel L, White JK, Wald LL (1980) The ultimate signal-to-noise ratio in realistic body models. Magn Reson Med 78:1969–1980. https://doi.org/10.1002/mrm.26564
9. Merkle EM, Dale BM (2005) Abdominal MRI at 3.0 T: the basics revisited. Am J Roentgenol 186(6):1524–1532. https://doi.org/10.2214/AJR.05.0932
10. Rooney WD, Johnson G, Li X, Cohen ER, Kim SG, Ugurbil K, Springer CS (2007) Magnetic field and tissue dependencies of human brain longitudinal ^1H_2O relaxation *in vivo*. Magn Reson Med 57(2):308–318. https://doi.org/10.1002/mrm.21122
11. Seehafer JU, Kalthoff D, Farr TD, Wiedermann D, Hoehm M (2010) No increase of the blood oxygenation level-dependent functional magnetic resonance imaging signal with higher field strength: implications for

brain activation studies. J Neurosci 30 (15):5234–5241. https://doi.org/10.1523/JNEUROSCI.0844-10.2010

12. Schenck JF (1995) Imaging of brain iron by magnetic resonance: T_2 relaxation at different field strengths. J Neurol Sci 134:10–18. https://doi.org/10.1016/0022-510X(95)00203-E
13. Duyn JH (2012) The future of ultra-high field MRI and fMRI for study of the human brain. NeuroImage 62:1241–1248. https://doi.org/10.1016/j.neuroimage.2011.10.065
14. Baldanchani P, Naidich TP (2015) Ultra-high-field MR neuroimaging. Am J Neuroradiol 36 (7):1204–1215. https://doi.org/10.3174/ajnr.A4180
15. Niendorf T, Pohlmann A, Reimann HM, Waiczies H, Peper E, Huelnhagen T, Seeliger E, Schreiber A, Kettritz R, Strobel K, Ku MC, Waiczies S (2015) Advancing cardiovascular, neurovascular, and renal magnetic resonance imaging in small rodents using cryogenic radiofrequency coil technology. Front Pharmacol 6:255. https://doi.org/10.3389/fphar.2015.00255
16. Schick F (2005) Whole-body MRI at high field: technical limits and clinical potential. Eur Radiol 15(5):946–959. https://doi.org/10.1007/s00330-005-2678-0
17. Van de Moortele PF, Akgun C, Adriany G, Moeller S, Ritter J, Collins CM, Smith MB, Vaughan JT, Ugurbil K (2005) B_1 destructive interferences and spatial phase patterns at 7 T with a head transceiver array RF coil. Magn Reson Med 54:1503–1518. https://doi.org/10.1002/mrm.20708
18. Niendorf T, Graessl A, Thalhammer C, Dieringer MA, Kraus O, Santoro D, Fuchs K, Hezel F, Waiczies S, Ittermann B, Winter L (2013) Progress and promises of human cardiac magnetic resonance at ultrahigh fields: a physics perspective. J Magn Reson 229:208–222. https://doi.org/10.1016/j.jmr.2012.11.015
19. Fiedler T, Ladd ME, Bitz AK (2017) SAR simulations & safety. NeuroImage 168:33–58. https://doi.org/10.1016/j.neuroimage.2017.03.035
20. Stockmann JP, Wald LL (2018) In vivo B_0 field shimming methods for MRI at 7T. NeuroImage 168:71–87. https://doi.org/10.1016/j.neuroimage.2017.06.013
21. Juchem C, de Graaf RA (2016) B_0 magnetic field homogeneity and shimming for *in vivo* magnetic resonance spectroscopy. Anal Biochem 529:17–29. https://doi.org/10.1016/j.ab.2016.06.003
22. Pan JW, Lo KM, Hetherington HP (2012) Role of very high order and degree B_0 shimming for spectroscopic imaging of the human brain at 7 Tesla. Magn Reson Med 68 (4):1007–1017. https://doi.org/10.1002/mrm.24122
23. Motyka S, Moser P, Hingerl L, Hangel G, Heckova E, Strasser B, Eckstein K, Robinson SD, Poser BA, Gruber S, Trattnig S, Bogner W (2019) The influence of spatial resolution on the spectral quality and quantification accuracy of whole-brain MRSI at 1.5T, 3T, 7T, and 9.4T. Magn Reson Med 82(2):551–565. https://doi.org/10.1002/mrm.27746
24. Meyer A, Stolz K, Dreher W, Bergemann J, Thimmashetty VH, Lueschen N, Azizi Z, Khobragade V, Maedler K, Kuestermann E (2015) Manganese-mediated MRI signals correlate with functional β-cell mass during diabetes progression. Diabetes 64(6):2138–2147. https://doi.org/10.2337/db14-0864
25. Gruber B, Froeling M, Leiner T, Klomp DWJ (2018) RF coils: a practical guide for nonphysicists. J Magn Reson Imaging 48:590–604. https://doi.org/10.1002/jmri.26187
26. Doty FD, Entzminger G, Kulkarni J, Pamarthy K, Staab JP (2007) Radio frequency coil technology for small-animal MRI. NMR Biomed 20:304–325. https://doi.org/10.1002/nbm.1149
27. Lopez Rios N, Pouliot P, Papoutsis K, Foias A, Stikov N, Lesage F, Dehaes M, Cohen-Adad J (2018) Design and construction of an optimized transmit/receive hybrid birdcage resonator to improve full body images of medium-sized animals in 7T scanner. PLoS One 13(2): e0192035. https://doi.org/10.1371/journal.pone.0192035
28. Chang D, Wang YC, Xu TT, Peng XG, Cai Y, Wang L, Bai YY, Ju S (2017) Noninvasive identification of renal hypoxia in experimental myocardial infarctions of different sizes by using BOLD MR imaging in a mouse model. Radiology 286(1):129–139. https://doi.org/10.1148/radiol.2017161998
29. Wallner BK, Edelman RR, Bajakian RL, Kleefield J, Atkinson DJ, Mattle HP (1990) Signal normalization in surface-RF coil MR imaging. Am J Neuroradiol 11(6):1271–1272
30. Hayes CE, Axel L (1985) Noise performance of surface RF coils for magnetic resonance imaging at 1.5 T. Med Phys 12(5):604–607. https://doi.org/10.1118/1.595682
31. Garwood M, DelaBarre L (2001) The return of the frequency sweep: designing adiabatic pulses for contemporary NMR. J Magn Reson 153 (2):155–177. https://doi.org/10.1006/jmre.2001.2340

32. Hueper K, Schmidbauer M, Thorenz A, Bräsen JH, Gutberlet M, Mengel M, Hartung D, Chen R, Meier M, Haller H, Wacker F, Rong S, Gueler F (2017) Longitudinal evaluation of perfusion changes in acute and chronic renal allograft rejection using arterial spin labeling in translational mouse models. J Magn Reson Imaging 46(6):1664–1672. https://doi.org/10.1002/jmri.25713
33. Gareis D, Wichmann T, Lanz T, Melkus G, Horn M, Jakob PM (2007) Mouse MRI using phased-array RF coils. NMR Biomed 20 (3):326–334. https://doi.org/10.1002/nbm.1156
34. Zubkov M, Hurshkainen AA, Brui EA, Glybovski SB, Gulyaev V, Anisimov NV, Volkov DV, Pirogov YA, Melchakova IV (2018) Small-animal, whole-body imaging with metamaterial-inspired RF coil. NMR Biomed 31:e3952. https://doi.org/10.1002/nbm.3952
35. Hoult DI, Lauterbur PC (1979) The sensitivity of the zeugmatographic experiment involving human sample. J Magn Reson 34(2):425–433. https://doi.org/10.1016/0022-2364(79)90019-2
36. Edelstein WA, Glover GH, Hardy CJ, Redington RW (1986) The intrinsic signal-to-noise ratio in NMR imaging. Magn Reson Med 3 (4):604–618. https://doi.org/10.1002/mrm.1910030413
37. Marques JP, Simonis FFJ, Webb AG (2019) Low-field MRI: an MR physics perspective. J Magn Reson Imaging 49:1528–1542. https://doi.org/10.1002/jmri.26637
38. Kovacs H, Moskau D, Spraul M (2005) Cryogenically cooled probes—a leap in NMR technology. Prog Nucl Magn Reson Spectrosc 46:131–155. https://doi.org/10.1016/j.pnmrs.2005.03.001
39. Ratering D, Baltes C, Nordmeyer-Massner J, Marek D, Rudin M (2008) Performance of a 200-MHz cryogenic RF probe designed for MRI and MRS of the murine brain. Magn Reson Med 59:1440–1447. https://doi.org/10.1002/mrm.21629
40. Baltes C, Radzwill N, Bosshard S, Marek D, Rudin M (2009) Micro MRI of the mouse brain using a novel 400MHz cryogenic quadrature RF probe. NMR Biomed 22:834–842. https://doi.org/10.1002/nbm.1396
41. Xie L, Layton AT, Wang N, Larson PEZ, Zhang JL, Lee VS, Liu C, Johnson GA (2016) Dynamic contrast-enhanced quantitative susceptibility mapping with ultrashort echo time MRI for evaluating renal function. Am J Physiol Ren Physiol 310(2):F174–F182. https://doi.org/10.1152/ajprenal.00351.2015
42. Poirier-Quinot M, Ginefri JC, Girard O, Robert P, Darrasse L (2008) Performance of a miniature high-temperature superconducting (HTS) surface RF coil for in vivo microimaging of the mouse in a standard 1.5T clinical whole-body scanner. Magn Reson Med 60 (4):917–927. https://doi.org/10.1002/mrm.21605
43. Hu R, Kleimaier D, Malzacher M, Hoesl MAU, Paschke NK, Schad LR (2019) X-nuclei imaging: current state, technical challenges, and future directions. J Magn Reson Imaging 51(2):355–376. https://doi.org/10.1002/jmri.26780
44. Nagel AM, Umathum R, Rösler MB, Ladd ME, Litvak I, Gor'kov PL, Brey WW, Schepkin VD (2016) ^{39}K and ^{23}Na relaxation times and MRI of rat head at 21.1T. NMR Biomed 29:759–766. https://doi.org/10.1002/nbm.3528
45. Schepkin VD, Brey WW, Gor'kov PL, Grant SC (2010) Initial *in vivo* rodent sodium and proton MR imaging at 21.1 T. Magn Reson Imaging 28(3):400–407. https://doi.org/10.1016/j.mri.2009.10.002
46. Schepkin VD, Elumalai M, Kitchen JA, Qian C, Gor'kov PL, Brey WW (2014) In vivo chlorine and sodium MRI of rat brain at 21.1 T. MAGMA 27:63–70. https://doi.org/10.1007/s10334-013-0387-2
47. Waiczies S, Rosenberg JT, Kuehne A, Starke L, Ramos Delgado P, Millward JM, Prinz C, Periquito J, Pohlmann A, Niendorf T (2019) Fluorine19 MRI at 21.1 T: enhanced spin–lattice relaxation of perfluoro15crown5ether and sensitivity as demonstrated in *ex vivo* murine neuroinflammation. MAGMA 32:37–49. https://doi.org/10.1007/s10334-018-0710-z
48. Waiczies S, Millward JM, Starke L, Ramos Delgado P, Huelnhagen T, Prinz C, Marek D, Wecker D, Wissmann R, Koch S, Boehm-Sturm P, Waiczies H, Niendorf T, Pohlmann A (2017) Enhanced fluorine-19 MRI sensitivity using a cryogenic radiofrequency probe: technical developments and *ex vivo* demonstration in a mouse model of neuroinflammation. Sci Rep 7:9808. https://doi.org/10.1038/s41598-017-09622-2
49. Sack M, Wetterling F, Sartorius A, Ende G, Weber-Fahr W (2014) Signal-to-noise ratio of a mouse brain ^{13}C CryoProbe™ system in comparison with room temperature coils: spectroscopic phantom and *in vivo* results. NMR Biomed 27:709–715. https://doi.org/10.1002/nbm.3110

50. Boska MD, Meyerhoff DJ, Twieg DB, Karczmar GS, Matson GB, Weiner MW (1990) Image-guided ^{31}P magnetic resonance spectroscopy of normal and transplanted human kidneys. Kidney Int 38:294–300. https://doi.org/10.1038/ki.1990.199

51. Klemm A, Rzanny R, Fünfstück R, Werner W, Schubert J, Kaiser WA, Stein G (1998) ^{31}P-magnetic resonance spectroscopy (^{31}P-MRS) of human allografts after renal transplantation. Nephrol Dial Transplant 13 (12):3147–3152. https://doi.org/10.1093/ndt/13.12.3147

52. Maril N, Margalit R, Mispelter J, Degani H (2004) Functional sodium magnetic resonance imaging of the intact rat kidney. Kidney Int 65:927–935. https://doi.org/10.1111/j.1523-1755.2004.00475.x

53. Kalayciyan R, Wetterling F, Neudecker S, Haneder S, Gretz N, Schad LR (2013) Bilateral kidney sodium-MRI: enabling accurate quantification of renal sodium concentration through a two-element phased array system. J Magn Reson Imaging 38(3). https://doi.org/10.1002/jmri.24024

54. Pohlmann A, Schreiber A, Ku MC, Waiczies H, Kox S, Kettritz R, Waiczies S, Niendorf T (2014) Assessment of renal inflammatory cell infiltration in a murine ANCA-induced glomerulonephritis model by 19F-MRI. In: Joint Annual Meeting ISMRM-ESMRMB 2014, Milan, Italy. https://doi.org/10.13140/RG.2.1.4143.4326

55. Ruiz-Cabello J, Barnett BP, Bottomley PA, Bulte JWM (2011) Fluorine (^{19}F) MRS and MRI in biomedicine. NMR Biomed 24 (2):114–129. https://doi.org/10.1002/nbm.1570

56. Hitchens TK, Ye Q, Eytan DF, Janjic JM, Ahrens ET, Ho C (2011) ^{19}F MRI detection of acute allograft rejection with in vivo perfluorocarbon labeling of immune cells. Magn Reson Med 65(4):1144–1153. https://doi.org/10.1002/mrm.22702

57. Hu L, Chen J, Yang X, Senpan A, Allen JS, Yanaba N, Caruthers SD, Lanza GM, Hammerman MR, Wickline SA (2014) Assessing intrarenal nonperfusion and vascular leakage in acute kidney injury with multinuclear ^{1}H/^{19}F MRI and perfluorocarbon nanoparticles. Magn Reson Med 71:2186–2196. https://doi.org/10.1002/mrm.24851

58. Pedersen M, Ursprung S, Jensen JD, Jespersen B, Gallagher F, Lautsten C (2019) Hyperpolarised ^{13}CMRI metabolic and functional imaging: an emerging renal MR diagnostic modality. MAGMA 33(1):23–32. https://doi.org/10.1007/s10334-019-00801-y

59. Gordon CJ (2017) The mouse thermoregulatory system: its impact on translating biomedical data to humans. Physiol Behav 179:55–66. https://doi.org/10.1016/j.physbeh.2017.05.026

60. Reimann HM, Hentschel J, Marek J, Huelnhagen T, Todiras M, Kox S, Waiczies S, Hodge R, Bader M, Pohlmann A, Niendorf T (2016) Normothermic mouse functional MRI of acute focal thermostimulation for probing nociception. Sci Rep 6:17230. https://doi.org/10.1038/srep17230

61. Hitt BA, Mazze RI, Cook TL, Beppu WJ, Kosek JC (1977) Thermoregulatory defect in rats during anesthesia. Anesth Analg 56 (1):9–15. https://doi.org/10.1213/00000539-197701000-00006

62. Niles DJ, Gordon JW, Fain SB (2016) Effect of anesthesia on renal R_2* measured by blood oxygen level-dependent MRI. NMR Biomed 28(7):811–817. https://doi.org/10.1002/nbm.3314

63. Nikken JJ, Krestin GP (2007) MRI of the kidney-state of the art. Eur Radiol 17 (11):2780–2793. https://doi.org/10.1007/s00330-007-0701-3

10

MR Elastography of the Abdomen: Experimental Protocols

Suraj D. Serai and Meng Yin

Abstract

Application of MRE for noninvasive evaluation of renal fibrosis has great potential for noninvasive assessment in patients with chronic kidney disease (CKD). CKD leads to severe complications, which require dialysis or kidney transplant and could even result in death. CKD in native kidneys and interstitial fibrosis in allograft kidneys are the two major kidney fibrotic pathologies where MRE may be clinically useful. Both these conditions can lead to extensive morbidity, mortality, and high health care costs. Currently, biopsy is the standard method for renal fibrosis staging. This method of diagnosis is painful, invasive, limited by sampling bias, exhibits inter- and intraobserver variability, requires prolonged hospitalization, poses risk of complications and significant bleeding, and could even lead to death. MRE based methods can potentially be useful to noninvasively detect, stage, and monitor renal fibrosis, reducing the need for renal biopsy. In this chapter, we describe experimental procedure and step by step instructions to run MRE along with some illustrative applications. We also includes sections on how to perform data quality check and analysis methods.

This publication is based upon work from the COST Action PARENCHIMA, a community-driven network funded by the European Cooperation in Science and Technology (COST) program of the European Union, which aims to improve the reproducibility and standardization of renal MRI biomarkers.

Key words Magnetic resonance elastography (MRE), Stiffness, Kidney, Preclinical imaging, MRI, Fibrosis, Chronic kidney disease (CKD)

1 Introduction

1.1 Magnetic Resonance Elastography

Magnetic resonance elastography (MRE) based imaging techniques are now being routinely used for noninvasive assessment of tissue mechanical properties. In MRI, elastography encompasses imaging techniques that noninvasively estimate tissue elasticity and related mechanical properties through the application of external forces [1]. MRE induces harmonic vibrations of acoustic-range frequencies in the tissue of interest and images the propagation of these vibrations in the tissues to calculate quantitative values of mechanical parameters. The desired output is to measure the level of stiffness. The elastogram differentiate if the tissue is hard or soft can give diagnostic information about the presence of the disease. In liver, tissue stiffness has been shown to be elevated with advanced fibrosis and to correlate with the stage of fibrosis [2–4]. Renal fibrosis is a pathological process common to all chronic kidney diseases (CKD) and thereby represents an excellent treatment target. A large number of molecular pathways involved in renal fibrosis have been identified in preclinical studies, some of them being similar among different organs and some with available drugs in various phases of clinical testing [5]. CKD may lead to end-stage renal failure, with extensive morbidity, mortality, and increasing health costs. Primary and secondary prevention requires a better knowledge of mechanisms underlying renal scarring, the development of specific therapies to slow down the progression of the disease and the development of noninvasive diagnostic tools to characterize the process.

Among imaging methods, MRE, that has been successfully demonstrated in the liver, is an attractive alternative for staging of renal fibrosis. Application of MRE to kidney has been shown to be possible and initial results are encouraging. MRE methods are advantageous as compared to ultrasound based elastography methods because the kidneys are usually located deeply in the body and therefore there is no direct access to apply an external compression easily. An increase in the extracellular matrix synthesis, with excessive fibrillary collagens, characterizes the development of chronic lesions in the glomerular, interstitial, and vascular compartments, leading progressively to end-stage renal failure [6]. Mechanisms participating in these processes are increasingly identified and various therapeutic interventions have been shown to prevent or to favor regression of fibrosis in several experimental models. Therefore, development of new noninvasive MRE based methods for identification and quantification of fibrosis is worthwhile.

1.2 Modulus of Elasticity

The shear modulus (μ) and Young's modulus (E) are two parameters often used for describing tissue mechanical properties and are used as contrast parameters in elasticity imaging. Poisson's ratio (ν), another widely used parameter, is the ratio of lateral strain to longitudinal strain. Among these parameters, only two are independent. The shear modulus is known to be related to Young's modulus and one can be estimated from the other by knowing the Poisson's ratio. In general, soft tissues can be assumed to be incompressible and hence the Poisson's ratio can be assumed to be 0.5. The relationship between shear modulus and Young's modulus can be written as $E = 3\mu$, which means that the calculation of Young's modulus or shear modulus provides the same information. MRE is a dynamic elasticity imaging technique capable of calculating quantitative values of shear modulus of tissues and is clinically approved to be used for the assessment of liver fibrosis. MRE uses low-frequency (40–80 Hz) sound waves to induce shear waves in the liver, visualizes the shear waves by tracking tissue displacement using a modified phase-contrast sequence, and measures the speed of the propagating wave with specialized software called an inversion algorithm [7]. In the commercial version of MRE supplied by Resoundant, the mechanical waves are generated by a subwoofer ("active driver") outside the scan room and are transmitted to a plastic disk ("passive driver") via a plastic tube passing through a wave guide [8]. For preclinical imaging, the same subwoofer active driver may be used or alternatively a functional generator may be used for generating a low frequency sinusoidal mechanical motion (typical range: 20–400 Hz). When the shear stresses (amplitude of microns) are applied to the top surface of a material with certain frequency, the induced waves are propagating into the tissue and every point in the tissue reciprocates in this micromotion. During clinical MRE image acquisition, the passive driver is secured by an elastic band over the abdominal organ of interest [8, 9]. In general, most patients can feel the vibrations generated by the disk but do not find them uncomfortable. For clinical image postprocessing, identical MRE hardware and inversion algorithms are commercially available on scanners manufactured by major MR vendors [10, 11]. Several studies have shown that MRE is a robust, reliable, repeatable, and reproducible technique for detection and staging of liver fibrosis [10]. The accuracy of MRE ranges from 0.85 to 0.99 for differentiating different stages of liver fibrosis [2]. The performance of MRE for differentiating mild fibrosis (stage I) from normal liver or inflammation is lower and the performance is highest for diagnosis of cirrhosis (stage 4) [4, 10]. For preclinical MRE, an actuator, replicating the use of passive driver may be used to couple to the tissue of interest to generate propagating shear waves within a soft tissue material [12]. The electrical signal for the drivers is created by a signal generator synchronized with the MRI pulse sequence triggered and is amplified by an audio amplifier before being fed into the mechanical driver. After the mechanical excitation, a phase-contrast based pulse sequence is used to encode the shear wave motion into the MR phase signal by using a series of magnetic field gradients called motion-encoding gradients (MEG). The MEG, synchronized with the mechanical excitations, is applied after RF excitation [13]. Postprocessing may be done on the scanner or images may be taken offline for analysis. Details of data processing and image reconstruction are covered in the following sections.

1.3 Need for Preclinical MRE

Renal fibrosis causes a change in the structure of the kidney wherein there is an excess accumulation of interstitial extracellular matrix and reduction in the number of tubules. Increasing evidence has demonstrated that, unlike cirrhosis, the early stages of fibrosis are treatable and reversible if appropriate antifibrotic treatment is given [5, 14]. As antifibrotic therapies evolve, a reliable, noninvasive assessment of fibrosis is needed to manage patients with chronic disease. Being able to noninvasively monitor the progression of fibrosis would help in understanding the natural history in patients with chronic disease, determining which patients require antiviral therapy, predicting the approximate time to the development of high-grade fibrosis, and discovering new directions of scientific inquiry. Therefore, there are ongoing investigations using preclinical models with a reliable, noninvasive method to assess organ inflammation and fibrosis, not only to detect and stage the disease itself but also to monitor treatment efficacy and optimize dosing. The feasibility of MRE has been demonstrated on a mouse model of autosomal recessive polycystic kidney disease (ARPKD) which is an inherited disorder of the kidneys and liver caused by mutations in the PKHD1 gene and an important cause of congenital hepatic fibrosis in humans [3].

1.4 Quest for Renal MRE

Many different mechanisms induce glomerular injury, including glomerulonephritis, hypertensive nephrosclerosis and diabetic nephropathy. However, once renal damage reaches a certain threshold, progression of renal disease is consistent, and largely independent of the initial insult. This common pathway to end-stage renal failure is mainly due to tubulointerstitial damage characterized by tubular atrophy, loss of peritubular capillaries and interstitial fibrosis. Mechanisms leading to kidney failure via tubulointerstitial damage and development of fibrosis are mostly massive proteinuria and chronic hypoxia. Fibrosis further impairs oxygen diffusion and supply to tubular cells, rendering a vicious cycle. Thus, in the assessment of chronic renal failure, fibrosis is a major histological feature and may be an important surrogate endpoint for prognosis and monitoring of treatment response. Besides, some investigations suggest that fibrosis might be reversible, when the cause is treated, emphasizing the need for an early detection and quantification of this fibrosis [14–19]. Currently, the extent of interstitial fibrosis is evaluated by renal biopsy which has several drawbacks: it is a semiquantitative approach with wide interobserver variability, and it is prone to sampling errors and associated with significant morbidity. Thus a noninvasive, truly quantitative method of interstitial fibrosis monitoring would be desirable. Diffusion-weighted and blood oxygenation level dependent (BOLD) MRI findings have been shown to be correlated to renal function, but no data have been published as to their correlation with the degree of fibrosis. Blood or urinary markers of fibrosis are also currently evaluated but none is used in clinical practice yet. MRE based methods can estimate tissue stiffness (and thus, the degree of fibrosis) by measuring the velocity of shear waves traveling through the organ of interest. Clinically, they have been mostly used in liver. The ultrasound-based transient elastography (Fibroscan™ device) is able to discriminate the different stages of liver fibrosis with a quadratic trend of the curve plotting histologic scores versus elasticity measurements. Among patients with cirrhosis, stiffness thresholds predicting the onset of specific complications (ascites, esophageal bleeding, hepatocarcinoma, etc.) have been identified. However, this technique is limited by its 1D nature that does not allow the exploration of the entire liver. MRE has been successfully used to assess liver fibrosis. The shear stiffness of normal liver was found to be approximately 2.2 kPa by independent groups, using vibrating frequencies of 60 Hz [4]. As with ultrasound-based transient elastography, MRE can discriminate the different stages of liver fibrosis, with the same quadratic trend of the fibrosis/elasticity curve [2]. MRE has the advantage of being intrinsically a 2D technique and can be associated with conventional liver imaging at the same time. MRE has also been used for applications in the abdomen such as characterizing focal liver lesions, and in organs such as pancreas, breast, muscle, prostate, and kidney [9].

Currently, the most definitive means of assessing renal fibrosis is a kidney biopsy. The invasiveness of a biopsy coupled with its small sampling size have limited its utility in quantifying and monitoring changes in renal fibrosis, especially because fibrosis can be heterogeneously distributed. Accordingly, a noninvasive modality that assesses fibrosis on a kidney-wide scale would be of clinical utility. By replacing soft healthy tissue with stiff extracellular matrix, fibrosis stiffens organs, a phenomenon that has led multiple groups to explore whether tissue stiffness could be used as a surrogate measure for fibrosis. MRE based technique that measures tissue stiffness, would be a novel application for assessment of renal fibrosis. During MRE, the organ of interest is gently vibrated by applying acoustic waves through a pad placed on the overlying skin. The resulting microscopic vibrational waves passing through the organ generate shear waves that can be imaged with motion-synchronized MRI. The velocity of wave propagation is dependent on organ stiffness, with stiffer fibrotic tissue leading to more rapidly moving waves with longer wavelength. Capturing shear waves at multiple time points enables the reconstruction of a quantitative stiffness map. MRE is already a well-established, gold standard technique for liver fibrosis imaging, having been shown to accurately reflect biopsy-derived liver fibrosis measurements. In contrast, MRE for nonhepatic applications is still early in its development, and its technique has not yet been standardized. Small pilot studies of MRE have been performed in native kidneys and kidney allografts, attempting to correlate kidney stiffness with either fibrosis burden or kidney function. Although MRE in porcine kidneys showed a correlation between stiffness and fibrosis in the medulla, the results of small pilot human studies thus far have been conflicting, and no studies as yet have assessed whether stiffness measured by MRE predicts progression of kidney dysfunction. In this chapter, we provide recommended MRE protocols for applications in the abdomen with a focus on the kidney, and a few illustrative applications of MRE in preclinical imaging.

This introduction chapter is complemented by a separate chapter describing the concepts of MRE in the abdomen, which is part of this book.

This chapter is part of the book Pohlmann A, Niendorf T (eds) (2020) Preclinical MRI of the Kidney—Methods and Protocols. Springer, New York.

2 Materials

MRE is an MR-based elastography technique that uses mechanical shear waves to evaluate viscoelastic properties of tissues. Mechanical shear waves produced by an external driver are propagated into the organ of interest using a passive abdominal driver placed over the organ and in contact with the abdominal wall. Tissue displacements in the range of microns produced by propagating shear waves because phase shifts that can be detected with motion encoding gradients in the MRE sequence. The frequency of shear wave applied ranges from 40 to 400 Hz. In liver, the frequency of shear waves used for clinical liver MRE is 60 Hz. A lower frequency is used for organs that are situated deep in the body and a higher frequency may be used for regions of interest that may be closer to the body surface. A lower frequency wave has deeper penetration and spatial lower resolution. A higher frequency wave has higher attenuation and higher spatial frequency. Once decided on the resolution and frequency, these parameters must stay consistent for the duration of the study and must not be changed. Stiffness values measured with one particular frequency are not convertible with those measured with a different frequency. An inversion algorithm automatically produces stiffness maps using the phase shift information. Shear stiffness values can be obtained by drawing regions of interest over the tissue of interest in the stiffness maps and expressed in kiloPascals (kPa).

2.1 Animals

The experimental protocols in this section are tailored for rats (Wistar, Sprague-Dawley or Lewis) with a body mass of 250–350 g. Advice for adaptation to other smaller animals (e.g., mice) or larger animals (e.g., pigs) are given in the sections where necessary.

2.2 Lab Equipment

1. Anesthesia: For nonrecovery experiments urethane solution (Sigma-Aldrich, Steinheim, Germany; 20% in distilled water) can provide anesthesia for several hours with comparatively few side effects on renal physiology, which is an important issue. For an in-depth description and discussion of anesthesia please refer to the chapter by Kaucsar T et al. "Preparation and Monitoring of Small Animals in Renal MRI."
2. Gases: O_2, N_2, and compressed air, as well as a gas-mixing system (FMI Föhr Medical Instruments GmbH, Seeheim-Ober Beerbach, Germany) to achieve required changes in the

oxygen fraction of inspired gas mixture (FiO_2). Besides air, the following gas mixtures are required during the experiment: 10% O_2–90% N_2 for hypoxia and 100% O_2 for hyperoxia.

3. Device for FiO_2 monitoring in gas mixtures: for example Capnomac AGM-103 (Datex GE, Chalfont St Gils, UK).

2.3 MRI Hardware

The general hardware requirements for renal 1H MRI on mice and rats are described in the chapter by Ramos Delgado P et al. "Hardware Considerations for Preclinical Magnetic Resonance of the Kidney." The technique described in this chapter is tailored for a standard 1.5 T or a 3.0 T MR scanner using a head coil or small flex coil (for signal reception) or knee RF coil (transmit–receive) is given where necessary but advice for adaptation to other field strengths and systems (e.g., 9.4 T MR system Biospec 94/20, Bruker Biospin, Ettlingen, Germany). No special or additional hardware is required, except for the following:

1. A physiological monitoring system that can track the respiration, and which is connected to the MR system such that it can be used to trigger the image acquisition.
2. MRE hardware to generate shear waves in the abdomen, details explained in the following section. The experimental protocols are tailored for using a FDA approved and commercially available subwoofer-based system for generating shear waves (Resoundant, MN, USA). Advice for options on using other in-house custom-made MR conditional hardware is included where necessary.

2.3.1 Generating Propagating Shear Waves in the Abdomen: Hardware

MRE has received considerable attention due to the flexibility of MR in acquiring arbitrary 2D images and 3D volumes and its capability to measure motion in all three directions. Though the application of excitation to the tissue of interest could be either internal or external, and either static or dynamic, MRE typically uses dynamic vibrations of a single frequency (within the audio frequency range) induced by external drivers. The electrical signal for these drivers is created signal generator synchronized with MRI pulse sequence triggered and is amplified by an audio amplifier before being fed into the mechanical driver. The mechanical vibrations applied to tissue fall into three categories: transient, quasi-static, or harmonic. It is now well known that the MRE-measured shear modulus of soft tissue is dependent on the frequency of applied mechanical waves. That is why the term "shear stiffness" is often used to describe the shear modulus at a specific frequency. However, it should be fully understood that the formula that calculates the shear modulus from the measured velocity of the waves ($\mu = \rho c^2$, where μ = shear modulus, ρ = density of tissue, and c = wave speed) is valid only in purely elastic tissues. MRE

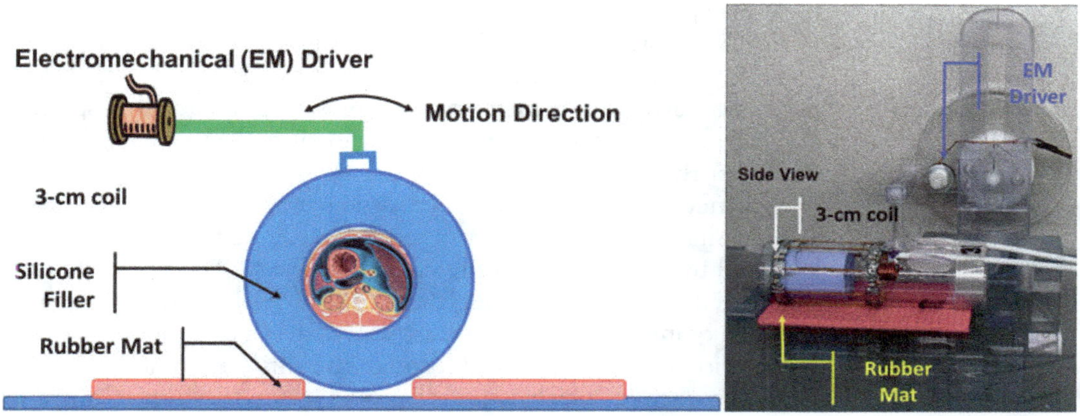

Fig. 1 For smaller animals, an electromechanical driver setup may be used for shear wave generation. Rotational vibrations generated by the electromechanical driver are transmitted into the entire body of the animal. The transmitted shear wave frequency range can be set between 50 and 400 Hz

typically uses harmonic vibrations generated by an external driver device to perturb the tissue. In harmonic excitation, a low-frequency acoustic wave (20–400 Hz) is transmitted within the tissue using a sinusoidal mechanical source. When performing MR elastography, the goal is to acquire tissue stiffness maps for each imaging slice, with a large area of the tissue of interest not covered by the 95% confidence map so that a large portion of the tissue can be measured. The confidence maps are calculated during the stiffness inversion, as the fit of a smooth polynomial to the phase images. In a typical MR elastography configuration, to create a sinusoidal mechanical motion, an active pneumatic wave driver, which is a subwoofer, is located outside the MR scanner room and is connected, by way of a flexible plastic (polyvinyl chloride) tube, to a passive driver that is fastened onto the abdominal wall or the organ or interest. For the most part, three kinds of active driver mechanical driving mechanisms have been used in the literature. They are electromechanical drivers, piezoelectric drivers, and acoustic speaker-based driver systems [20–22]. Electromechanical drivers were one of the initially developed driver systems (Fig. 1). They use the Lorentz force between the induced magnetic moment created by voice coils, and the static magnetic field of the main MRI magnet to create the motion [20]. Piezoelectric and needle-based drivers have commonly been used in preclinical or MRE of tissues [12, 21]. This is primarily because of the advantages of the ease of positioning of the driver in comparison to the electromechanical drivers and the avoidance of an additional magnetic field, leading to a reduction of artifacts [22]. Also, these drivers can create more reliable waveforms with less ringing effects, which becomes especially useful in situations where a single transient wave needs to be induced in the tissue or sample of interest. Acoustic speaker-based driver systems are commercially available and are commonly used for clinical MRE scans. The vibrations in the acoustic systems are again produced by the Lorentz force, but the static magnetic field is from a devoted permanent magnet present in an acoustic speaker. These speakers, with their own permanent magnets, that are much weaker than the static field B_0 of the MR system, are designed such that they are placed away from the main magnet. Thus, this system necessitates an additional component to couple the vibrations produced by the speakers to the tissue of interest. The active driver is coupled to a passive driver that is positioned on the abdominal organ of interest. The passive driver transfers a continuous acoustic vibration that is transmitted through the entire abdomen, at a fixed low frequency, which is typically 60 Hz for the liver. Choice of frequency is a balance between wave penetration and desired spatial resolution. A higher frequency improves spatial resolution while a low frequency improves wave penetration. The advantage of this system is that the passive drivers can be developed according to the application in different organs and can thus be used to effectively propagate shear waves within the desired organ of interest with comfort to the patient. For preclinical images in small animals such as mice or rats, a frequency of up to 400 Hz may be used to get the desired spatial resolution. A modified phase-contrast based pulse sequence with motion encoding gradient pairs synchronized to oscillate at the same frequency of mechanical waves created by the passive driver are used to encode the motion of the tissues in the phase of an MR image. This sequence is then used to image the micron-level cyclic displacements caused by the propagating shear waves to create a magnitude image, which provides anatomic information, and a phase image, which provides wave motion information. The phase or "wave" images, containing wave-propagation information, are then inverted to calculate quantitative stiffness maps (elastograms).

2.3.2 Pulse Sequence for MRE Motion Encoding: Software

The two main pulse sequence groups in MRI are spin echo (SE) and gradient recalled echo (GRE). In the early 1980s, the SE sequence was the main magnetic resonance sequence in clinical imaging [23]. Later, the GRE sequence proposed by Mansfield and Maudsley became an essential technique and a good alternative to SE sequences [24]. The two types of acquisition sequences currently in use to obtain abdomen organ stiffness values are the GRE based and the SE based with echo-planar readout; both of which have been shown to have excellent correlation on both 1.5 and 3.0 T MRI scanners [13, 25, 26]. The use of GRE-based sequence has demonstrated to correlate with histological grading of liver fibrosis in previous studies and a recent meta-analysis [10, 13]. However, the inherent limitations of GRE-based acquisition on field strengths of 3.0 T or higher in addition to enhanced sensitivity to susceptibility, is the signal drop off due to longer echo time (TE) and relatively shorter T2 relaxation time of the liver. GRE-based MRE also has relatively lower accuracy in obese patients due to the increased distance from the driver to the liver. Thicker layers of fat can result in signal loss and produce limitations for encoding shear waves in the deeper areas of the liver, hence reducing the resulting stiffness measurable area [25]. Since chronic liver disease is quite frequently associated with obesity, radiologists should be aware of the limitations of GRE-based acquisition in such cases. GRE-based MRE acquisition also require relatively longer periods of acquisition and have higher susceptibility to breathing motion. Clinically, the current GRE-based protocol, for MRE image acquisition requires a breath-hold of approximately 20 s for a single slice. Echo-planar imaging (EPI), on the other hand, is a fast magnetic resonance imaging technique that obtains all spatial-encoding information in a single radiofrequency (RF) pulse, allowing for faster acquisition times with less motion artifacts. SE-EPI MRE has several advantages over the GRE MRE sequence: (1) It allows for acquisition of multiple slices in a single breath-hold covering entire kidney as compared to GRE MRE, which allowed for acquisition of only a single slice per breath-hold; (2) Entire 3D acquisition with three motion encoding directions can be performed in three breath-holds, which enables completion of the study in patients who cannot perform more than three breath-holds and cannot lay flat for longer period of time in the scanner; (3) SE-EPI MRE can avoid problems such as data misregistration caused due to multiple breath-holds when acquiring multiple slices compared to GRE MRE. SE-EPI-based images are also advantageous because it enables measuring larger areas of the organ due to higher waves encoded per relaxation time (TR). Despite these advantages, use of SE-EPI MRE sequence has a few limitations such as it is prone to the distortion artifacts arising from the eddy currents caused by gradients switching on and off rapidly. These distortions may cause increase in the apparent wavelength of the waves propagating through the kidneys thereby causing an increase in the stiffness estimations. Care must be taken to correct for the distortions when observed. Additionally, SE-EPI MRE is also very sensitive to chemical shift and ghosting artifacts. Appropriate steps need to be taken during acquisition by application of spatial spectral frequency pulses and phase correction to correct for these artifacts, respectively for accurate estimate of MRE-derived stiffness values.

The tissue response to the applied harmonic excitation is represented in terms of waves propagating within the tissue. After the mechanical excitation, the phase-contrast based pulse sequence is used to encode the shear wave motion into the MR phase signal by using a series of magnetic field gradients called MEG. The MEG is typically applied after RF excitation pulses and before signal

2.4 Image Postprocessing: Generating Elastograms for Stiffness Estimation

acquisition. From the acquired wave images, inverse reconstruction algorithms are applied to convert the displacement data to mechanical properties [27]. The mechanical quantity that MRE characterizes typically is shear modulus (μ), which describes the proportionality relationship between the shear stress and strain. In MRE excitation is primarily shear and the displacements in MRE are very small (~microns). Therefore, it is a good approximation to model tissue as a linear, viscoelastic solid. It can be assumed that there is no volume change as layers of material move in shear, perpendicular to the direction of the wave propagation. The shear stiffness, μ, can be calculated if the wavelength, λ, is measured, as the frequency is known and the density of most soft tissues is close to the density of water (1000 kg/m^3). Assuming an isotropic material, this reduces to two independent quantities, the Lame constants λ and μ related to longitudinal and shear deformation respectively. If local homogeneity is assumed, λ and μ become single unknowns, and the equation for harmonic motion becomes an algebraic matrix equation that can be solved locally: $\mu\nabla 2u + (\lambda + \mu)\nabla(\nabla \cdot u) = -\rho\omega 2u$ [28], with ρ the density, ω the angular frequency of the mechanical oscillation, and u the displacement vector. Approaches such as local frequency estimation (LFE), phase gradient (PG), and direct inversion (DI) have been used to estimate the localized wavelength [28, 29]. The algorithms assume that the waves are propagating in a uniform, infinite, homogeneous medium. The LFE algorithm can estimate the spatial frequency of the propagating shear waves. LFE is a robust method for estimating isotropic tissue stiffness even in the presence of noise when compared to other methods, as it is performed in the k-space domain. However, it suffers from edge effects where the estimates values at the sharp boundaries can be inaccurate. Hence, if LFE is used, the ROIs on the elastograms must be drawn away from the edges. DI is another inversion algorithm where lower order polynomials are fit to the displacement field data to obtain its Laplacian; and solving the Helmholtz wave equation by plugging the Laplacian generates the stiffness map. However, DI is also sensitive to noise because of the Laplacian operator.

2.5 Periodic Quality Assurance (QA)

Recommended QA: Measurements of organ stiffness (magnitude of the complex shear modulus) obtained with MRE depend on the spatial fidelity of the acquired phase images. Therefore, the validity of the field of view and image linearity should be assessed and confirmed on an ongoing basis, as is already routine for all clinical scanners, using manufacturer-recommended procedures.

While other instrumental causes of drift in stiffness measurements have not been documented in the literature, technical failures such as faulty synchronization of the driver system or incorrect driver frequency settings can cause incorrect measurement.

Performing and documenting a routine QA process also helps in preparation of local institutional research guidelines.

Optional QA: Correct user setup and proper functioning of the MRE system can be confirmed using a phantom with known stiffness properties. These usually consist of a uniform, tissue-simulating material with known stiffness and known stability over time and storage conditions. An MRE phantom can be used to confirm proper functioning of the MRE system after initial installation and as a periodic test of correct functioning. There is as yet no consensus on recommendations for the frequency of phantom testing. Optional QA testing with a phantom should employ a protocol recommended by the phantom manufacturer.

3 Methods

3.1 Animal Setup on the Scanner

1. As described in Subheading 2, in a typical preclinical MRE study, animals are anesthetized by intraperitoneal injections of ketamine hydrochloride (50 mg/kg) and xylazine hydrochloride (5 mg/kg).
2. After shaving and preparation of the abdomen, animals are placed and fixed on a plastic table in the supine position. It is important to position the animal as close to the isocenter as possible to avoid any B_0 or B_1 inhomogeneity artifacts.
3. Start the temperature monitoring system, apply some surgical lubricant to the temperature probe and place it in the rectum of the animal.
4. Attach the respiration sensor to the upper abdomen of the animal using adhesive tape. Start and setup the respiratory monitoring system. If necessary, adjust the position of the respiration sensor until the amplitude of the respiration trace is sufficiently large for the system to reliably detect the trigger points at the beginning of expiration.
5. A silver needle (disposable silver acupuncture needles, Asahi Medical Instrument Co., Kawaguchi, Saitama, Japan) can be used in lieu of a passive driver and gently inserted gently into the target tissue through the anterior body wall (Figs. 2 and 3). The other end of the needle is attached to an electromechanical driver that generated longitudinally orientated sinusoidal vibrations at low frequency.

3.2 Scanner Adjustments and Anatomical Imaging

1. MR image acquisitions may be performed with a standard 1.5 T or a 3.0 T whole body MRI scanner using a receiving surface coil.
2. Acquire a fast pilot scan to obtain images in the three orthogonal planes x, y, and z.

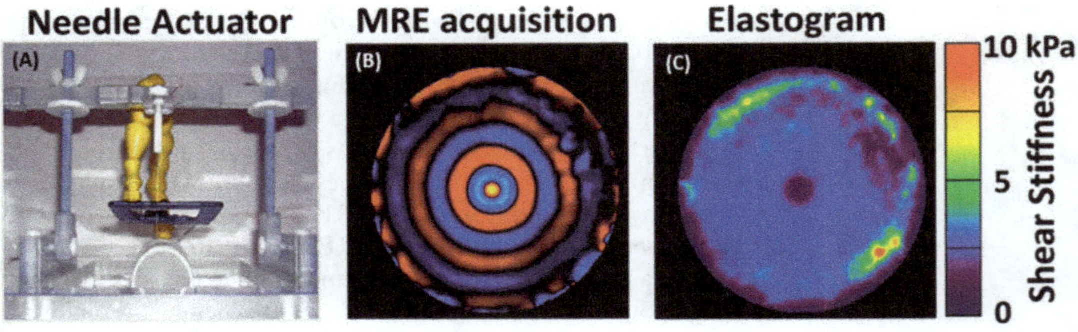

Fig. 2 (**a**) Drawing illustrates a typical experimental setup of a mouse or rat MR elastography configuration. A passive driver, a needle, is used to generate circular shear wave fields. A plastic connecting tube connects the passive driver to the active driver, which is located behind a wall outside the imaging room. This setup is relatively easy to apply for preclinical imaging. The active driver used may be a standard commercially available equipment. (**b**) Images acquired during a MRE phantom scan. Magnitude and phase images yield raw data: The magnitude images provide anatomic information, and the phase images provide wave motion information. After postprocessing, color wave images and (**c**) stiffness maps, also known as elastograms, are generated

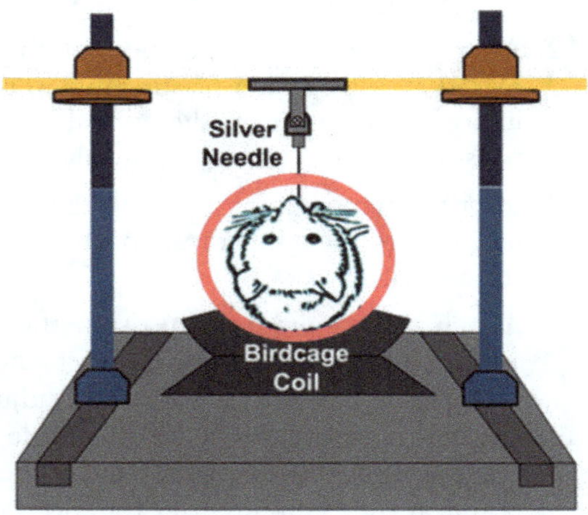

Fig. 3 A typical experimental setup for a mouse MRE study. A silver needle is used to generate circular shear wave field in the mouse liver in vivo

3. Acquire anatomical images in several oblique orientations to facilitate planning a coronal slice orientation with regards to the long axis of the kidney, as described in the chapter by Pohlmann A et al. "Essential Practical Steps for MRI of the Kidney in Experimental Research."
4. Perform localized shimming on the kidney as described in the chapter by Pohlmann A et al. "Essential Practical Steps for MRI of the Kidney in Experimental Research" (*see* **Note 16**).

Table 1
Recommended 2D MRE protocol parameters

Parameter	2D GRE MRE	2D SE-EPI MRE
TR (ms)	50	1000
TE (ms)	23.7	30
Matrix size	128 × 64 interpolated to 128 × 128	100 × 100 (true)
Voxel size (mm)	1.2 × 1.2	1.5 × 1.5
Slice thickness (mm)	6	6
Bandwidth (Hz/Px)	399	2380
No. of averages	1	1
No. of slices	4	4
MEG frequency (Hz)	60	60
MEG direction	*Z* axis (slice)	*Z* axis (slice)
Echo spacing (ms)	24.7	0.5
EPI factor	NA	100
Acceleration factor	2	2
Scan time (min: s)	1:00	0:11

3.3 MRE Imaging

1. A gradient echo (GRE) MRE sequence may be used for wave image acquisition with the following parameters: matrix size of 256 × 64, TR/TE of 33.3 ms/17.8 ms, flip angle of 30°, slice thickness of 5 mm, field of view of 10 cm × 10 cm, one pair of 1.76 G/cm trapezoidal motion-encoding gradients (MEG) at 120 Hz (8.33 ms duration). The repetition time is typically set as an integer multiple of the mechanical wave period to allow for continuous shear wave motion during the scan via the customary synchronized trigger pulses. Details of protocol parameters for relevant acquisition sequence choices are provided in Tables 1, 2 and 3.
2. It should be noted that the trigger pulses are moved during the scan to obtain images at four different phase offsets between the motion and the MEG, equally spaced over one cycle of the motion.
3. Perpendicular to the driving needle, several sequential imaging planes containing tissue of interest should be chosen for MRE wave data collection. The number of slices to be acquired depends on the size of the organ of interest, but is typically 2–4.
4. The MEG should be set to sensitize the shear motion along the through-plane direction (i.e., the anterior–posterior or slice-select direction for these coronal images). Typically, respiratory

Table 2
Recommended imaging protocol for propagating shear waves in the abdomen (small animal 3D MRE protocol parameters)

Parameter	3D MRE
Pulse sequence type	2D SE-EPI
Matrix	128 × 128
No. of averages	1–16
No. of EPI shots	1
TR (ms)	1000
TE (ms)	Minimum
No. of slices	12–20
Slice thickness (mm)	1
Gap (mm)	0, Interleave
No. of phases	3–4
MEG frequency (Hz)	200–400
MEG direction	*X*, *Y*, and *Z* axes
MEG Power per axis	25 G/cm
Field of view (cm)	3–4

If available on the scanner, it is strongly recommended to use 3D MRE protocol parameters
GRE gradient recalled echo, *SE-EPI* spin-echo echo-planar imaging, *2D* two dimensional, *MRE* magnetic resonance elastography, *MEG* motion encoding gradients, *msec* milliseconds, *mm* millimeters, *Hz* hertz, *mT/m* milliTesla/meter, *Px* pixel, *min* minutes, *s* seconds, *NA* not applicable

or cardiac gating is not needed for lower abdomen organs such as liver and kidneys but this may be added if significant motion is observed. With a fixed needle inserted into the liver tissue, anaesthetized animals only performed shallow and fast upper-chest breathing instead of deep and slow diaphragm breathing. Therefore, the tissue do not move much during respiration. In addition, the phase-encoding direction is chosen to be right-left (frequency-encoding direction superior-inferior), which prevents possible motion artifacts from the chest wall and the heart from corrupting the tissue signal. In preclinical setting, motion artifacts can also be minimized by using multiple averages. As a reference for mice MRE imaging, preclinical MRE studies on ten ARPKD mice, with ages ranging from 3 to 12 months were used in the study by Yin et al. [3].

An accurate and reproducible stiffness measurement of the kidney, given its small size, and deeply seated location, requires

Table 3
Recommended 3D MRE imaging protocol parameters for clinical renal imaging

Parameter	3D MRE
Pulse sequence type	2D SE-EPI
Matrix	96 × 96
No. of averages	1
No. of EPI shots	1
TR (ms)	2400
TE (ms)	Minimum
No. of slices	42
Slice thickness (mm)	3.6
Gap (mm)	0, Interleave
No. of phases	3
MEG frequency (Hz)	120
Wave frequency (Hz)	60/90
MEG direction	*X*, *Y*, and *Z* axes
No. of breath-holds	6
Acceleration factor	3
Driver amplitude range	30–50%

3D analysis of wave field data. For this reason, if available on the scanner, 3D MRE is recommended to be utilized for renal imaging. In 3D MRE, the propagating shear waves are imaged with a 2D multislice spin-echo echo-planar imaging (SE-EPI) pulse sequence modified to include the motion encoding gradients (MEG) in the *X*, *Y*, and *Z* directions. MEGs can be applied in one or more directions to encode the motion in those specific directions. This is different from the 2D MRE typically utilized for commercial MRE imaging in which motion is encoded only in a single direction.

A typical small animal preclinical 3D MRE protocol is shown in Table 2.

Figures 4, 5, and 6 show cross sectional spin echo anatomical images of the animal abdomen, more specifically of the mouse liver region and its respective wave displacement images along the *x*, *y*, and *z* directions and the absolute values of the complex shear modulus.

In 3D MRE, the propagating shear waves are imaged with a 2D multislice spin-echo echo-planar imaging (SE-EPI) pulse sequence

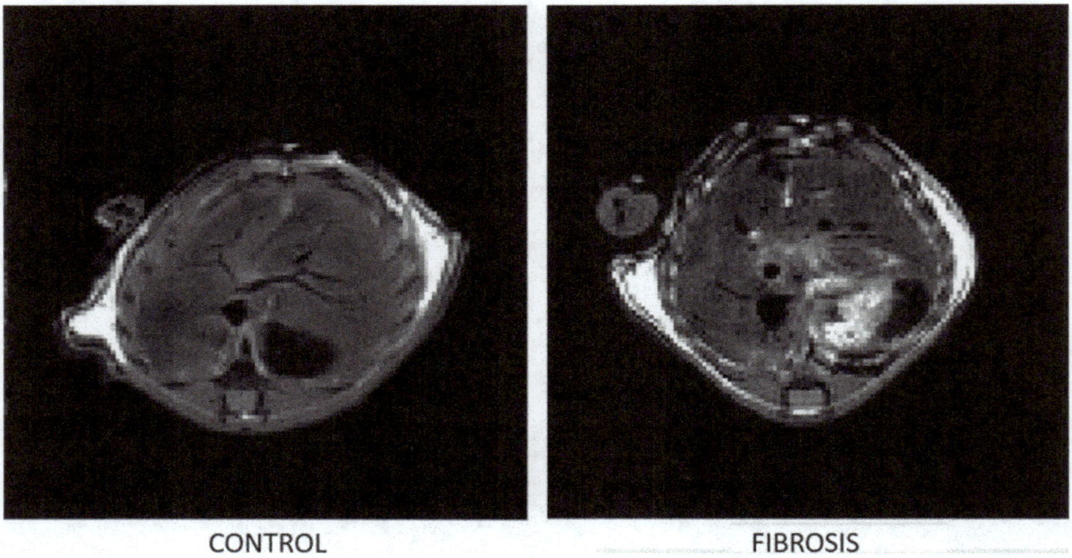

Fig. 4 Cross-sectional spin-echo anatomical images of the mouse abdomen, more specifically of the liver region (Image courtesy of Dr. S. Majumdar and Dr. D. Klatt from the Motion-encoding MRI Lab at the University of Illinois at Chicago, Chicago, Illinois, USA)

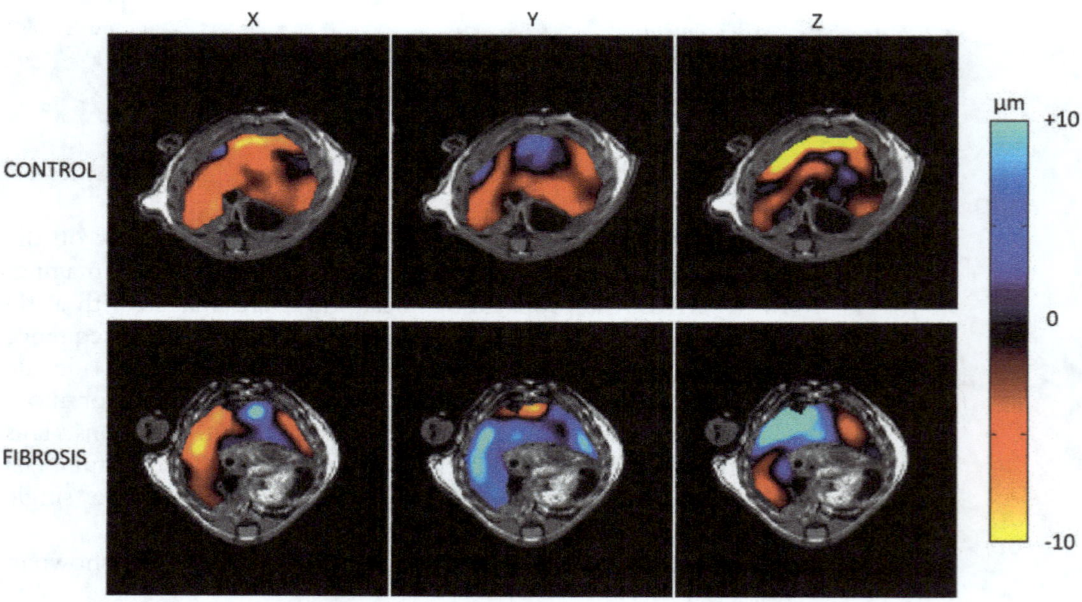

Fig. 5 Wave-displacement images along the *x*, *y*, and *z* directions (Image courtesy of Dr. S. Majumdar and Dr. D. Klatt from the Motion-encoding MRI Lab at the University of Illinois at Chicago, Chicago, Illinois, USA)

modified to include the motion encoding gradients (MEG) in the *X*, *Y*, and *Z* directions. Since kidney is a viscoelastic material, the stiffness varies with excitation frequency (i.e., stiffness increases with an increase in frequency). Once decided, it is important to keep the MEG frequency consistent for the duration of the study.

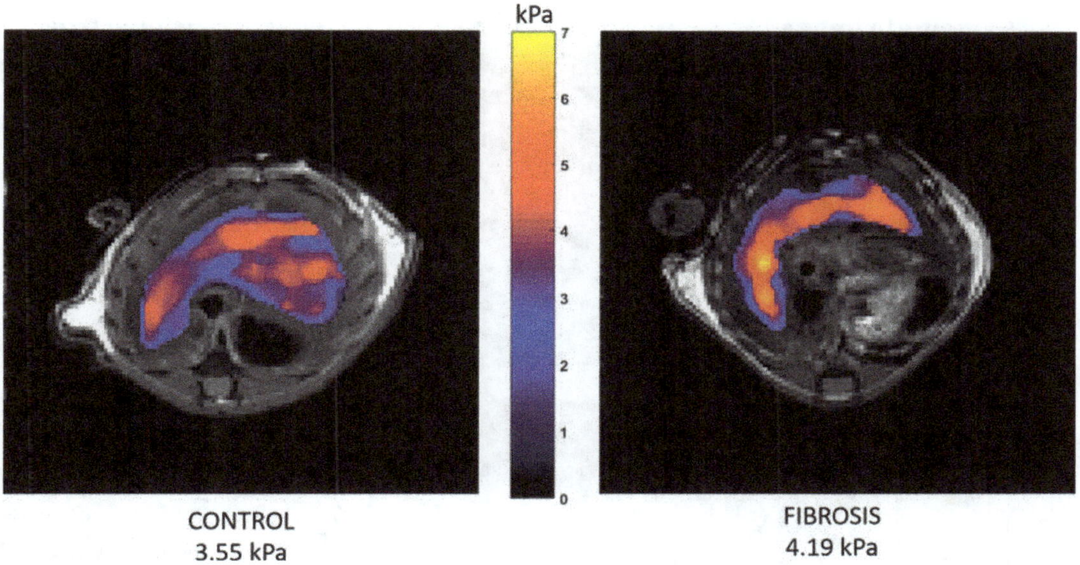

Fig. 6 |G*| or the absolute value of the complex shear modulus (Image courtesy of Dr. S. Majumdar and Dr. D. Klatt from the Motion-encoding MRI Lab at the University of Illinois at Chicago, Chicago, Illinois, USA)

At a frequency of 60 Hz, the average kidney stiffness range of 3.5–5 kPa has been reported on normals in the literature by multiple groups [30, 31]. At a frequency of 90 Hz, a higher kidney stiffness range of 5–7.5 kPa was measured.

3.4 Image Review to Ensure Technical Success

The raw magnitude and phase images obtained from the MRE acquisition should be reviewed on the scanner console at the time of the exam. The magnitude images should show signal loss in the subcutaneous fat just below the passive driver placement, confirming that mechanical waves are being applied. The signal loss is due to the phase images (also known as wave images) should demonstrate shear waves in the specific abdominal organ of interest. In the color phase images, red to blue region is a wavelength and this wavelength becomes longer in the presence of a stiff region for a given excitation frequency. Then these wave images are converted into spatial stiffness maps using an inversion algorithm known as elastograms. If no waves are seen in the tissue of interest, then the driver system should be checked. A phantom scan of known stiffness may be performed if needed to validate driver system. Shear wave images represent an instantaneous snapshot of the mechanical waves propagating through the tissue. After the magnitude and phase images are created, an inversion algorithm is applied to processes these raw data images to create several additional images and maps.

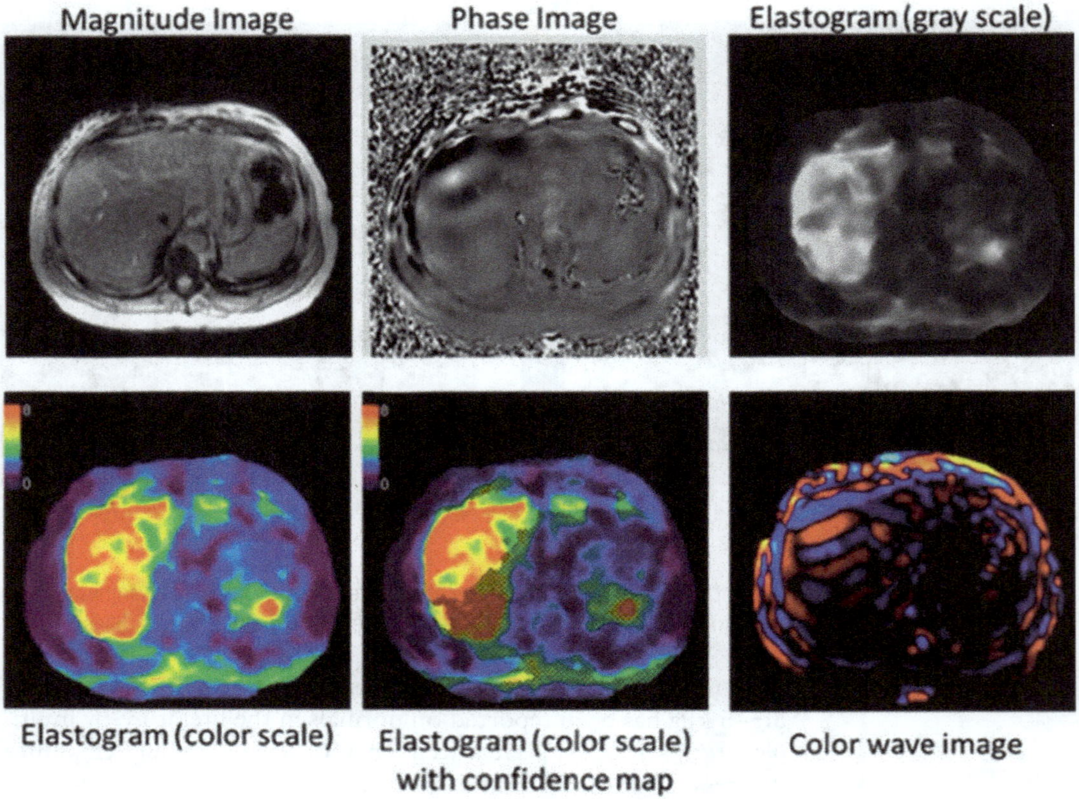

Fig. 7 Representation of typical postprocessed images generated in a clinical liver MRE study. Additional postprocessed images may be generated offline depending on the software version of the pulse sequence installed on the scanner

3.5 Color Display of Images

This section is tailored for images acquired using an FDA approved and commercially available subwoofer-based system for generating shear waves (Resoundant, MN, USA). For images generated using other in-house developed hardware and software, image display should be optimized as recommended by the manufacturer.

For image viewing purposes, the following information should preferably be generated (Fig. 7).

1. Unwrapped wave images clearly depicting the propagation of shear waves through the abdomen. Phase wrapping occurs when the shear wave motion is large. Since MRE is a phase-based technique, the displacement data typically must be unwrapped before subsequent processing is performed.
2. A gray-scale elastogram without a superimposed 95% confidence map.

3. A gray-scale elastogram with a super imposed 95% confidence map. The confidence map displayed is a statistical derivation used to overlay a "checkerboard" on the stiffness map to exclude regions that have less reliable (i.e., noisy and discontinuous) stiffness data so that a high-quality and valid stiffness measurement can be obtained.
4. A color elastogram without a superimposed 95% confidence map. The color elastogram, typically generated in JPEG format is generally used for qualitative stiffness evaluation and visual purposes. However, if the color elastograms are generated in DICOM format, then they can also be used to obtain quantitative measurements.
5. And a color elastogram with a superimposed 95% confidence map.

The gray-scale elastogram, generated and saved in DICOM format is commonly used to obtain quantitative stiffness measurement, in kiloPascals (kPa). The color elastogram used clinically has a stiffness display range of 0–8 kPa. A 0–20 kPa color elastogram display range may also be created and is useful for appreciating tissue stiffness heterogeneity across the larger region. For research purposes, the range may be adjusted as desired.

3.6 Drawing Regions of Interest to Measure Stiffness

Mean shear stiffness of the organ is calculated using manually specified regions of interest (ROIs). Skilled interpretation of the magnitude and wave images is currently required to select a ROI from which the average hepatic stiffness can be calculated from the elastogram. Areas with wave interference and noise, as well as partial volume effects and hepatic blood vessels, can bias the stiffness calculation and need to be avoided when selecting this ROI. The ROIs are drawn manually in the largest possible area of organ parenchyma in which coherent shear waves are visible. To avoid areas of incoherent waves, avoid regions immediately under the paddle and stay ~1 cm inside the organ boundary and contain a minimum of 500 pixels per slice. ROIs should be placed in individual slices. The ROI should also exclude areas of low confidence, as seen by the checkerboard pattern in the masked elastogram images. The procedure needs to be repeated for every slice, with magnitude, phase, and elasticity images all needing to be analyzed. The confidence maps calculated during the stiffness inversion as the fit of a smooth polynomial to the phase images may be helpful in guiding the ROIs across multiple slices. The mean value is calculated from all slices and reported as stiffness in kPa. In practice, the ROIs may be drawn in a single step, keeping these principles in mind. If available, an automated tool capable of deriving ROIs from MRE images and accurately calculating stiffness may be helpful to reduce measurement variability [32, 33].

3.7 Image Interpretation

Overall mean stiffness of organ is reported by recording the mean stiffness value of each ROI and then calculating the mean value, weighted by ROI size.

Example: Slice 1: mean stiffness = 2.42 kPa and ROI size = 2000 mm^2; Slice 2: mean stiffness = 2.55 kPa and ROI size = 1800 mm^2; Slice 3: mean stiffness = 2.92 kPa and ROI size = 800 mm^2; and Slice 4: mean stiffness = 4.22 kPa and ROI size = 1000 mm^2; then the weighted mean = $((2.42 \times 2000) + (2.55 \times 1800) + (2.92 \times 800) + (4.22 \times 1000))/(2000 + 1800 + 800 + 1000) = 2.85$ kPa.

3.8 Role of Preclinical MRE

Since MRE is a relatively new, multistep MR technique, there is room for improvement of efficacy, expansion and exploration. There is evidently a need for preclinical applications of the method, primarily to validate the technique against invasive measures and better understand changes in different diseases. Preclinical work helps to realize some of this potential with the exploration of novel driving and contrast mechanisms to improve the efficiency of MRE and to test and provide clinical capabilities that are otherwise unavailable.

3.9 Application to Renal Disease Models

Acute kidney injury (AKI) is a sudden episode of kidney failure or kidney damage that happens within a few hours or a few days of an insult such as administration of nephrotoxins. AKI is common in patients who are hospitalized, have underlying kidney disease and especially in older adults. Medullary hypoxic injury plays a major role in the pathogenesis of AKI [34], as has been studied by MRE.

A typical hardware setup for pig MRE is shown in Fig. 8. In a study by Warner et al., the authors tested the hypothesis that renal blood flow (RBF) is an important determinant of renal stiffness as measured by MRE [35]. In this study, in six anesthetized pigs with renal artery stenosis, MRE studies were performed to determine cortical and medullary elasticity during acute graded decreases in RBF (by 20%, 40%, 60%, 80%, and 100% of baseline) achieved by a vascular occlusion (Figs. 9 and 10). Three sham-operated swine, that served as control pigs, were anesthetized (telazol 5 mg/kg and xylazine 2 mg/kg) and maintained with mechanical ventilation of 1–2% isoflurane in room air. An ear vein catheter was introduced for saline infusions (5 mL/min). MRE studies were performed on a standard clinical 3.0 T MRI system (GE Healthcare, Waukesha, WI) using a standard multichannel phased array coil. After localization, a renal volume series was performed in the axial plane with a T2 weighted fast spin echo sequence using the following parameters: TR/TE = 2000 ms/88 ms; Flip angle = 90; FOV = 35 cm; imaging matrix = $384 \times 320 \times 40$; thickness = 2.5 mm; NEX = 1. The MRE acquisition sequence used was SE-EPI method. Shear waves were induced by two cylindrical passive pneumatic drivers aligned along the posterior body wall. Continuous vibrations at a

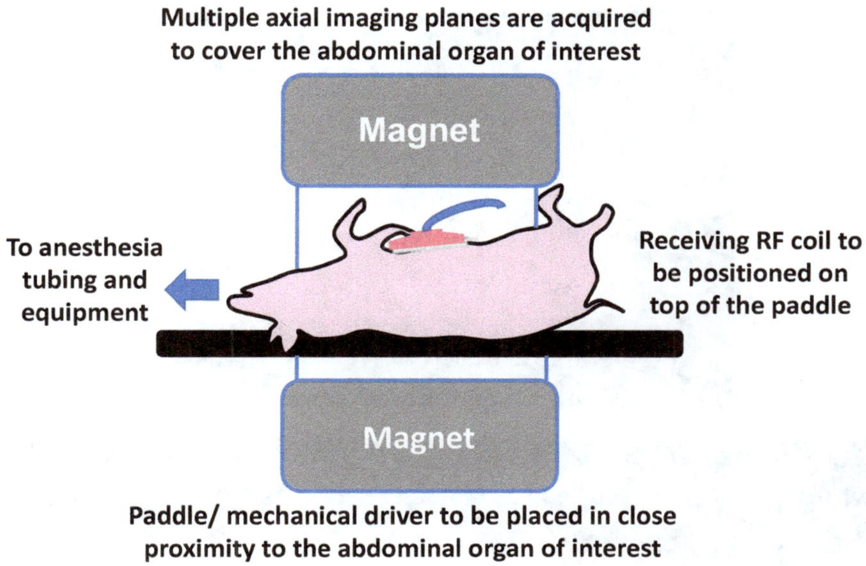

Fig. 8 A typical experimental setup for a pig MRE study

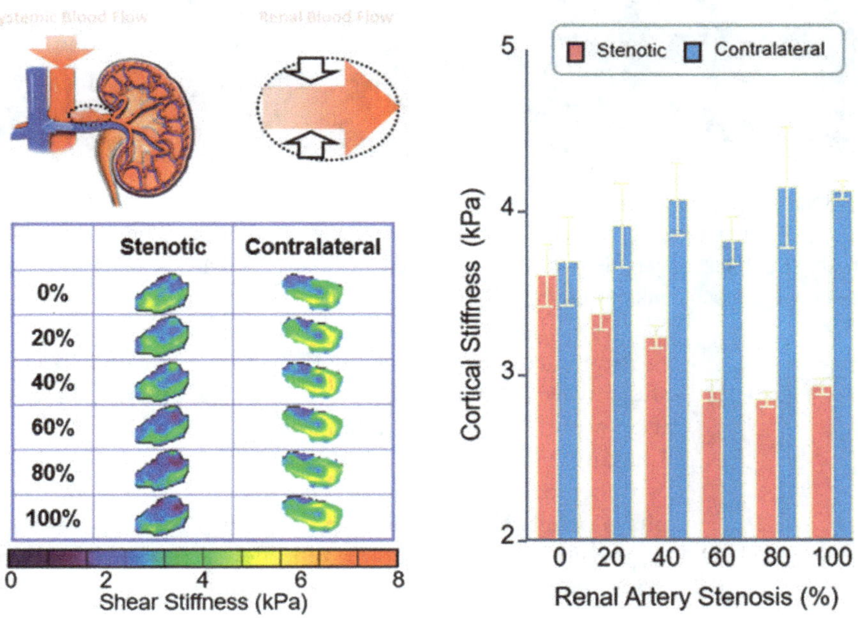

Fig. 9 A representative example from one of the pigs' kidney MRE is shown. The stenosis extent changed gradually from 0% to 100%. Meanwhile, the systemic blood pressure also rose during the acute decrements in renal blood flow from 75 ± 3 to 96 ± 3 mmHg. The kidney's elastograms at six different extents of acute stenosis are shown. The chart summarizes the mean kidney stiffness measurements in stenotic and contralateral sides respectively. From the left elastograms and the right chart, the authors observed that the renal cortex stiffness decreased progressively as the degree of stenosis increased. It is another evidence that less perfusion causes reduced stiffness. Conversely, the contralateral kidney slightly increased in the stiffness during the same period. It is caused by increased systemic blood pressure

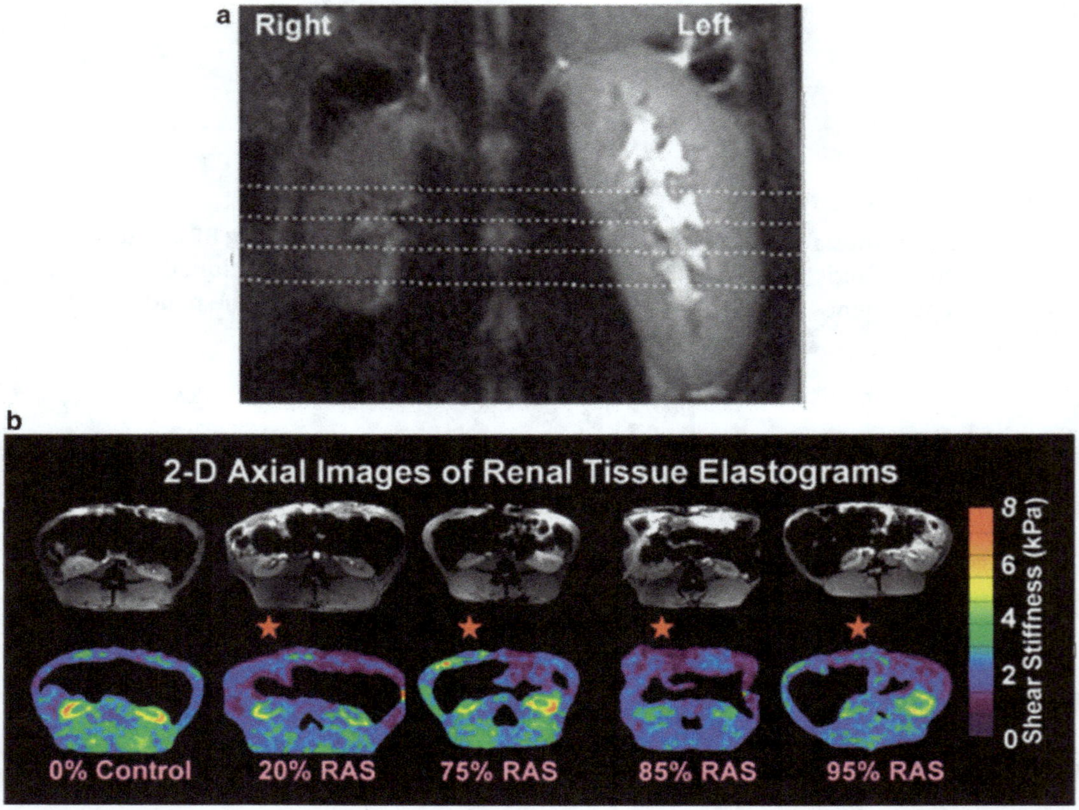

Fig. 10 (**a**) Right (stenotic) and left (contralateral) kidneys in experimental renal artery stenosis. (**b**) 2D axial magnitude and elastograms for normal (control) and variable renal artery stenosis at 10 weeks. The elastogram shear stiffness legend is on the far right. Red stars indicate stenotic kidneys. The images were oriented to show the stenotic kidney on the left

motion encoding gradient (MEG) frequency of 120 Hz generated shear waves throughout the abdominal tissues. MRI parameters used were: TR/TE = 2334 ms/48 ms; FOV = 35 × 35 cm^2; Imaging Matrix = 96 × 96; Slice thickness = 3 mm; NEX = 1; Number of shots = 2; parallel imaging ASSET factor = 2; four phase offsets through one cycle of motion, six pairs of tetrahedral trapezoidal motion encoding gradients in three orthogonal directions with one motion encoding gradient on each side of the refocusing pulse synchronized with motion. The main finding of their study was that acute decreases in renal blood flow with no fibrosis lead to a decrease in renal cortical shear stiffness. Similarly, in chronic renal arterial stenosis the decrease in renal blood flow offsets a likely increase in stiffness secondary to development of renal fibrosis. Decreased renal stiffness may therefore mask the presence of renal fibrosis, but nevertheless stiffness is a marker of renal hypoperfusion.

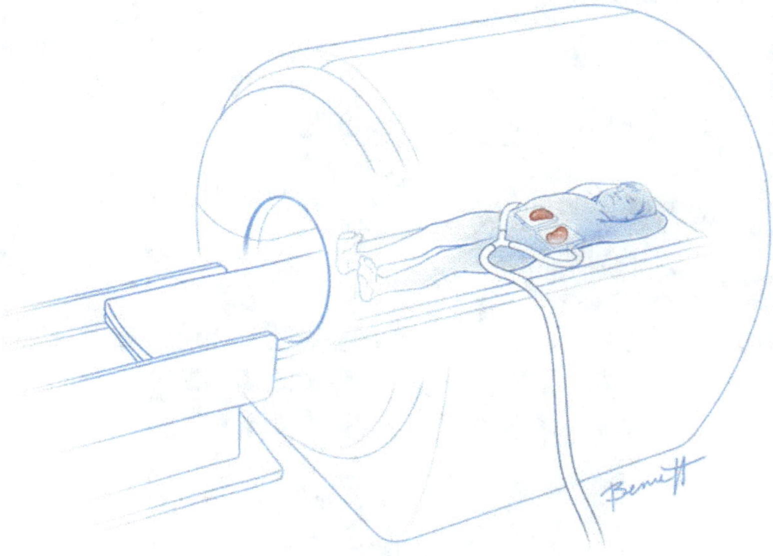

Fig. 11 MRE paddle placement on dorsal side

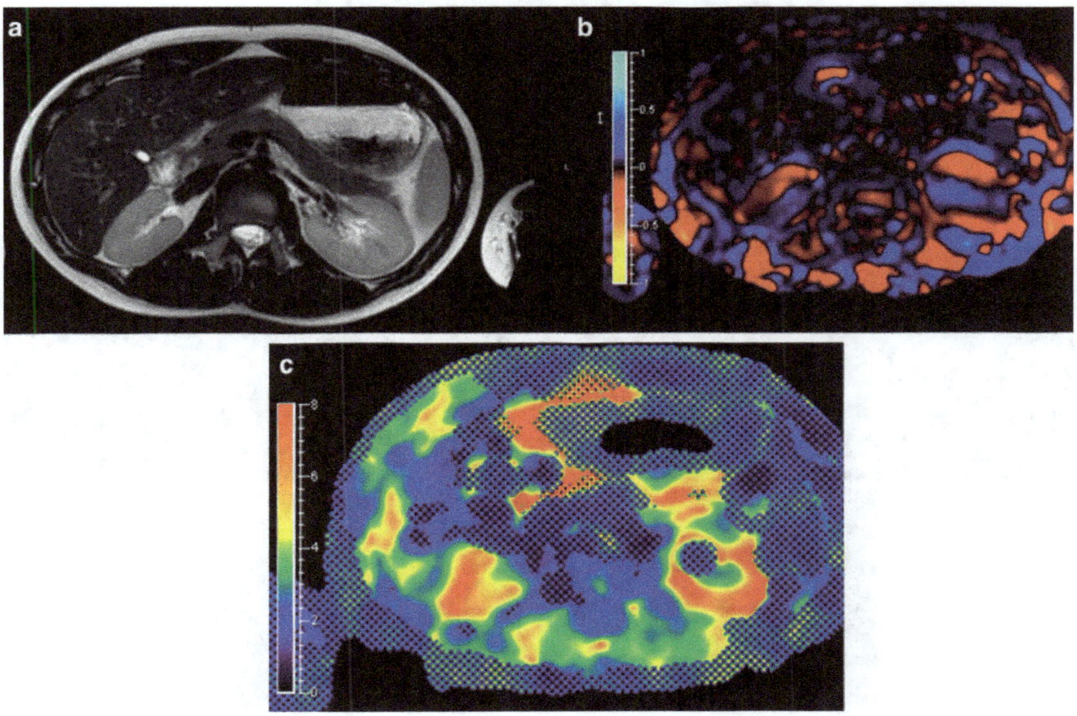

Fig. 12 MRE of the kidneys in a normal 15-year-old male volunteer. (**a**) T2W images in axial plane. (**b**) Wave illumination and (**c**) corresponding stiffness map. Note good illumination of waves in both kidneys (Image courtesy of Dr. Jonathan R. Dillman, Cincinnati, Ohio, USA)

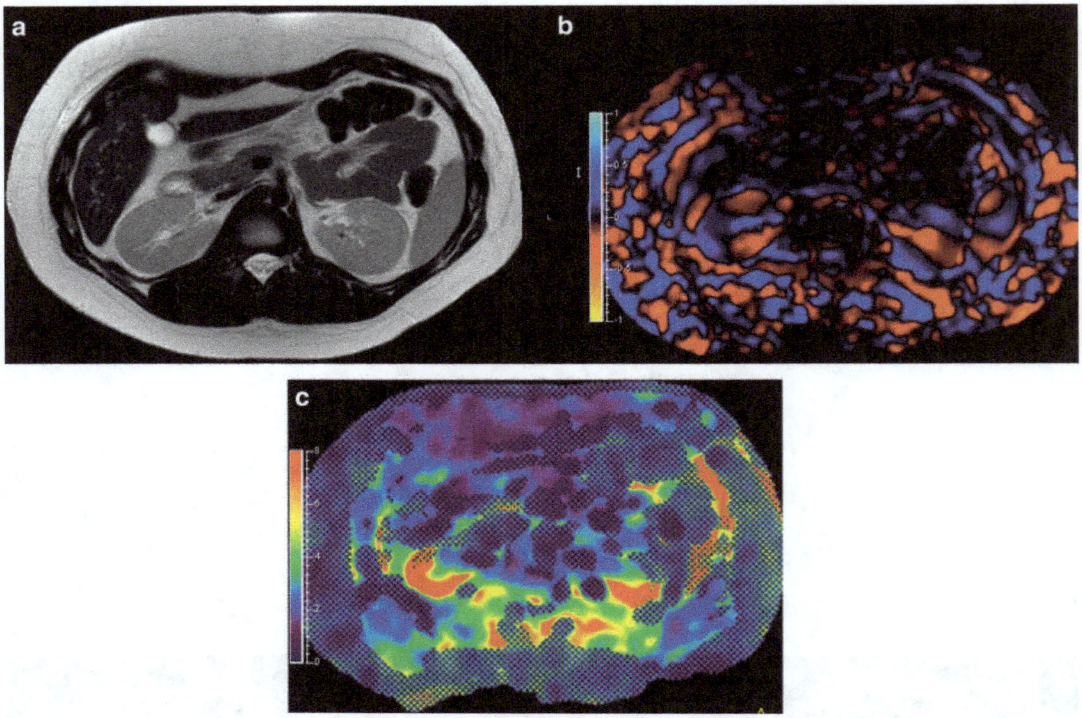

Fig. 13 MRE of the kidneys of a 13-year-old female patient with loss of corticomedullary differentiation; chronic kidney disease. (**a**) T2W images in axial plane. (**b**) Wave illumination and (**c**) corresponding stiffness map (Image courtesy of Dr. Jonathan R. Dillman, Cincinnati, Ohio, USA)

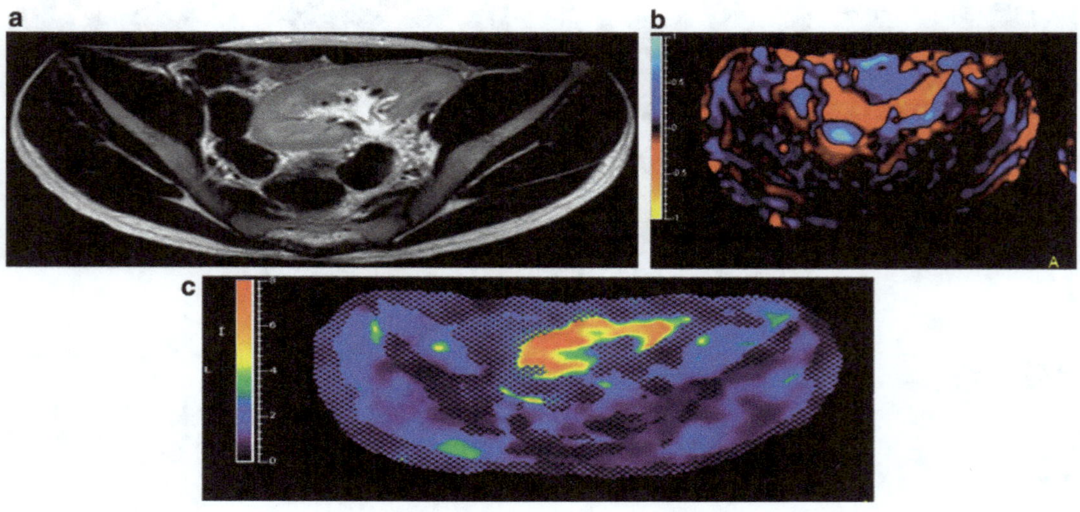

Fig. 14 MRE of the kidneys in a 20-year-old patient with transplant rejection. (**a**) T2W images in axial plane. (**b**) Wave illumination and (**c**) corresponding stiffness map (Image courtesy of Dr. Jonathan R. Dillman, Cincinnati, Ohio, USA)

Renal MRE has also been demonstrated to provide clinical utility in humans. In clinical renal MRE, the paddle is recommended to be placed on the dorsal side with the patient lying in supine position (Fig. 11). Preliminary results show successful transmission of waves by placing the driver in this position (Figs. 12, 13, and 14). In a recent study by Kirpalani et al., the authors examined whether MRE could noninvasively estimate allograft fibrosis and predict progression of allograft dysfunction [36]. In this study, renal MRE was performed on a standard clinical 3.0 T MRI scanner (Skyra, Siemens Healthineers, USA). Patients were positioned head first and supine, and they were imaged with a standard 18-channel torso phased array coil centered over the allograft. The mechanical vibrations required for MRE were supplied by an active pneumatic driver system. MRE acquisitions were performed using a MEG of 60 Hz vibrations and a free-breathing, flow-compensated two-dimensional gradient echo coronal MRE pulse sequence to derive magnitude images and a corresponding stiffness map. The imaging orientation was standardized to the coronal plane, with the frequency encoding direction superior to inferior. Other imaging parameters were as follows: field of view, 32×40 cm^2; acquisition matrix, 128×128 reconstructed to 1.48×1.48 mm^2 in-plane resolution; no parallel imaging; five two-dimensional slices through the allograft, with each slice being 5-mm thick with a 1-mm inter-slice gap; TR/TE = 50 ms/21 ms. Four time points of the motion and three mutually perpendicular directions of the vector motion were sampled. The acquisition time per scan was reported to be approximately 5 min. This study is based on the hypothesis that fibrosis stiffens organs as soft healthy tissue is replaced by stiff extracellular matrix and suggests the potential of renal MRE as a new noninvasive way to assess whole-allograft fibrosis burden; one that may predict future changes in kidney function.

Renal fibrosis causes an increase in the interstitial extracellular matrix and reduction in the number of tubules, thereby making the kidneys stiffer. Previous studies suggest that renal fibrosis is a distinctive feature of progressive kidney diseases such as chronic kidney disease (CKD), a change that increases the risk of cardiovascular diseases. Therefore, renal fibrosis is an important hallmark for diagnosing CKD. Noninvasive MRE is attractive for clinical use in humans.

Existing imaging technologies have been very successful in the noninvasive assessment of many focal diseases of the kidneys, but they have been somewhat less helpful for evaluating diffuse (medical) renal disease such as glomerulonephritis, and renal biopsy remains the diagnostic tool of choice in many situations. It is now feasible to quantitatively image the shear stiffness of both kidneys with an MRE employing a large, posteriorly located passive acoustic driver. Wave images and the corresponding elastograms can be relatively easily acquired in axial, coronal, and sagittal planes.

Preliminary results provide a basis and motivation for investigating the potential to use MRE as a diagnostic tool for characterizing renal parenchyma in diffuse and focal diseases of the kidneys.

References

1. Muthupillai R, Ehman RL (1996) Magnetic resonance elastography. Nat Med 2 (5):601–603
2. Yin M, Talwalkar JA, Glaser KJ, Manduca A, Grimm RC, Rossman PJ, Fidler JL, Ehman RL (2007) Assessment of hepatic fibrosis with magnetic resonance elastography. Clin Gastroenterol Hepatol 5(10):1207–1213.e1202. https://doi.org/10.1016/j.cgh.2007.06.012
3. Yin M, Woollard J, Wang X, Torres VE, Harris PC, Ward CJ, Glaser KJ, Manduca A, Ehman RL (2007) Quantitative assessment of hepatic fibrosis in an animal model with magnetic resonance elastography. Magn Reson Med 58 (2):346–353. https://doi.org/10.1002/mrm.21286
4. Xanthakos SA, Podberesky DJ, Serai SD, Miles L, King EC, Balistreri WF, Kohli R (2014) Use of magnetic resonance elastography to assess hepatic fibrosis in children with chronic liver disease. J Pediatr 164 (1):186–188. https://doi.org/10.1016/j.jpeds.2013.07.050
5. Klinkhammer BM, Goldschmeding R, Floege J, Boor P (2017) Treatment of renal fibrosis—turning challenges into opportunities. Adv Chronic Kidney Dis 24 (2):117–129. https://doi.org/10.1053/j.ackd.2016.11.002
6. El Nahas M (2005) The global challenge of chronic kidney disease. Kidney Int 68 (6):2918–2929. https://doi.org/10.1111/j.1523-1755.2005.00774.x
7. Venkatesh SK, Ehman RL (2014) Magnetic resonance elastography of liver. Magn Reson Imaging Clin N Am 22(3):433–446. https://doi.org/10.1016/j.mric.2014.05.001
8. Serai SD, Towbin AJ, Podberesky DJ (2012) Pediatric liver MR elastography. Dig Dis Sci 57 (10):2713–2719. https://doi.org/10.1007/s10620-012-2196-2
9. Venkatesh SK, Ehman RL (2015) Magnetic resonance elastography of abdomen. Abdom Imaging 40(4):745–759. https://doi.org/10.1007/s00261-014-0315-6
10. Serai SD, Obuchowski NA, Venkatesh SK, Sirlin CB, Miller FH, Ashton E, Cole PE, Ehman RL (2017) Repeatability of MR elastography of liver: a meta-analysis. Radiology 285 (1):92–100. https://doi.org/10.1148/radiol.2017161398
11. Trout AT, Serai S, Mahley AD, Wang H, Zhang Y, Zhang B, Dillman JR (2016) Liver stiffness measurements with MR elastography: agreement and repeatability across imaging systems, field strengths, and pulse sequences. Radiology 281(3):793–804. https://doi.org/10.1148/radiol.2016160209
12. Othman SF, Curtis ET, Plautz SA, Pannier AK, Butler SD, Xu H (2012) MR elastography monitoring of tissue-engineered constructs. NMR Biomed 25(3):452–463. https://doi.org/10.1002/nbm.1663
13. Serai SD, Dillman JR, Trout AT (2017) Spin-echo echo-planar imaging MR elastography versus gradient-echo MR elastography for assessment of liver stiffness in children and young adults suspected of having liver disease. Radiology 282(3):761–770. https://doi.org/10.1148/radiol.2016160589
14. Schuppan D, Ashfaq-Khan M, Yang AT, Kim YO (2018) Liver fibrosis: direct antifibrotic agents and targeted therapies. Matrix Biol 68-69:435–451. https://doi.org/10.1016/j.matbio.2018.04.006
15. Alukal JJ, Thuluvath PJ (2019) Reversal of NASH fibrosis with pharmacotherapy. Hepatol Int 13(5):534–545. https://doi.org/10.1007/s12072-019-09970-3
16. Ismail MH, Pinzani M (2009) Reversal of liver fibrosis. Saudi J Gastroenterol 15(1):72–79. https://doi.org/10.4103/1319-3767.45072
17. Lee SY, Kim SI, Choi ME (2015) Therapeutic targets for treating fibrotic kidney diseases. Transl Res 165(4):512–530. https://doi.org/10.1016/j.trsl.2014.07.010
18. Tampe D, Zeisberg M (2014) Potential approaches to reverse or repair renal fibrosis. Nat Rev Nephrol 10(4):226–237. https://doi.org/10.1038/nrneph.2014.14
19. Bledsoe G, Shen B, Yao Y, Zhang JJ, Chao L, Chao J (2006) Reversal of renal fibrosis, inflammation, and glomerular hypertrophy by kallikrein gene delivery. Hum Gene Ther 17 (5):545–555. https://doi.org/10.1089/hum.2006.17.545
20. Braun J, Braun K, Sack I (2003) Electromagnetic actuator for generating variably oriented shear waves in MR elastography. Magn Reson

Med 50(1):220–222. https://doi.org/10.1002/mrm.10479

21. Chan QC, Li G, Ehman RL, Grimm RC, Li R, Yang ES (2006) Needle shear wave driver for magnetic resonance elastography. Magn Reson Med 55(5):1175–1179. https://doi.org/10.1002/mrm.20856
22. Tse ZT, Chan YJ, Janssen H, Hamed A, Young I, Lamperth M (2011) Piezoelectric actuator design for MR elastography: implementation and vibration issues. Int J Med Robot Comput Assist Surg 7(3):353–360. https://doi.org/10.1002/rcs.405
23. Mansfield P (1977) Multi-planar image formation using NMR spin echoes. J Phys C Solid State Phys 10(3):L55. https://doi.org/10.1088/0022-3719/10/3/004
24. MAUDSLEY PMAA (1977) Planar spin imaging by NMR. J Magn Reson Imaging 27:101–119
25. Calle-Toro JS, Serai SD, Hartung EA, Goldberg DJ, Bolster BD Jr, Darge K, Anupindi SA (2019) Magnetic resonance elastography SE-EPI vs GRE sequences at 3T in a pediatric population with liver disease. Abdom Radiol. https://doi.org/10.1007/s00261-018-1884-6
26. Gandhi D, Kalra P, Raterman B, Mo X, Dong H, Kolipaka A (2019) Magnetic resonance elastography of kidneys: SE-EPI MRE reproducibility and its comparison to GRE MRE. NMR Biomed 32(11):e4141. https://doi.org/10.1002/nbm.4141
27. Doyley MM (2012) Model-based elastography: a survey of approaches to the inverse elasticity problem. Phys Med Biol 57(3): R35–R73. https://doi.org/10.1088/0031-9155/57/3/r35
28. Oliphant TE, Manduca A, Ehman RL, Greenleaf JF (2001) Complex-valued stiffness reconstruction for magnetic resonance elastography by algebraic inversion of the differential equation. Magn Reson Med 45(2):299–310. https://doi.org/10.1002/1522-2594(200102)45:2<299::aid-mrm1039>3.0.co;2-o
29. Manduca A, Oliphant TE, Dresner MA, Mahowald JL, Kruse SA, Amromin E, Felmlee JP, Greenleaf JF, Ehman RL (2001) Magnetic resonance elastography: non-invasive mapping of tissue elasticity. Med Image Anal 5 (4):237–254. https://doi.org/10.1016/s1361-8415(00)00039-6
30. Low G, Owen NE, Joubert I, Patterson AJ, Graves MJ, Glaser KJ, Alexander GJ, Lomas DJ (2015) Reliability of magnetic resonance elastography using multislice two-dimensional spin-echo echo-planar imaging (SE-EPI) and three-dimensional inversion reconstruction for assessing renal stiffness. J Magn Reson Imaging 42(3):844–850. https://doi.org/10.1002/jmri.24826
31. Gandhi D, Kalra P, Raterman B, Mo X, Dong H, Kolipaka A (2019) Magnetic resonance elastography-derived stiffness of the kidneys and its correlation with water perfusion. NMR Biomed 33(4):e4237. https://doi.org/10.1002/nbm.4237
32. Dzyubak B, Venkatesh SK, Glaser K, Yin M, Talwalkar J, Chen J, Manduca A, Ehman RL (2013) Stable automated segmentation of liver MR elastography images for clinical stiffness measurement. Proceedings of SPIE—the international society for optical engineering 8672. https://doi.org/10.1117/12.2006943
33. Dzyubak B, Venkatesh SK, Manduca A, Glaser KJ, Ehman RL (2016) Automated liver elasticity calculation for MR elastography. J Magn Reson Imaging 43(5):1055–1063. https://doi.org/10.1002/jmri.25072
34. Hultstrom M, Becirovic-Agic M, Jonsson S (2018) Comparison of acute kidney injury of different etiology reveals in-common mechanisms of tissue damage. Physiol Genomics 50 (3):127–141. https://doi.org/10.1152/physiolgenomics.00037.2017
35. Warner L, Yin M, Glaser KJ, Woollard JA, Carrascal CA, Korsmo MJ, Crane JA, Ehman RL, Lerman LO (2011) Noninvasive in vivo assessment of renal tissue elasticity during graded renal ischemia using MR elastography. Investig Radiol 46(8):509–514. https://doi.org/10.1097/RLI.0b013e3182183a95
36. Kirpalani A, Hashim E, Leung G, Kim JK, Krizova A, Jothy S, Deeb M, Jiang NN, Glick L, Mnatzakanian G, Yuen DA (2017) Magnetic resonance elastography to assess fibrosis in kidney allografts. Clin J Am Soc Nephrol 12(10):1671–1679. https://doi.org/10.2215/cjn.01830217

11

Quantitative Analysis of Renal Perfusion by Arterial Spin Labeling

Kai-Hsiang Chuang, Frank Kober, and Min-Chi Ku

Abstract

The signal intensity differences measured by an arterial-spin-labelling (ASL) magnetic resonance imaging (MRI) experiment are proportional to the local perfusion, which can be quantified with kinetic modeling. Here we present a step-by-step tutorial for the data post-processing needed to calculate an ASL perfusion map. The process of developing an analysis software is described with the essential program code, which involves nonlinear fitting a tracer kinetic model to the ASL data. Key parameters for the quantification are the arterial transit time (ATT), which is the time the labeled blood takes to flow from the labeling area to the tissue, and the tissue T_1. As ATT varies with vasculature, physiology, anesthesia and pathology, it is recommended to measure it using multiple delay times. The tutorial explains how to analyze ASL data with multiple delay times and a T_1 map for quantification.

This chapter is based upon work from the COST Action PARENCHIMA, a community-driven network funded by the European Cooperation in Science and Technology (COST) program of the European Union, which aims to improve the reproducibility and standardization of renal MRI biomarkers. This analysis protocol chapter is complemented by two separate chapters describing the basic concept and experimental procedure.

Key words Magnetic resonance imaging (MRI), Kidney, Rodent, ASL, Blood flow, Perfusion

1 Introduction

The signal intensity differences measured by an arterial-spin-labelling (ASL) magnetic resonance imaging (MRI) experiment are proportional to the local perfusion, which can be quantified with kinetic modeling. To calculate the perfusion map, an additional T_1 relaxation map should be obtained from inversion recovery data acquired with the same image acquisition method (eg, Spin-Echo EPI or RARE) and geometry setting.

Creation of perfusion maps involves nonlinear fitting of a tracer kinetic model to the ASL data. Depending on the type of ASL sequence—pulsed or (pseudo)continuous—the model is slightly different. Two key parameters in the quantification are the arterial transit time (ATT), which is the time the labeled blood taken to flow from the labeling area to the tissue, and the tissue T_1. As ATT varies with vasculature, physiology, anesthesia, and pathology, it is recommended to measure it using multiple delay times (i.e., multiple TI in pulsed ASL, or multiple postlabeling delays in continuous ASL). In the kidney, the cortex and medulla have different T_1. T_1 could also change depending on the pathological conditions. Therefore acquiring a T_1 map is desirable. This chapter focuses on how to analyze ASL data with multiple delay times and a T_1 map for quantification.

This analysis protocol chapter is complemented by two separate chapters describing the basic concept and experimental procedure, which are part of this book.

This chapter is part of the book Pohlmann A, Niendorf T (eds) (2020) Preclinical MRI of the Kidney—Methods and Protocols. Springer, New York.

2 Materials

2.1 Software Requirements

The method described in this chapter provides a detailed description for a solution in MATLAB, but can be adopted to other platforms:

1. A programming environment capable of applying fitting models, such as Python, Octave, R or MATLAB®.
2. A software to convert the data format from DICOM or vendor proprietary format (eg, Bruker 2dseq) to the NifTi format, such as dcm2nii (for DICOM; https://people.cas.sc.edu/rorden/mricron/dcm2nii.html), or Bru2Nii (for Bruker 2dseq; https://github.com/neurolabusc/Bru2Nii).
3. An image viewing software such as Fiji (www.fiji.sc) or MRIcro (https://www.mccauslandcenter.sc.edu/crnl/mricro).
4. A software for motion correction, such as SPM, FSL, or AFNI.

2.2 Source Data: Format Requirements

2.2.1 Input Requirements

To be able to calculate perfusion maps, ASL data with interleaved control and label images and multiple delay times, and a T_1 mapping acquired with inversion recovery are needed. For more details on the basic concept of ASL please refer to the chapter by Ku M-C et al. "Noninvasive Renal Perfusion Measurement Using Arterial Spin Labeling (ASL) MRI: Basic Concept." The data acquisition is described in a step-by-step manner in the chapter by Chuang K-H et al. "Renal Blood Flow Using Arterial Spin Labeling (ASL) MRI: Experimental Protocol and Principles."

2.2.2 Intensity Scaling of Multiple Delay ASL Data

If the ASL data of multiple delay times was acquired by separate scans (eg, one delay time for one scan) but not all within the same scan, there could be a difference in the intensity scaling among separate scans due to changes in receiver gain and/or internal scaling factor during image reconstruction. Such a difference could lead to artifactual intensity among delay times leading to bias in the model fitting and inaccurate perfusion quantification.

On Bruker MRI systems, the default intensity scaling is set to maximize the dynamic range of the output format. Therefore scans with lower signal would be magnified. The intensity scaling method in the "Reconstruction" class should be changed to "User Scaling" with a scaling factor of 1 for all the scans.

To ensure the same intensity scaling of the ASL data, the receiver gain may be extracted from the header information ("RG" variable in the "acqp" file) and used to rescale the data.

2.2.3 Format Conversion

Convert all data into 4D NifTi format. Consider magnifying the voxel size by 10 in the image header if motion correction tools designed for humans (eg, FSL or SPM) will be used (*see* **Note 1**).

3 Methods

3.1 Quality Control/ Data Exclusion

During the ASL image acquisition, movement of the body or kidney itself can occur. Artifacts may also arise from ASL labeling pulses. In order to construct accurate perfusion maps, it is important to ensure that the scan series don't show severe movement, spikes, banding artifacts, or sudden changes in SNR. Scans with poor quality or large movement should be discarded.

1. Open each dataset by a NifTi image viewer.
2. Adjust the window/level (or reduce the maximum intensity range) to visualize the image better.
3. Scroll through each time frame to visually check whether there are sudden changes in intensity or movement.

3.2 Motion Correction

ASL perfusion imaging, due to its subtraction between label and control images, is very sensitive to movement. Despite respiratory trigger, slight movement between scans could still be present. Motion artifact maybe reduced by rigid-body motion correction tools in many software packages. Since most motion correction algorithms (regardless correlation or square error based cost function) rely on intensity changes for detecting movement, the intensity changes between control and label images and between scans of different delay times (particularly for FAIR ASL) could lead to pseudo motion. Besides, the T_1 mapping data should also be coregistered to the ASL data. Therefore, it is recommended to realign images to the same reference target, (e.g., the M_0 image or an averaged image). Additionally, use "cost functions" that are less dependent on the global intensity difference, such as normalized correlation or mutual information, and avoid using least square error (*see* **Note 2**).

1. Use FSL mcflirt to do motion correction on the ASL data (ASL_DATA_TI1.nii) using the mean image as the reference target, normalized correlation as the cost function, and spline for interpolation:
   mcflirt -in ASL_DATA_TI1.nii -out rASL_DATA_TI1 -cost normcorr -meanvol -spline_final.
2. Do motion correction on another ASL data set (ASL_DATA_TI2.nii). This time using the mean image generated from the first step as the reference target:
   mcflirt -in ASL_DATA_TI2.nii -out rASL_DATA_TI2 -cost normcorr -reffile ASL_DATA_TI1_meanvol.nii -spline_final.
3. Repeat the same procedures until all the ASL data are coregistered.
4. Similarly, do motion correction on T_1 mapping data (T1MAP.nii) also using the mean image generated from the first step as the reference target:
   mcflirt -in T1MAP.nii -out rT1MAP -cost normcorr -reffile ASL_DATA_TI1_meanvol.nii -spline_final.

3.3 Quantification of M_0 and T_1

3.3.1 Model Equations

Both M_0 and T_1 are important parameters needed in ASL kinetic model. Besides, the inversion efficiency will be used for FAIR ASL quantification to correct its "labeling efficiency."

The most common method to obtain these parameters is to fit the model of an inversion recovery experiment to the signal intensity data of each pixel at various TI, M(TI), using the following equation:

$$M(\mathrm{TI}) = \mathrm{abs}\left[M_0\left(1 - 2\alpha e^{-\frac{TI}{T_1}}\right)\right], \tag{1}$$

where M_0 is the fully relaxed magnetization signal which is a scaling factor that includes many parameters such as the proton density together with the coil sensitivity and the signal gain of the system. α is the inversion efficiency of the inversion pulse ($\alpha = 1$ for a perfect inversion), and T_1 is the longitudinal relaxation time.

3.3.2 Starting Values

An important step of the curve fitting process is the choice of suitable starting values for each parameter that will be determined by the fitting algorithm (NB: different starting values may lead to different results!). Here we describe how to derive starting values from the SI of each pixel.

1. Step through all pixels in the images using for loops for the pixel coordinates x and y.
2. Store the SI of that pixel at all TIs in a vector (in Matlab: SI_vector = imgData_forFitting(xPix, yPix,:)).

3. As starting value for the parameter M0 use the largest SI (in Matlab: startVal_M0 = max(SI_vector)).
4. For estimating a starting value for T1, one can exploit the fact that the null point of an inversion recovery, where the SI is 0, is $TI = \ln 2 \times T_1 = 0.693 \times T_1$. Estimate the starting T_1 value by finding the TI whose SI is minimal:
5. Find the index of the smallest value in the vector (in Matlab: [min_Value,min_Index] = min(SI_vector)).
6. Get the respective TI using the index from the last step and divide by ln2 to estimate T_1 (in Matlab: startVal_T1 = TI_forFitting(min_Index)/0.693).

As for a starting value for α, one can assume that is close to 1 (in Matlab: startVal_alpha = 1).

3.3.3 Fitting Algorithm

Least squares algorithms, such as the Levenberg–Marquardt and Trust-region methods, are the most commonly used curve fitting algorithms for T_1-mapping. They work by minimizing a cost function, which describes the deviation of the fitted curve from the data points. With starting values near the optimal solution they quickly converge, but with starting values far away from the solution, the Levenberg–Marquardt algorithm will slow down significantly. Also, there is the risk that it may converge to a local minimum (rather than the global minimum) and hence produce a wrong result.

In contrast, the Trust-region method (a further development of the Levenberg–Marquardt algorithm) will quickly converge, even with suboptimal starting values, and it will always find the global minimum. However, it does require the definition of lower and upper limits for the parameters to be fitted. Hence, for T_1-mapping, where such limits can easily be defined, the Trust-region method is well suited (*see* **Note 3**).

1. Create for loops for pixel coordinates x and y to step through all pixels of the image.
2. Store the SI of that pixel at all TIs in a vector (in Matlab: SI_vector = imgData_forFitting(xPix, yPix,:)).
3. Define the model for the function using Eq. 1 (in Matlab: T1model = fittype('abs(a*(1-2*c*exp.(−x*b)))', 'independent', 'x', 'dependent', 'y')).
4. Initialize the fitting options in Matlab: opts = fitoptions (T1model);
5. Choose the function for the fitting algorithm, that is, Trust-region or, if not available, then Levenberg–Marquardt (in Matlab: opts.Algorithm = 'Trust-Region').
6. Provide the starting values for M_0 and T_1 (in Matlab, e.g., opts. StartPoint = [startVal_M0 startVal_T1 startVal_alpha]).

7. Define lower and upper limits for the fit parameters. Use T1 [1 9000], α [0 1] and for M_0 the possible range of SI in the image data (this depends on the system; for 16-bit integer it may be [1 65536]). In Matlab, for example, opts.Lower = [1 1 0]; opts.Upper = [65536 9000 1].
8. Execute the curve fitting for each pixel data (in Matlab: [fitresult, gof] = fit(TI_forFitting, SI_vector, T1model, opts);).
9. Save the fit result for each variable in parameter maps: mapM0 (xPix, yPix) = fitresult.a; mapT1(xPix, yPix) = fitresult.b; mapAlpha(xPix, yPix) = fitresult.c; rsquare(xPix, yPix) = gof.rsquare.

Besides using Matlab, inversion recovery T_1 curve fitting can be done by using ImageJ. QuickVol II (http://www.quickvol.com/launch2.html) is a powerful ImageJ plugin that supports fitting the inversion recovery data and other user defined equation. The reader should refer to the user's manual on how to use the plugin.

3.3.4 Visual Display

1. Display the parameter map, which is a matrix with floating point numbers, as an image (in Matlab: imagesc(mapT1);).
2. Remove axis labels and ensure that the axes are scaled equally, so that pixels are square and not rectangular (in Matlab: axis off; axis equal;).
3. Select the color map and display a color bar (in Matlab: colormap(jet(256)); colorbar;) (*see* **Note 4**).
4. Set the display range for the color coding, for example, for T_1 [0 2000]; (in Matlab: caxis([0 2000]);).

3.4 Quantification of Perfusion

3.4.1 Model Equation for FAIR-ASL

The pairwise subtracted perfusion-weighted signals at different TIs, ΔM(TI), can be fitted to the following kinetic function [1] (*see* Fig. 1):

$$\Delta M(\mathrm{TI}) = 2M_0\alpha f/\lambda\left[\frac{\exp\left(-\mathrm{TI}/T_{1\mathrm{app}}\right) - \exp\left(-\mathrm{TI}/T_{1\mathrm{a}}\right)}{\left(1/T_{1\mathrm{a}} - 1/T_{1\mathrm{app}}\right)}\right] \quad (2)$$

where $1/T_{1\mathrm{app}} = 1/T_1 + f/\lambda$, f is the quantified perfusion in ml/100 g/min, λ is the blood–tissue partition coefficient. In the above equation, M_0 represents the equilibrium magnetization derived from T_1 mapping, T_1 the tissue longitudinal relaxation time, and α (the inversion efficiency) are all determined from the curve fitting of the inversion recovery T_1 mapping data. λ is a value typically derived from literature which ranges between 0.52 and 0.94 have been reported in [2]. Here, $\lambda = 0.9$ ml/g can be used based on studies in the brain [3]. However, the suitable value for the kidney remains to be determined. $T_{1\mathrm{a}}$ is the longitudinal relaxation time of arterial blood, which is field strength dependent. A

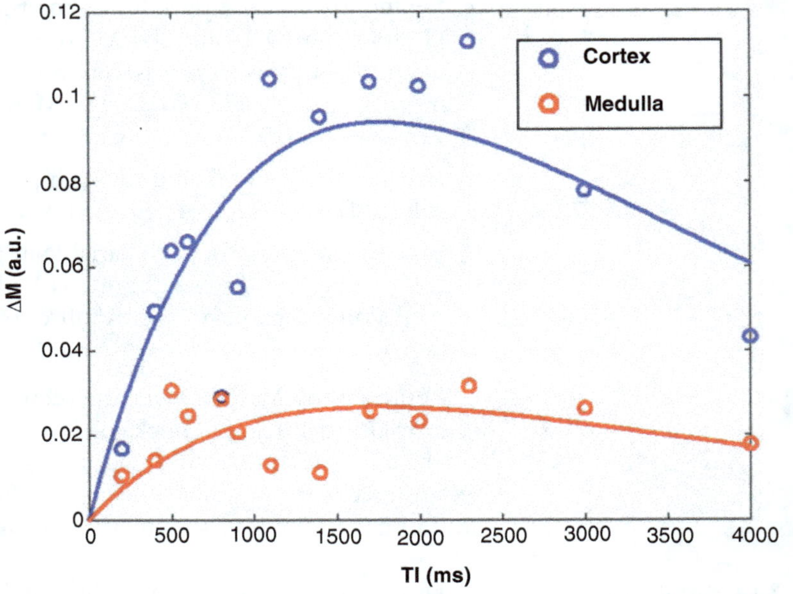

Fig. 1 Fitting perfusion-weighted signal from ROIs in the renal cortex and medulla to the FAIR-ASL kinetic model described in Eq. 2

value of 2.21 s can be used at 7 T [4]. And the blood T_1 at other field strength can be calculated using the equation in [4] (*see* **Note 5**).

3.4.2 Pairwise Subtraction

The first step is to generate the ΔM image of each TI, and then concatenate the results of different TI together to form a 4D time-series data:

1. Use the following FSL command to do pairwise subtraction:

```
asl_file --data = rASL_DATA_TI1 --ntis = 1 --iaf = tc --diff
--out = rASL_DeltaM_TI1 --mean = rASL_DeltaM_TI1_mean
```

   Note that the --iaf option is to specify the order of label–control pair where tc means the label (tag) image is acquired first and then followed by control image. Use --iaf = ct if the data is acquired with the opposite order.

2. Concatenate the mean difference images of all the TIs together:

```
fslmerge -t rASL_DeltaM_mean rASL_DeltaM_TI1_mean rASL_DeltaM_TI2_mean ... rASL_DeltaM_TIn_mean
```

   where *n* is the number of TI.

3. If the data is acquired with varying TIs in one scan, the command could be:

```
asl_file --data = rASL_DATA --ntis = n --iaf = tc --diff --out = rASL_DeltaM --mean = rASL_DeltaM_mean
```

   The resulted rASL_DeltaM_mean image will then be used in the following fitting process.

3.4.3 Starting Values

Deriving the starting value of perfusion from the SI of each pixel is not trivial. Therefore one can just use a literature value (e.g., 300 ml/100 g/min).

1. The starting value for perfusion (startVal_f = 300).

3.4.4 Fitting Algorithm

Similar to T_1 fitting, the Trust-region method can be used.

1. Create for loops for pixel coordinates *x* and *y* to step through all pixels of the image.
2. Store the SI of that pixel at all TIs in a vector (in Matlab: SI_vector = imgData_forFitting(xPix, yPix,:)).
3. Change T_1 value from millisecond to second (in Matlab: mapT1(xPix,yPix) = mapT1(xPix,yPix)/1000).
4. The model for the function using Eq. 2 (in Matlab: FAIRmodel = fittype('mapM0(xPix,yPix) * mapAlpha(xPix,yPix) * a * (exp(−x * (1/mapT1(xPix,yPix) + a)) – exp.(−x/0.221))/(1/0.221 – (1/mapT1(xPix,yPix) + a)) ', 'independent', 'x', 'dependent', 'y')).
5. Initialize the fitting options in Matlab: opts = fitoptions (FAIRmodel);
6. Choose the function for the fitting algorithm, that is, Trust-region or, if not available, then Levenberg–Marquardt (in Matlab: opts.Algorithm = 'Trust-Region').
7. Provide the starting values for perfusion (in Matlab, e.g., opts.StartPoint = [startVal_f]).
8. Define lower and upper limits for the fit parameters. Assuming perfusion will be below 900 ml/100 g/min, use for f [0 900/6000]. In Matlab, for example, opts.Lower = [0]; opts.Upper = [0.15] (*see* **Note 6**).

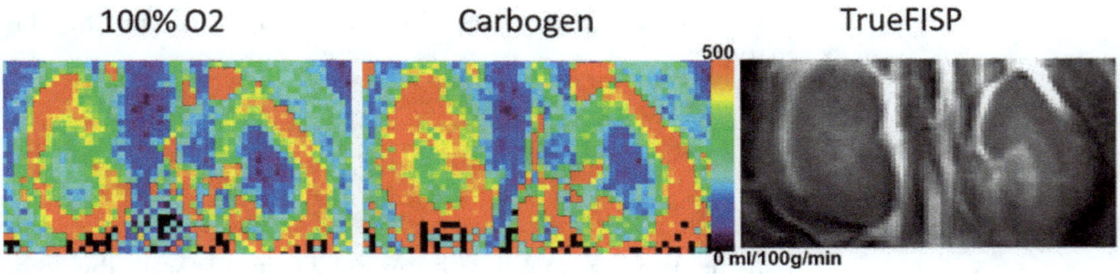

Fig. 2 Quantitative perfusion maps show lower perfusion under hyperoxia than that under carbogen (5% CO_2 + 95% O_2). Anatomical image was acquired with TrueFISP showing contrast between the cortex (dark) and medulla

9. Execute the curve fitting for each pixel data (in Matlab: [fitresult, gof] = fit(TI_forFitting, SI_vector, FAIRmodel, opts);).
10. Save the fit result in parameter maps and rescale by $2/\lambda$ and unit conversion factor: mapF(xPix, yPix) = fitresult.a * 0.9/2 * 6000; rsquare(xPix, yPix) = gof.rsquare (*see* **Note 6**).

3.4.5 Visual Display

1. Display the parameter map, which is a matrix with floating point numbers, as an image (in Matlab: imagesc(mapF);) (*see* Fig. 2).
2. Remove axis labels and ensure that the axes are scaled equally, so that pixels are square and not rectangular (in Matlab: axis off; axis equal;).
3. Select the color map and display a color bar (in Matlab: colormap(jet(256)); colorbar;) (*see* **Note 4**).
4. Set the display range for the color coding, for example, for perfusion [0 500] (in Matlab: caxis([0 500]);).

3.5 Regional Analysis

To obtain quantitative medulla and cortex perfusion, the kidney can be manually or automatically segmented based on the T_1 map or other kinds of structural images.

3.6 Results Validation

3.6.1 Comparison with Tissue Values Under Hypercapnia or Hyperoxia

Further validation of imaging derived results can be performed using datasets acquired under physiological manipulations that alter blood flow, such as hypercapnia or hyperoxia. As CO_2 is a potent vasodilator, the blood flow under hypercapnia condition should be higher than that in normal gas condition. Hyperoxia is expected to lead to the opposite result with O_2 acting like a vasoconstrictor (*see* Fig. 2).

3.6.2 Comparison with Reference Values from the Literature

Obtained values for both cortex and medulla tissue segmentation can be compared against reference values, shown in Table 1. It should be noted that blood flow is also modulated by anesthesia. For example, the commonly used isoflurane is a vasodilator and can increase blood flow depending on dosage. Therefore, the

Table 1
Comparison of renal blood flow measured by ASL-MRI in rodents

Cortex (ml/100 g/min)	Medulla (ml/100 g/min)	Animal strain, anesthesia and gas	Reference
338–452	123–240	C57BL/6 mouse, 1–1.5% isoflurane in 100% O_2	[5]
550–750	140–230	C57BL/6J mouse, 1.5% isoflurane (gas unknown)	[6]
344–575	ND	C57BL/6N mouse, isoflurane (dose and gas unknown)	[7]
288.4 ± 51.3	ND	Spraque-Dawley rat, 1.5% isoflurane (gas unknown)	[8]
750 ± 80	ND	Fisher 344 rat, thiobutabarbitural, 69-135 mg/kg (gas unknown)	[9]

comparison with literature values should be done with comparable anesthesia dosage.

4 Notes

1. Processing is typically performed in software packages such as MATLAB (The MathWorks, MA) or open source platforms as R programming language (http://r.org). The data can either be processed as DICOM images or if available as the raw data format from the scanner. As some motion correction tools (e.g., FSL, SPM) works on NiFti format, the data may need to be converted to that format during the processing. At the end of the processing pipeline, finalizing the data in the DICOM format would allow for further analysis and comparison to other image data on clinical viewers.
2. To correct for respiratory induced motion, resulted ASL images can be coregistered using Elastix (open source software, http://elastix.isi.uu.nl/) and a rigid registration algorithm.
3. An approach that is frequently used to increase the speed of the curve fitting, is to fit a linear model to the log of the SI data. This only requires a few simple modifications to the protocol described here. We recommend using exponential fitting (unless speed is very important), because the log-scaling leads to the noise error at each TI being scaled differently and this will impact on the fitted curve. If you do want to use linear fitting it would be good to initially perform both, exponential and linear fitting, on a few data sets and compare the results so as to better appreciate the impact of this choice.
4. Pseudocolor representations can be extremely useful for analyzing T_1-maps or perfusion maps, since they generally enhance

the perception of differences within the value range of the parameter. But one needs to be careful when choosing a color map. Parameter maps displayed as images in pseudocolor can potentially be misleading. Small differences in the underlying values may be artificially emphasized by a change in color hue, or a significant parameter difference that can easily be seen in a gray-scale image may be flattened or hidden if there is little change of hue or brightness over a certain range of the color-scale. It is recommended to always use the same color map and scale to improve comparability.

5. The transit time is ignored in the above equation as the delivery of spins is almost instantaneous with a small gap between the imaging and inversion slices used in FAIR ASL. Whether the transit time is negligible can be verified by adding the transit time into the kinetic model.
6. To get the correct unit, the T_1, T_{1a} and T_{1app} should be expressed in "second" and the perfusion value, *f*, will need to be multiplied by 6000 to convert to per 100 g/min.

Acknowledgments

This chapter is based upon work from COST Action PARENCH IMA, supported by European Cooperation in Science and Technology (COST). COST (www.cost.eu) is a funding agency for research and innovation networks. COST Actions help connect research initiatives across Europe and enable scientists to enrich their ideas by sharing them with their peers. This boosts their research, career, and innovation.

PARENCHIMA (renalmri.org) is a community-driven Action in the COST program of the European Union, which unites more than 200 experts in renal MRI from 30 countries with the aim to improve the reproducibility and standardization of renal MRI biomarkers.

References

1. Pell GS, Thomas DL, Lythgoe MF, Calamante F, Howseman AM, Gadian DG et al (1999) Implementation of quantitative FAIR perfusion imaging with a short repetition time in time-course studies. Magn Reson Med 41 (4):829–840
2. Kudomi N, Koivuviita N, Liukko KE, Oikonen VJ, Tolvanen T, Iida H et al (2009) Parametric renal blood flow imaging using [15O]H2O and PET. Eur J Nucl Med Mol Imaging 36 (4):683–691
3. Herscovitch P, Raichle ME (1985) What is the correct value for the brain–blood partition coefficient for water? J Cereb Blood Flow Metab 5 (1):65–69
4. Dobre MC, Ugurbil K, Marjanska M (2007) Determination of blood longitudinal relaxation time (T1) at high magnetic field strengths. Magn Reson Imaging 25(5):733–735
5. Rajendran R, Lew SK, Yong CX, Tan J, Wang DJ, Chuang KH (2013) Quantitative mouse renal perfusion using arterial spin labeling. NMR Biomed 26(10):1225–1232

6. Duhamel G, Prevost V, Girard OM, Callot V, Cozzone PJ (2014) High-resolution mouse kidney perfusion imaging by pseudo-continuous arterial spin labeling at 11.75T. Magn Reson Med 71(3):1186–1196
7. Hueper K, Gutberlet M, Rong S, Hartung D, Mengel M, Lu X et al (2014) Acute kidney injury: arterial spin labeling to monitor renal perfusion impairment in mice-comparison with histopathologic results and renal function. Radiology 270(1):117–124
8. Romero CA, Cabral G, Knight RA, Ding G, Peterson EL, Carretero OA (2018) Noninvasive measurement of renal blood flow by magnetic resonance imaging in rats. Am J Physiol Renal Physiol 314(1):F99–F106
9. Wang JJ, Hendrich KS, Jackson EK, Ildstad ST, Williams DS, Ho C (1998) Perfusion quantitation in transplanted rat kidney by MRI with arterial spin labeling. Kidney Int 53(6):1783–1791

12

Data Preparation Protocol for Low Signal-to-Noise Ratio Fluorine-19 MRI

Ludger Starke, Thoralf Niendorf, and Sonia Waiczies

Abstract

Fluorine-19 MRI shows great promise for a wide range of applications including renal imaging, yet the typically low signal-to-noise ratios and sparse signal distribution necessitate a thorough data preparation.

This chapter describes a general data preparation workflow for fluorine MRI experiments. The main processing steps are: (1) estimation of noise level, (2) correction of noise-induced bias and (3) background subtraction. The protocol is supplemented by an example script and toolbox available online.

This chapter is based upon work from the COST Action PARENCHIMA, a community-driven network funded by the European Cooperation in Science and Technology (COST) program of the European Union, which aims to improve the reproducibility and standardization of renal MRI biomarkers. This analysis protocol chapter is complemented by two separate chapters describing the basic concept and experimental procedure.

Key words Magnetic resonance imaging (MRI), Fluorine, Data preparation, Mice, Rats

1 Introduction

Fluorine-19 (^{19}F) MR methods have found their application in a wide range of biomedical research areas including renal imaging [1–8]. The sensitivity constraints, low signal-to-noise ratio (SNR) and sparse signal distribution typical of fluorine-19 MRI necessitate a thorough data preparation. The main processing steps are: (1) estimation of noise level, (2) correction of noise-induced bias and (3) background subtraction. While variations on this theme are common in fluorine MRI studies, a standardized method of data preparation and analysis with well-documented implementation will improve accuracy and reproducibility of reported results.

Estimating the noise level is a prerequisite for all subsequent processing steps. Assuming data from a single channel RF coil, the signal in MR magnitude images follows a Rician distribution [9, 10] (*see* **Note 1** for information on multichannel RF coils). At SNR $>$ 10, this distribution closely resembles a Gaussian distribution. Yet, when analyzing low SNR fluorine MRI data, its diverging properties need to be taken into account. The MRI magnitude signal is computed from complex data, which contain signal with positive and negative values, and is corrupted by zero mean Gaussian noise. Mapping positive and negative signals to the positive magnitude results in a pronounced upward bias at low SNRs. Additionally, the standard deviation of the measured signal is reduced (Fig. 1a). To ensure accurate measurement of signal intensities, the noise-induced bias must be corrected. It is also essential to consider the signal level-dependence of the measured standard deviation for correct noise level estimation.

Background subtraction is the process of classifying image voxels as either signal or noise. Most fluorine MRI studies are dealing with signals that are close to the detection threshold; in this case the background subtraction method strongly influences the sensitivity of the measurement and most importantly the reliability and reproducibility of the obtained results. Ideally, reporting of the used background subtraction method should include the expected false positive rate (FPR).

In this chapter we present a data preparation protocol for low SNR fluorine MRI data (Fig. 2). An open source toolbox is used for bias correction (Fig. 2b) of the magnitude data (Fig. 2a). We expand upon the common method of SNR-based thresholding [2, 4, 11] (Fig. 2c) by proposing an additional outlier removal processing step (Fig. 2d). The shown example is based on a dataset with fluorine nanoparticle labeled immune cells showing the sites of inflammation in a mouse model of multiple sclerosis (*see* Setup 4 in Starke et al. [12] for details). The data preparation protocol is equally applicable to low SNR ^{19}F MRI of the kidney.

A self-contained script reproducing Fig. 2 and illustrating the data preparation step-by-step, from noise level estimation to generation of a proton/fluorine-19 overlay is provided online together with the example data.

This analysis protocol chapter is complemented by separate chapters describing the basic concept and experimental procedure, which are part of this book.

2 Materials

2.1 Software Requirements

The processing steps outlined in this protocol require:

1. A software development environment. The provided code examples follow the syntax of *MATLAB*® (The MathWorks, Natick, Massachusetts, USA; mathworks.com) and *Octave* (gnu.org/software/octave). The code could also be adapted for other scientific software development environments like *Python* (python.org/) or *Julia* (julialang.org/).

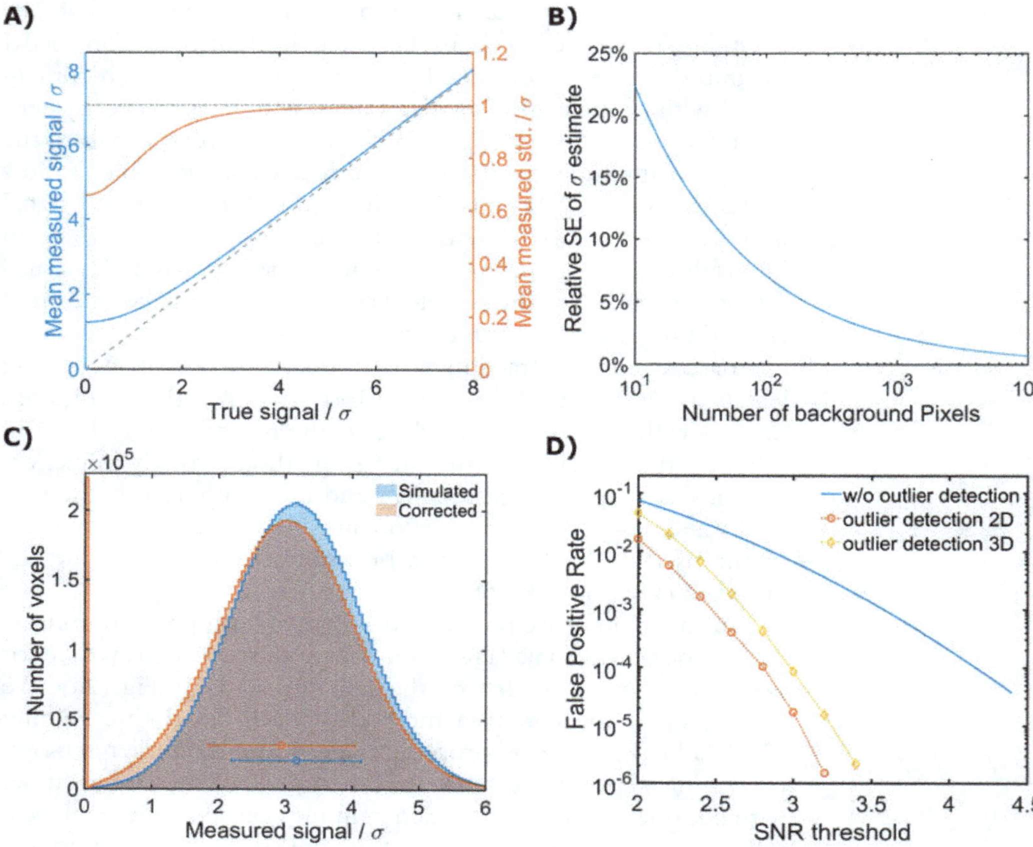

Fig. 1 (**a**) Mean measured signal and mean measured standard deviation (std.) of MR magnitude data. σ denotes the signal level independent standard deviation of the Gaussian noise in the underlying complex data. (**b**) The size of the used background region determines the uncertainty of the standard deviation estimate. The relative standard error (SE) shown here is defined as the standard deviation of the standard deviation estimate divided by σ itself. Note the logarithmic scale of the *x*-axis. (**c**) Histogram of simulated Rician data for true signal $= 3\sigma$ (blue). The corrected data was computed using the tool described in Subheading 3.3 (red). The circles and bars indicate the mean and standard deviations of the two distributions. (**d**) Expected false positive rate (FPR) for different SNR thresholds with and without outlier detection. The FPR is defined as number of false positive voxels divided by number of true negative voxels. Without outlier detection background subtraction is performed by simple thresholding. The expected FPR can be computed by the steps in **Note 5**. Outlier detection is performed by removing all groups of less than three connected signal voxels after SNR based thresholding. In 2D 8-connectivity is used and in 3D 18-connectivity. Here simulated data is shown

2. A MATLAB / Octave tool for noise bias correction downloadable from github.com/LudgerS/MRInoiseBiasCorrection. This tool includes detailed documentation to facilitate adaptation for other software development environments or use with multichannel RF coil data.

3. A collection of data preparation specific MATLAB / Octave subfunctions found under github.com/LudgerS/19fMRIdataPreparation. It is provided together with a script

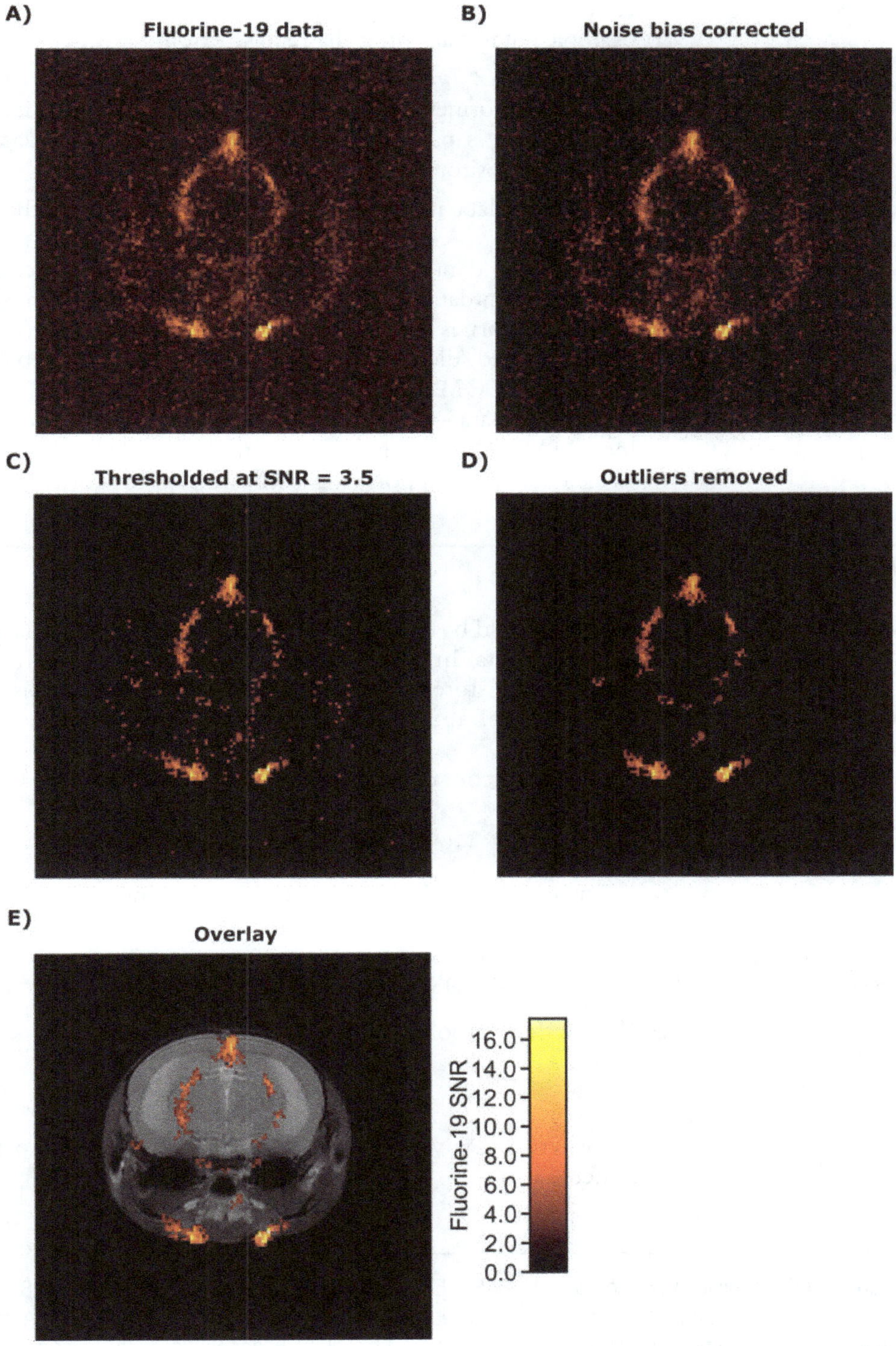

Fig. 2 Example analysis for fluorine-19 MRI data acquired in a mouse model of multiple sclerosis. Immune cells were labeled in situ with fluorine-19 nanoparticles such that fluorine signal shows sites of inflammation.

collecting all processing steps of this protocol as well as an example dataset allowing the reproduction of Fig. 2.

4. The MATLAB *Image Processing* toolbox is needed to run the function fluorineOverlay.m which creates proton/fluorine overlays and is part of the aforementioned 19fMRIdataPreparation repository.
5. A tool for data import. This tool will depend on the data format:

   DICOM data—MATLAB contains a built-in function to import dicom data: dicomread. For Octave, Python and Julia, dicom support is offered by supplemental packages (octave.sourceforge.io/dicom/, pydicom.github.io/, github.com/JuliaIO/DICOM.jl).

   Bruker data—Bruker also offers a toolbox to import data into MATLAB directly. To obtain Bruker's *pvtools*, contact Bruker software support (mri-software-support@bruker.com).

3 Methods

3.1 Data Import and Scaling

These steps should be executed for both the fluorine MRI data and the noise scan data. In the following sections it is assumed that the fluorine data was stored in variable `imageData` and the noise scan in variable `noiseData`.

3.1.1 DICOM Data

1. To import dicom data execute the command

```
data = dicomread('filePath');
```

   where `'filePath'` is a string containing the relative or absolute path of the .dcm file.

3.1.2 Bruker Data

For a Linux or MacOS system, substitute the file separator \ by /.

1. Ensure that pvtools is on the search path:

```
addpath(genpath('...\pvtools'))
```

   where `'...\pvtools'` specifies the path of the pvtools folder.

Fig. 2 (continued) Acquisition parameters: 2D-RARE, ETL $= 32$, $[20 \times 20]$ mm^2 FOV, 128×128 matrix, 3.2 mm slice thickness. The noise level was determined from a corresponding noise scan. Details regarding the animal model and acquisition can be found in Starke et al. [12] under Setup 4. (**a**) Fluorine-19 MRI magnitude data. (**b**) Data after application of the Rician noise bias correction. (**c**) Thresholding was performed at SNR $= 3.5$. (**d**) Removal of groups of <3 connected pixels. (**e**) Overlay of the fluorine data on an anatomical image

2. Store the path to the scan you want to load in variable `scanFolder`.
3. Read the visu_pars parameter file:

```
visuPars = readBrukerParamFile([scanFolder, '\visu_pars']);
```

4. Load the Paravision reconstruction:

```
[data, ~] = readBruker2dseq([scanFolder, '\pdata\1\2dseq'],
visuPars);
```

3.2 Correct Data Scaling

There are vendor-specific conventions regarding the averaging of multiple image acquisitions. In some cases, for example in Bruker data, the individual acquisitions are simply added instead of computing the mean. To ensure comparability between different scan times, determine the employed convention (*see* **Note 2**) and if necessary divide the data by the number of averages. This processing step will be required if a pure noise scan has been employed to determine the noise level.

1. Assuming `nAverages` is the number of averages acquired for the fluorine data and the noise scan was acquired with a single average, simply execute

```
imageData = imageData/nAverages;
```

3.3 Noise Level Estimation

The amount of random variation in MR magnitude images, as measured by the standard deviation, is signal level dependent (Fig. 1a). By convention, the noise level is reported as the asymptotic standard deviation at high SNR, which we denote by σ [13, 14]. This value is equal to the standard deviation of the Gaussian noise in the underlying complex data. While a larger number of noise level estimation methods has been proposed [13], two are of practical relevance for fluorine MRI: estimation based on a background region, which is known to be without signal, or estimation based on a dedicated pure noise scan. Although the former yields adequate results for most applications, we strongly recommend the use of a noise scan due to its independence of user input and improved accuracy. The uncertainty of the standard deviation estimate depends on the number of samples n. For $n > 10$, we can approximate the standard error as $SE_\sigma \approx \frac{\sigma}{\sqrt{2n}}$ (Fig. 1b) [15].

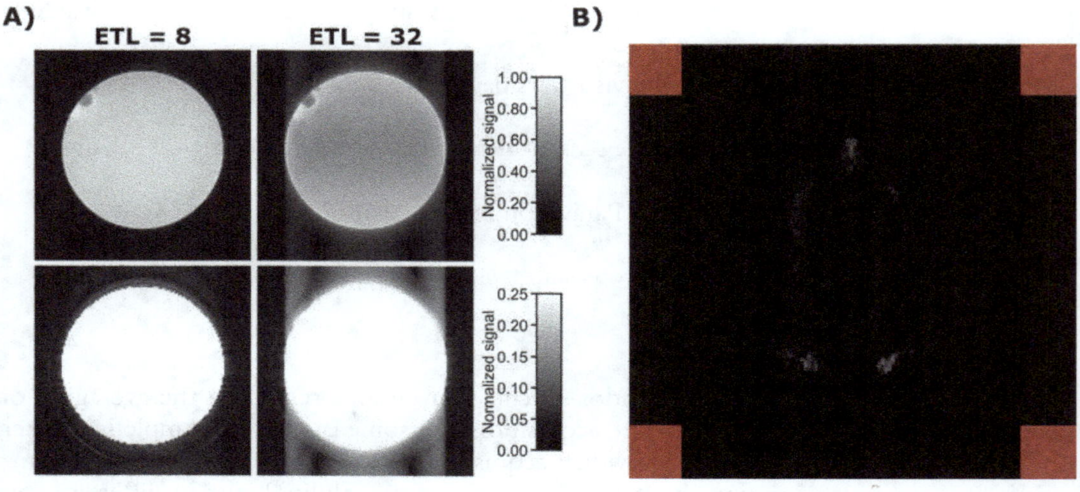

Fig. 3 (**a**) Point spread function artifacts can corrupt background regions without being visually obvious. In this water phantom example, the RARE image with echo train length 8 (ETL = 8, top left) does not show artifacts. However rescaling (bottom left) shows that a noise level estimate based on a background region would lead to erroneous values if the region is not chosen just in the corners of the image. The example on the right (ETL = 32) shows an exaggerated case where the effect is obvious in the image itself. (**b**) The red regions show a background mask that would yield reliable values for the example shown in Fig. 2

3.3.1 Estimation Based on a Background Region

The largest possible background region free of major signal artifacts should be used to improve accuracy (also *see* **Note 3**). However, point spread function artifacts can corrupt image regions even distal from signal features without being necessarily visible (Fig. 3a). We recommend using quadratic regions in all four corners of the image.

1. Create a mask of the background region for logical indexing

```
backgroundMask = createBackgroundMask(size(imageData),
cornerSize);
```

   The argument `size(imageData)` determines the dimensions of the mask and `cornerSize` sets the size of the four corners (Fig. 3b).

2. The noise level can then be computed as

```
sigma = std(imageData(backgroundMask))/0.6551;
```

   where the factor 0.6551 accounts for the ratio between the background standard deviation and σ (Fig. 1a) [13]. It needs to be adjusted for data from multichannel RF coils (*see* **Note 4**).

3.3.2 Estimation Based on a Noise Scan

In this case the complete noise image constitutes the background region. It is not necessary to acquire the noise scan with multiple averages, as the dependence of the noise level on the number of averages is well understood mathematically (*see* **Note 5** for further comments on noise scan acquisition).

1. If the noise scan was acquired with a single average and the number of averages of the image data is given by `nAverages`, the noise level can be computed as

```
sigma = std(noiseData(:))/(0.6551*sqrt(nAverages));
```

3.4 Bias Correction

Rician noise leads to a systematic upward bias in MR magnitude images at low SNR. Signal intensities need to be multiplied with a correction factor <1 to achieve correct signal estimation on average (Fig. 1a, c). While the expected measured signal $E[M]$ for a given true signal level A and noise level σ is known, there is no established inverse function $A(E[M], \sigma)$ [9, 10, 14]. The provided toolbox thus uses a lookup table to compute the correction factor [9]. Signal intensities below the mean background level are set to zero (Fig. 1c). Alternatively, the correction scheme of Koay and Basser could be used [14]. *See* **Note 6** for a comment on averaging over regions of interest (ROIs).

1. After determining the noise level, the corrected image (Fig. 2b) can simply be computed as

```
correctedImage = correctNoiseBias(imageData, sigma, 1);
```

   where the last argument specifies the number of receive elements in the RF coil (*see* **Note 1**).

3.5 Background Subtraction

In fluorine MRI, background subtraction commonly involves thresholding by removing all voxels below a certain SNR (Fig. 2c). However, the threshold necessary to prevent the occurrence of false positives could compromise sensitivity, especially for larger datasets such as those from 3D MR data (Fig. 1d, *see* **Note 7** for an analytical formula). Based on the assumption that all relevant fluorine features should at least comprise a minimum of three connected voxels, we recommend an additional outlier correction that excludes isolated voxels (Fig. 2d). To determine features with a minimum of three connected voxels, we recommend to use 8-connected neighborhoods (connection via edges or corners) for 2D images and 18-connected neighborhoods (connection via faces or edges but not corners) for 3D images. This additional processing step drastically reduces the expected FPR. In the 2D case, for example, thresholding at SNR = 2.74 with outlier detection reduces the FPR to the same level as thresholding at SNR = 4 without outlier detection (Fig. 1d).

1. Copy the bias corrected image to a new variable

```
thresholdedImage = correctedImage;
```

2. Set all voxels below the chosen threshold `snrThreshold` to zero

```
thresholdedImage(thresholdedImage < snrThreshold*sigma) = 0;
```

3. Then apply the provided function for outlier removal on the thresholded image:

```
cleanedImage = removeIsolatedVoxels(thresholdedImage, 3);
```

The second argument specifies the minimum size of preserved features.

3.6 Proton/Fluorine-19 Overlays

In order to locate the source of fluorine signal within an in vivo context, it will need to be coregistered with an anatomical image. While it might be appealing to overlay transparent fluorine images to avoid concealing of anatomical detail, we advise against this practice for quantification purposes, as manipulation of the data will result in ambiguous readings. If no external standard is used to determine fluorine concentrations, it is best practice to show the fluorine signal in terms of the SNR as this also conveys a standard means of information. For the provided function the anatomical image should be acquired with the same field of view as the fluorine MR image.

1. An overlay of fluorine on proton MR images (Fig. 2e) can be achieved simply by calling

```
fluorineOverlay(anatomyData, cleanedImage, colorMap, resizeF, fileName)
```

`anatomyData` is the anatomical image, `colorMap` specifies the fluorine color map in the conventional MATLAB format, `resizeF` is a factor by which the image size is increased to ensure faithful display and `fileName` the file name of the saved image.

2. To complement the fluorine image with a corresponding color bar (Fig. 2e) execute

```
plotFluorineColorBar(colorMap, fileNameCB, max(cleanedImage(:))/sigma, 'Fluorine-19 SNR')
```

`fileNameCB` states the path and file name of the saved color bar image. The third argument specifies the range of the color map. Dividing the maximum of the fluorine image by σ establishes the SNR scaling. The fourth argument determines the label of the color bar.

4 Notes

1. In the case of multichannel RF coil data and sum-of-squares reconstruction, the MR signal follows a noncentral chi distribution instead of a Rician distribution. This case is described thoroughly in Constantinides et al. [16]. The bias correction toolbox used in this protocol also handles the more general case. It should be noted that the bias effects become more pronounced with increasing number of receive elements.
2. To determine the employed convention of averaging, acquire high SNR phantom data with varying numbers of averages while keeping all other parameters fixed. Import the data as described in Subheading 3.1. If all scans show the same signal magnitude, the scaling step described in Subheading 3.1 should be omitted. However, if, for example, doubling the number of averages also doubles the signal amplitude, rescaling should be performed.
3. Be aware that some vendors include heavy filtering and/or background masking into the automated reconstruction pipeline. This has a major impact on the background noise or sets background values to zero and hence renders estimation based on a background region not suitable for noise assessment.
4. Assuming a sum-of-squares reconstruction, the factor 0.6551 should be replaced by 0.6824, 0.6953, 0.7014 or 0.7043 for 2, 4, 8 or 16 receive element RF coil data [16].
5. A pure noise scan is acquired by setting the excitation flip angle and reference power to zero so that no excitation occurs and pure noise is acquired. The receiver gain needs to be set identical to all other scans for which the noise level should be determined. The number of averages can be reduced to one, as the resulting change in noise level is easily compensated. Instead of setting the reference power to zero in preparation of the noise scan, the output of the RF power supply can be disconnected following the system adjustments.
6. In a background region without true signal, the Rice distribution reduces to the Rayleigh distribution [10], which is equivalent to a chi-squared distribution. Thus the expected FPR can be computed via the cumulative distribution function of the chi-squared distribution. First calculate the expected signal [17] for the chosen SNR cutoff snrThreshold

   thresholdExpectation = sigma × sqrt(pi/2) × laguerreL (1/2,0,-snrThreshold.^2./(2 × sigma^2)).

   Then calculate the expected FPR as

   FPR = 1 − gammainc((thresholdExpectation/sigma)^2/2, 1, 'lower').

   This formula is valid for simple thresholding without outlier removal and data from single receive element RF coils.

7. Often fluorine-MRI studies involve calculating signal-to-noise ratios for specific regions of interest (ROIs). Averaging over all pixels in the region should be performed before applying the noise bias correction. This is particularly relevant for phantom studies where the number of voxels in the assumed to be homogeneous ROI is large enough to obtain accurate values even for regions with SNR < 2. *See* **Note 8** for a comment on the uncertainty of SNR estimates.

8. SNR is conventionally reported as the bias corrected signal level divided by the asymptotic standard deviation σ [14]. The uncertainty of the SNR estimate is determined by the signal level, the size of the ROI and the uncertainty of the noise level. A convenient formula for the standard error is $\frac{\mathrm{SE_{SNR}}}{\mathrm{SNR}} \approx \sqrt{\frac{1}{m \cdot \mathrm{SNR}^2} + \frac{1}{2n}}$, where m denotes the number of voxels in the ROI and n the number of voxels in the background region used to estimate the noise level. At high SNRs the uncertainty of the SNR estimate is dominated by the uncertainty of the noise level estimate.

   Derivation: The standard errors of the mean ROI signal $\bar{S}$ and noise level σ are $\mathrm{SE}_{\bar{S}} = \frac{\sigma}{\sqrt{m}}$ and $\mathrm{SE}_\sigma \approx \frac{\sigma}{\sqrt{2n}}$ [15]. Assuming independence of $\bar{S}$ and σ, the variance formula [18] for the standard error of $\frac{\bar{S}}{\sigma}$ yields

$$\mathrm{SE_{SNR}} \approx \sqrt{\left(\frac{1}{\sigma} \cdot \frac{\sigma}{\sqrt{m}}\right)^2 + \left(\frac{\bar{S}}{\sigma^2} \cdot \frac{\sigma}{\sqrt{2n}}\right)^2} = \sqrt{\frac{1}{m} + \frac{\mathrm{SNR}^2}{2n}} .$$

Acknowledgment

This study was funded, in part (Sonia Waiczies, Thoralf Niendorf; DFG WA2804, DFG PO1869), by the Deutsche Forschungsgemeinschaft and, in part (T.N. and S.W.), by the German Research Foundation (Gefoerdert durch die Deutsche Forschungsgemeinschaft (DFG), Projektnummer 394046635, SFB 1365, RENOPROTECTION. Funded by the Deutsche Forschungsgemeinschaft (DFG, German Research Foundation), Project number 394046635, SFB 1365, RENOPROTECTION).

This chapter is based upon work from COST Action PARENCH IMA, supported by European Cooperation in Science and Technology (COST). COST (www.cost.eu) is a funding agency for research and innovation networks. COST Actions help connect research initiatives across Europe and enable scientists to enrich their ideas by sharing them with their peers. This boosts their research, career, and innovation.

PARENCHIMA (renalmri.org) is a community-driven Action in the COST program of the European Union, which unites more than 200 experts in renal MRI from 30 countries with the aim to improve the reproducibility and standardization of renal MRI biomarkers.

References

1. Ruiz-Cabello J, Barnett BP, Bottomley PA, Bulte JW (2011) Fluorine (19F) MRS and MRI in biomedicine. NMR Biomed 24 (2):114–129
2. Ahrens ET, Helfer BM, O'Hanlon CF, Schirda C (2014) Clinical cell therapy imaging using a perfluorocarbon tracer and fluorine-19 MRI. Magn Reson Med 72(6):1696–1701
3. Prinz C, Delgado PR, Eigentler TW, Starke L, Niendorf T, Waiczies S (2019) Toward (19)F magnetic resonance thermometry: spin-lattice and spin-spin-relaxation times and temperature dependence of fluorinated drugs at 9.4 T. Magma 32(1):51–61
4. Waiczies S, Rosenberg JT, Kuehne A et al (2019) Fluorine-19 MRI at 21.1 T: enhanced spin-lattice relaxation of perfluoro-15-crown-5-ether and sensitivity as demonstrated in ex vivo murine neuroinflammation. Magma 32(1):37–49
5. Kuethe DO, Caprihan A, Fukushima E, Waggoner RA (1998) Imaging lungs using inert fluorinated gases. Magn Reson Med 39 (1):85–88
6. Hu LZ, Chen JJ, Yang XX et al (2014) Assessing intrarenal nonperfusion and vascular leakage in acute kidney injury with multinuclear H-1/F-19 MRI and perfluorocarbon nanoparticles. Magn Reson Med 71(6):2186–2196
7. Hitchens TK, Ye Q, Eytan DF, Janjic JM, Ahrens ET, Ho C (2011) 19F MRI detection of acute allograft rejection with in vivo perfluorocarbon labeling of immune cells. Magn Reson Med 65(4):1144–1153
8. Moore JK, Chen J, Pan H, Gaut JP, Jain S, Wickline SA (2018) Quantification of vascular damage in acute kidney injury with fluorine magnetic resonance imaging and spectroscopy. Magn Reson Med 79(6):3144–3153
9. Henkelman RM (1985) Measurement of signal intensities in the presence of noise in MR images. Med Phys 12(2):232–233
10. Gudbjartsson H, Patz S (1995) The Rician distribution of noisy MRI data. Magn Reson Med 34(6):910–914
11. van Heeswijk RB, Pilloud Y, Flögel U, Schwitter J, Stuber M (2012) Fluorine-19 magnetic resonance angiography of the mouse. PLoS One 7(7):e42236
12. Starke L, Pohlmann A, Prinz C, Niendorf T, Waiczies S (2019) Performance of compressed sensing for fluorine-19 magnetic resonance imaging at low signal-to-noise ratio conditions. Magn Reson Med 84(2):592–608
13. National Electrical Manufacturers Association (2001) Determination of signal-to-noise ratio (SNR) in diagnostic magnetic resonance imaging. NEMA standards publication MS 1-2001. NEMA, Arlington, VA
14. Koay CG, Basser PJ (2006) Analytically exact correction scheme for signal extraction from noisy magnitude MR signals. J Magn Reson 179(2):317–322
15. Ahn S, Fessler A (2003) Standard errors of mean, variance, and standard deviation estimators. EECS Department, The University of Michigan, Ann Arbor, MI. http://web.eecs.umich.edu/fessler/papers/files/tr/stderr.pdf
16. Constantinides CD, Atalar E, McVeigh ER (1997) Signal-to-noise measurements in magnitude images from NMR phased arrays. Magn Reson Med 38(5):852–857
17. Aja-Fernández S, Vegas-Sánchez-Ferrero G (2016) Statistical analysis of noise in MRI. Springer International Publishing, Cham
18. Ku HH (1966) Notes on the use of propagation of error formulas. J Res Natl Bur Stand 70 (4):263–273

13

Analysis Protocol for the Quantification of Renal pH using Chemical Exchange Saturation Transfer (CEST) MRI

Hahnsung Kim, Yin Wu, Daisy Villano, Dario Livio Longo, Michael T. McMahon, and Phillip Zhe Sun

Abstract

The kidney plays a major role in maintaining body pH homeostasis. Renal pH, in particular, changes immediately following injuries such as intoxication and ischemia, making pH an early biomarker for kidney injury before the symptom onset and complementary to well-established laboratory tests. Because of this, it is imperative to develop minimally invasive renal pH imaging exams and test pH as a new diagnostic biomarker in animal models of kidney injury before clinical translation. Briefly, iodinated contrast agents approved by the US Food and Drug Administration (FDA) for computed tomography (CT) have demonstrated promise as novel chemical exchange saturation transfer (CEST) MRI agents for pH-sensitive imaging. The generalized ratiometric iopamidol CEST MRI analysis enables concentration-independent pH measurement, which simplifies in vivo renal pH mapping. This chapter describes quantitative CEST MRI analysis for preclinical renal pH mapping, and their application in rodents, including normal conditions and acute kidney injury.

This publication is based upon work from the COST Action PARENCHIMA, a community-driven network funded by the European Cooperation in Science and Technology (COST) program of the European Union, which aims to improve the reproducibility and standardization of renal MRI biomarkers. This analysis protocol chapter is complemented by two separate chapters describing the basic concepts and experimental procedure.

Key words Chemical exchange saturation transfer (CEST), Magnetic resonance imaging (MRI), pH, Rats, Mice, Iopamidol, Kidney, Contrast agents, pH imaging

1 Introduction

Chemical exchange saturation transfer (CEST) MRI provides a sensitive means to image microenvironment properties such as tissue pH, temperature, metabolites, and enzyme activities via dilute labile protons [1–12]. Endogenous CEST MRI has been increasingly adopted for imaging a host of disorders including acute ischemic stroke [13–22], tumor [23–27], and epilepsy [28, 29]. In addition, CEST MRI contrast agents have been developed for exogenous CEST imaging that may provide more sensitive

CEST detection which is specific to the administered agents [30–34]. This is because the labile proton exchange rate and chemical shifts can be designed/preselected to optimize these for exogenous CEST MRI contrast [35–38]. There has been an emerging library of iodinated-based CEST agents such as iopamidol, iobitridol, iopromide, and iodixanol, which have been approved by the U.S. Food and Drug Administration (FDA) for computed tomography (CT) head and body imaging applications [39–47]. Such FDA-approved iodinated contrast agents are promising for translational CEST imaging to characterize renal dysfunction, diagnose regional kidney injury before symptom onset, and help guide treatment before irreversible damage [48–50].

Because the CEST MRI effect depends on not only pH-dependent exchange rates but also on the labile proton ratio, relaxation rates and experimental conditions such as magnetic field strength, saturation power, and duration, CEST-weighted MRI contrast is often complex [51–55]. As such, it remains challenging to quantify CEST MRI toward tissue indices such as absolute pH and/or total protein concentration. Persistent progress has been achieved toward simplified and quantitative in vivo pH mapping [56–61]. In particular, ratiometric CEST MRI refers to a specific type of CEST MRI analysis that takes multiple CEST measurements, the ratio of which normalizes common confounding factors such as tissue labile proton concentration and relaxation effects, therefore enabling quantitative in vivo CEST mapping [42, 56, 62–67]. Although pH imaging is more straightforward at high magnetic fields ($B_0 \geq 7$ T) due to the large frequency shift difference between labile and bulk tissue water protons, it is important to extend pH MRI to magnetic fields such as 3 and 4.7 T [68, 69]. Due to the complexity of the source of the MRI CEST signal, multiple approaches have been established for a better quantification of the CEST contrast [54, 60]. In this chapter, we describe variant ratiometric pH CEST MRI analysis techniques, image down-sampling expedited adaptive least-squares (IDEAL) fitting algorithm, smoothing splines interpolation algorithm and use of iodinated CEST agents for mapping renal pH in vivo [50, 70].

This analysis protocol chapter is complemented by two separate describing the basic concepts and experimental procedure, which are part of this book.

This chapter is part of the book Pohlmann A, Niendorf T (eds) (2020) Preclinical MRI of the Kidney—Methods and Protocols. Springer, New York.

2 Materials

2.1 Software Requirements

2.1.1 Essential Tools

1. Matlab/Python: The method described in this chapter requires MATLAB (MathWorks, Natick, MA, https://www.mathworks.com/products/matlab.html) for data analysis of applying fitting models and measuring ratiometric. Because Matlab functions used in the data processing can also be implemented in python (https://www.python.org/), python can be used instead.
2. An image processing software (e.g., Image J, we recommend using Fiji, which is ImageJ with a wide range of plugins already included, https://fiji.sc/, open-source), as a practical tool for the image quality check or to measure SNR.

2.1.2 Optional Tools

A statistical analysis software (e.g., SPSS, SPSS Inc., Chicago, IL or Prism, GraphPad, USA) as a practical tool for the statistical significance calculation.

2.2 Source Data: Format Requirements and Data Preprocessing

2.2.1 Input Requirements

The CEST images can be retrieved directly from the MRI scanner as raw binary images or in DICOM format (*see* **Note 1**). To be able to perform CEST analysis different scans are needed:

- Anatomical image (optional).
- Unsaturated image (optional).
- CEST images or Z-spectra.
- CEST images (Z-spectra) before and after contrast agent (CA) injection for in vivo acquisitions.

Information about some scan acquisition parameters is also necessary as is the frequency offsets vector.

2.2.2 Background Removal

In order to avoid the analysis outside the object of interest and to shorten the analysis duration a first segmentation between the background and the imaged object is suggested. Manual thresholding or automatic thresholding (as by the Otsu method) can be easily applied within the Matlab environment.

3 Methods

3.1 Motion Correction

If needed, postprocessing motion correction can be applied to coregister images to correct for motion artifacts.

3.2 Z-Spectra Analysis

Z-spectra can be analyzed as mean contribution inside one or more regions of interest, that can be drawn on an anatomical image reference, or preferentially, by a voxel-by-voxel analysis. Different approaches for Z-spectra analysis will be described in detail.

3.2.1 Multi Pool Lorentzian Fitting

The Z-spectra are numerically described using a multipool Lorentzian model [24, 71–74]:

$$Z(\omega) = 1 - \frac{M_z}{M_0} = \sum_{i=1}^{N} L_i(\omega) \tag{1}$$

where ω is the frequency offset from the water resonance, N is the total number of proton pools, and L_i is the Lorentzian spectrum of the ith pool. The Lorentzian lineshape is represented by the following equation:

$$L(\omega) = \frac{A}{1 + 4\left(\frac{\omega-\omega_0}{\sigma}\right)^2} \tag{2}$$

where A, ω_0, and σ are the amplitude, center frequency, and linewidth of the ith saturation transfer effects, respectively.

1. Map B_0 inhomogeneity with water saturation shift referencing (WASSR) using external acquired B_0 maps, by field maps or by interpolation procedures looking to the minimum of the Z-spectrum (internal B_0 mapping) [75–79].
2. Shift CEST MRI Z-spectrum based on the field inhomogeneity, per voxel, for correction.
3. Normalize the Z-spectra (i_z) by the signal without RF irradiation (M_0).
4. Fit the Z-spectrum using a five pool Lorentzian model (two pools for iopamidol amide groups at 4.3 and 5.5 ppm, one for bulk tissue water (0 ppm), and two pools for the hydroxyl groups at 0.8 and 1.8 ppm) [80, 41]. Representative multipool Lorentzian fitting is described in Fig. 1.

3.2.2 Image Down-Sampling Expedited Adaptive Least-Squares (IDEAL) Fitting Algorithm

1. Initially down-sample the B_0 field inhomogeneity-corrected CEST images to one or a few pixels and calculate the global Z-spectrum by averaging the Z-spectra of all voxel within an ROI to substantially improve the signal-to-noise ratio (SNR) for the numerical fitting.
2. Set the boundaries to be between 1% and 100 times of the initial values for the amplitude and linewidth of each chemical pool, with their peak frequency shift within ± 0.2 ppm of the initial chemical shift. The relaxed boundary constraints ensure that the initial fitting provides a reasonable estimation of the multiple Lorentzian pools under the condition of sufficiently high SNR.
3. Fit the down-sampled image exploiting.
4. Resample the CEST images to 2×2 matrix size.

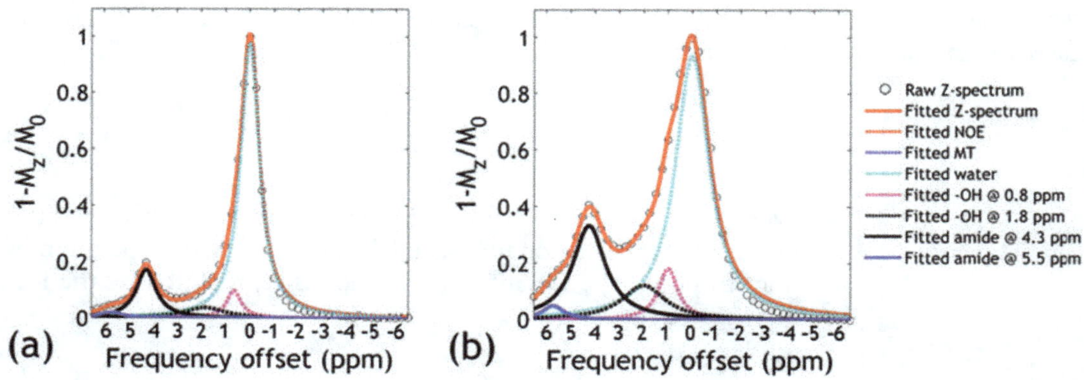

Fig. 1 Multipool Lorentzian fitting of representative CEST Z-spectra from a 40 mM iopamidol solution vial with a pH of 7.0. CEST Z-spectrum obtained from under (**a**) $B_1 = 1$ μT and (**b**) 2 μT under body temperature. A five-pool Lorentzian model was used to describe the CEST spectrum [Adapted with permission from *Magnetic Resonance in Medicine* 2018 (A generalized ratiometric chemical exchange saturation transfer (CEST) MRI approach for mapping renal pH using Iopamidol, Volume: 79, Issue: 3, Pages: 1553–1558, DOI: https:/doi.org/10.1002/mrm.26817)]

5. Take the initial values for the fitting of each voxel of the resampled image from the results of the previous image with lower spatial resolution.
6. Set the boundary constraints relatively loose albeit narrower than the initial fitting, to be 10% and ten times of the initial values.
7. Use a nonlinearly constrained fitting algorithm with twofold overweighting applied for Z-spectra between 4.0 and 5.8 ppm to increase the fitting accuracy of Iopamidol CEST effects at 4.3 and 5.5 ppm.
8. Resample the CEST images, 4 × 4, 8 × 8, 12 × 12, 24 × 24 until the original resolution of 48 × 48 or voxel-wise multipool Lorentzian fitting and repeat from **step 5** until you get the desired final resolution.
9. Figure 2 shows the flowchart of the IDEAL fitting algorithm.

3.2.3 Smoothing Splines Interpolation

The cubic smoothing splines estimate the interpolating function *f*, minimizing the following expression, linearly composed by two parts:

$$p\sum_{j=1}^{N}\left|y_j - f(x_j)\right|^2 + (1-p)\int\left|D^2 f(t)\right|^2 \mathrm{d}t \qquad (3)$$

The first addend represents the mean square error between data y_j and the interpolating cubic spline $f(x_j)$ calculated in x_j measure

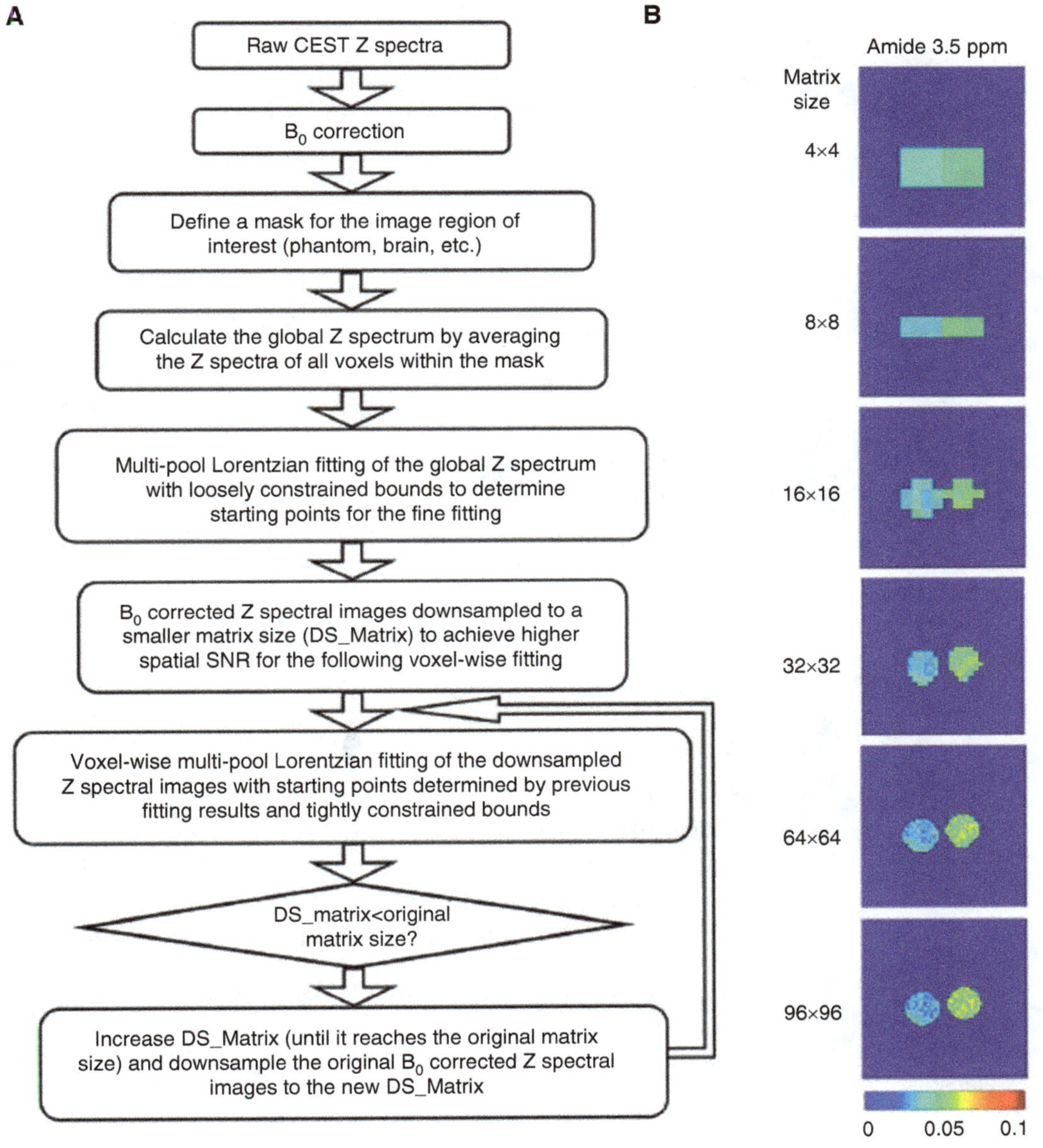

Fig. 2 Illustration of the Image Downsampling Expedited Adaptive Least Squares (IDEAL) CEST analysis algorithm. (**a**) Flow chart of data processing steps of the IDEAL fitting algorithm. (**b**) The intermediate fitting results of iteratively less downsampled images from a two-compartment CEST phantom [Adapted with permission from *Scientific Reports*. 2017 (Quantitative chemical exchange saturation transfer (CEST) MRI of glioma using Image Downsampling Expedited Adaptive Least-squares (IDEAL) fitting, Volume: 7, Issue: 1, Pages: 84, DOI: https:/doi.org/10.1038/s41598-017-00167-y)]

points. The second term consists of the integral of the squared second-order derivative of f and is a measure of function flexibility.

p is a smoothing parameter and determines the relative weight you would like to place on the contradictory demands of having

f be smooth *vs* having f be close to the data. Its value ranges between 0 and 1. For $p = 1$, the curvature constraint is nullified, f passes for all data points and converges to the interpolating spline, while, at the other extreme, for $p = 0$, f curvature is minimized and f results in a linear least square fit.

1. Normalize pre- and postinjection Z-spectra to the maximum intensity value of the free water signal, generally corresponding to the most distant offset or to the unsaturated image (M_0) [79].
2. Interpolate each voxel Z-spectra data with a cubic spline function paying action to regularization factor selection (*see* **Note 2**) and ignoring the background pixels/voxels (in Matlab use csasp function).
3. Find in the fitted spectra the absolute minimum corresponding to bulk water frequency offset (in Matlab use fnmin function).
4. Use the minimum position (corresponding to water peak shift from zero) to correct B_0 inhomogeneity shifting the frequency offsets vector.
5. Save minimum position in a matrix to construct the B_0 shift map.

To exclude noisy data points from the analysis a filtration step is suggested:

6. Construct R^2 matrix evaluating the distance of the interpolating function to data in each pixel.
7. Define a R^2 threshold (in our application R^2 ranges between 0.97 and 0.99).
8. Ignore pixel for which the R^2 value is lower than the threshold.

Smoothing spline algorithm workflow is described in Fig. 3.

3.3 CEST Quantification

After having fitted the Z-spectra by smoothing splines or Lorenzian fitting, CEST contrast quantification can be evaluated and ratiometric values (ratio between two CEST contrast quantifications to remove the concentration effect) can be calculated.

3.3.1 CEST Ration Calculation by Asymmetry Analysis

The CEST ratio (CESTR) is calculated by asymmetry analysis:

$$\mathrm{CESTR}(\omega) = \frac{M_z(-\omega) - M_z(\omega)}{M_0} \tag{4}$$

where ω is the labile proton chemical shift from the bulk water resonance (for Iopamidol $\omega = 4.2$ ppm and 5.5 ppm). For the in vivo images, contrast was calculated by subtracting contrast after CA injection from the contrast before the injection at the different frequency offsets.

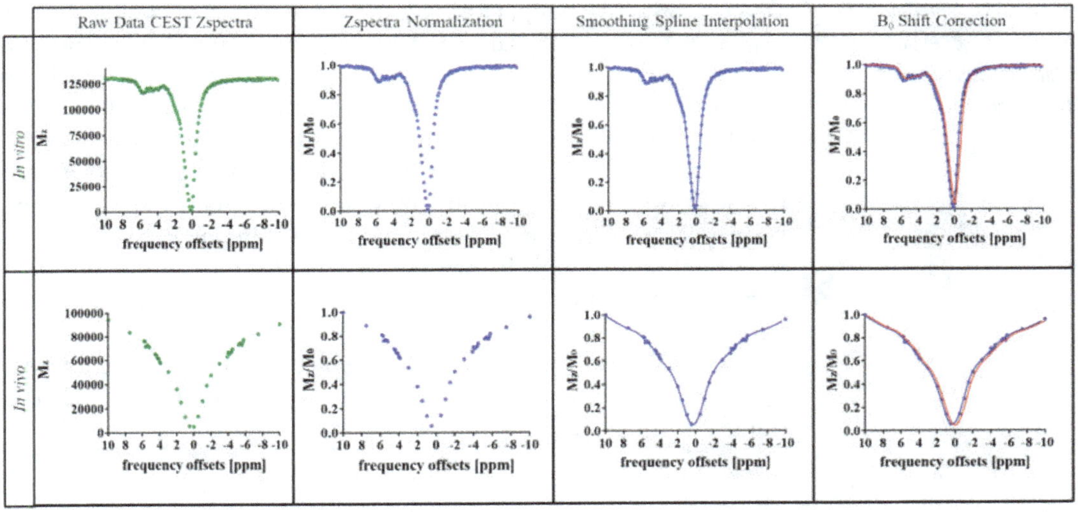

Fig. 3 Representative z-spectra from in vitro (bottom) and in vivo (top) images showing the analysis steps for data normalization, smoothing splines interpolation and B_0 shift correction (from left to right)

1. Calculate CEST contrast according to Eq. 4 for the two pools of Iopamidol (4.2 and 5.5 ppm).

3.3.2 CEST Ratio Calculation from Lorentzian Fitting

1. Calculate CEST contrast from the amplitude obtained from the Lorentzian fitting according to Eq. 4 for the two pools of Iopamidol (4.2 and 5.5 ppm).

3.3.3 Chemical Shift-Based Ratiometric CEST Analysis

Because the direct saturation is relatively small at the magnetic field at or above 7 T, the coupling between multiple CEST effects is relatively small, and a ratiometric analysis of two CEST effects obtained under the same RF irradiation power level can be calculated for pH calibration, as

$$R_{\mathrm{ST}}(\mathrm{pH}) = \frac{\mathrm{CESTR}(\delta 1)}{\mathrm{CESTR}(\delta 2)} \tag{5}$$

3.3.4 RF Power-based Ratiometric CEST Analysis

For CEST agent of a single labile proton group, the conventional ratiometric analysis does not apply. It has been shown that the ratiometric analysis can be generalized by taking the ratio of CEST effects obtained under two RF power levels as [42].

$$R_{\mathrm{ST}}(\mathrm{pH}) = \frac{\mathrm{CESTR}(B_{1b})}{\mathrm{CESTR}(B_{1a})} \tag{6}$$

If the direct water saturation is not negligible, the saturation effect can be calculated/removed to improve the precision of RF power-based ratiometric analysis [56, 64].

3.3.5 The Generalized RF Power- and Chemical Shift-Hybrid Ratiometric CEST Analysis

When CEST MRI is performed at lower magnetic field strengths ($B_0 < 7.0$ T) or the RF saturation power induces nonnegligible direct saturation effect, the coupling between multiple CEST effects (i.e., CEST and direction water saturation) become nonnegligible. Under such conditions, the routine ratiometric analysis (chemical shift- and RF power-based methods) may be susceptible to the coupling. In addition, the coupling depends on the transverse relaxation rate, which may be the difference between phantom calibration and in vivo experiments. To minimize such confounding coupling effect, the CEST effect can be decoupled with the multipool Lorentzian model, and their ratio is more reproducible and specific to pH. As such, the ratiometric analysis is generalized to a ratio of CEST effects of different chemical shift obtained under different saturation power levels.

$$R_{\mathrm{ST}}(\mathrm{pH}) = \frac{\mathrm{CESTR}(\delta 1, B_{1b})}{\mathrm{CESTR}(\delta 2, B_{1a})} \tag{7}$$

1. Calculate the ratiometric values following one of the previously described Eqs. 5–7.

3.4 Set-Up of pH Calibration Curve

To investigate the relation between the R_{ST} value and the pH a calibration is needed. In the following steps the calibration done for Iopamidol on a pH varying phantom is described. Two examples of pH calibration curves obtained at 7 T and at 4.7 T are shown in Fig. 4.

1. Acquire CEST spectra images of the pH varying phantom;
2. Draw the ROI including only the pH compartment;
3. Evaluate mean CESTR at 4.2 and 5.5 ppm inside each compartment;
4. Calculate R_{ST};
5. Fit the R_{ST} as function of the titrated pH (usually a polynomial fit of the third order is selected).

It is worth to observe that by decoupling the CEST effects at 4.2 and 5.5 ppm, the generalized ratiometric CEST MRI index provides an extended range of pH measurement at 4.7 T (Fig. 4b). Note that such a calibration experiment is important to ensure that the pH dynamic range is sufficient to cover tissue pH of interest. The polynomial regression enables the derivation of the absolute pH map of renal images.

6. From the calculated ratiometric value derives the pH value according to the used calibration curve.

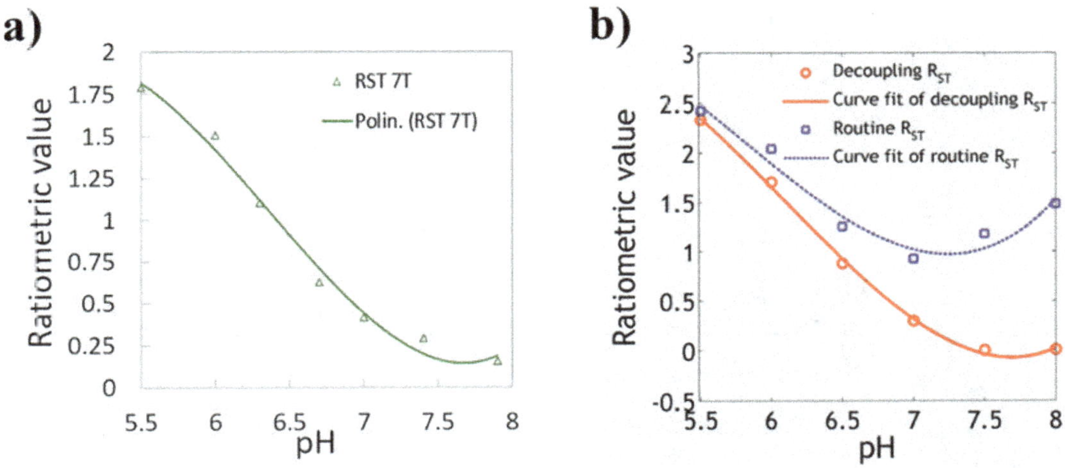

Fig. 4 Comparison of ratiometric analysis of Iopamidol at high magnetic field of 7 T (**a**) and at sub-high magnetic field of 4.7 T (**b**). Note that the routine R_{ST} of 5.5 and 4.3 ppm provides a limited pH MRI range below pH = 7 due to the CEST MRI effect coupling at high pH. In comparison, the modified approach extends the pH imaging range to 7.5 [Adapted with permission from *Magnetic Resonance in Medicine* 2018 (A generalized ratiometric chemical exchange saturation transfer (CEST) MRI approach for mapping renal pH using lopamidol, Volume: 79, Issue: 3, Pages: 1553–1558, DOI: https:/doi.org/10.1002/mrm.26817)]

3.5 *In Vivo Application for pH Mapping*

3.5.1 pH Mapping by Lorentzian Fitting or IDEAL Approach

1. Obtain two representative in vivo CEST Z-spectra from a normal rat (or mouse) kidney during Isovue infusion under two RF saturation power levels of 1 and 2 μT at 4.7 T as shown in Fig. 5.
2. Apply the IDEAL algorithm and perform Lorentzian decoupling to resolve Iopamidol CEST effects at 4.3 and 5.5 ppm.
3. Outline the renal cortex, medulla, and calyx based on T_2-weighted MRI.
4. Z-spectra are broadened at a higher RF power level due to more prominent direct RF saturation effect. Notably, the CEST effect increases from the cortex, medulla to calyx. This is because pH gradually reduces from the cortex, medulla to the calyx, which causes a persistent reduction in the Iopamidol CEST exchange rate. As such, the saturation efficiency increases when the exchange rate becomes comparable to the saturation field. In addition, the kidney concentrates and excretes Isovue, resulting in a concentration gradient across the kidney.
5. Describe the CEST effect by a six-pool Lorentzian model (i.e., five-pool model plus semisolid macromolecule magnetization transfer (MT) effect in tissue). Corresponding parametric images for CEST contrast and pH mapping in rat kidneys are shown in Fig. 6.

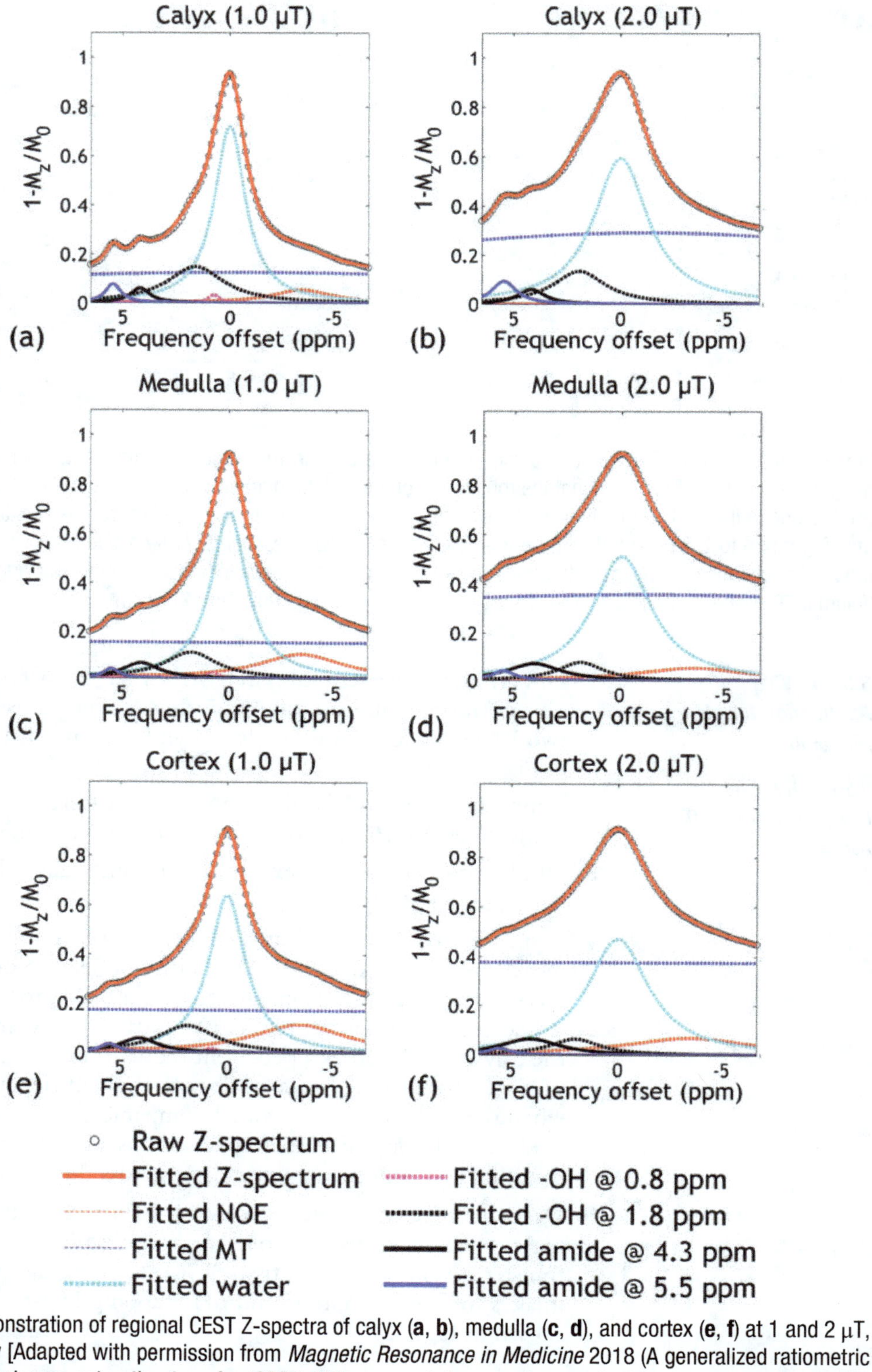

Fig. 5 Demonstration of regional CEST Z-spectra of calyx (**a**, **b**), medulla (**c**, **d**), and cortex (**e**, **f**) at 1 and 2 μT, respectively [Adapted with permission from *Magnetic Resonance in Medicine* 2018 (A generalized ratiometric chemical exchange saturation transfer (CEST) MRI approach for mapping renal pH using lopamidol, Volume: 79, Issue: 3, Pages: 1553–1558, DOI: https:/doi.org/10.1002/mrm.26817)]

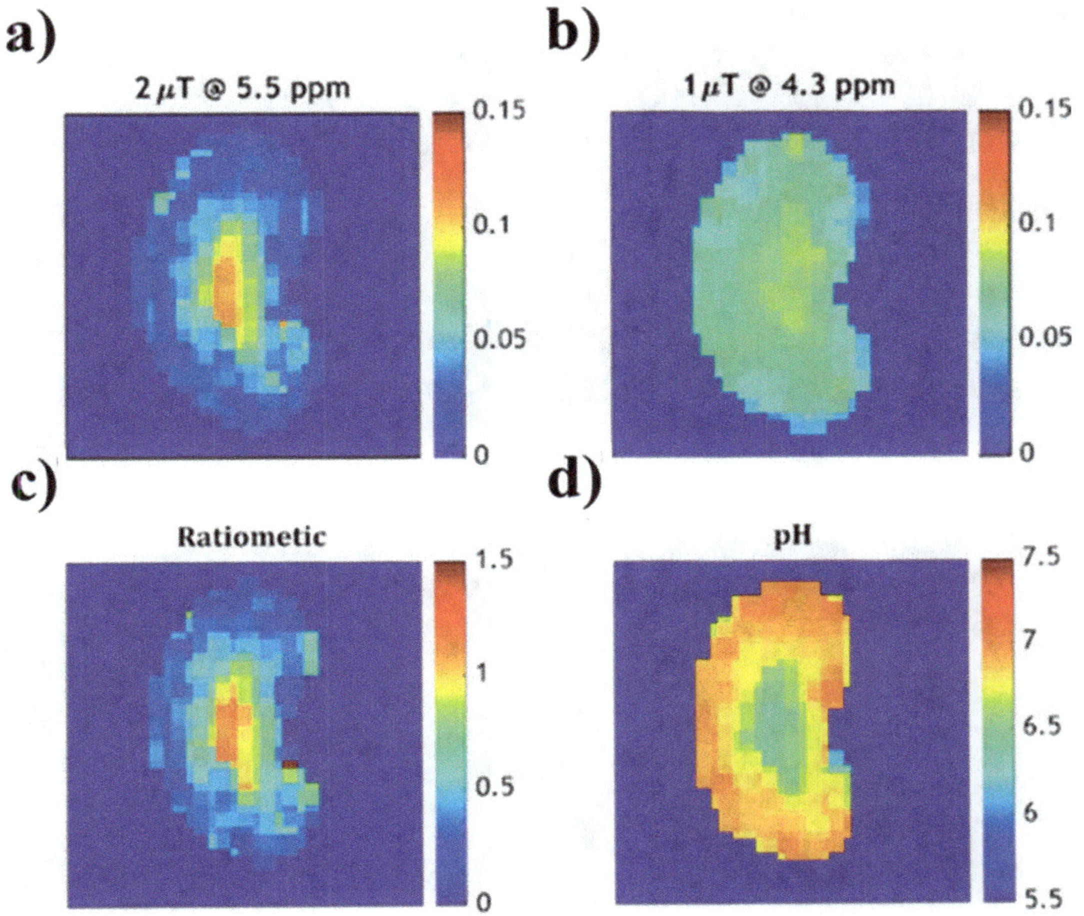

Fig. 6 Demonstration of a renal pH map from a representative rat following Iopamidol injection at 4.7 T. The resolved maps of ST effects at 5.5 ppm (**a**) and 4.3 ppm (**b**) were obtained with the IDEAL fitting algorithm, from which the ratiometric map was obtained (**c**). (**d**) pH map overlaid on the corresponding T_2-weighted image show the renal pH gradually decreasing from the cortex, medulla to calyx

3.5.2 pH Mapping by Using the Smoothing Splines Approach

1. Import your scans (anatomical image, pre- and postinjection CEST images) and save them in a matrix.
2. Use cubic spline algorithm to interpolate both pre- and post-injection Z-spectra as described in Subheading 3.2.3.
3. Use cubic spline interpolated Z-spectra to calculate CESTR at specific ω (+4.2 and +5.5 ppm for Iopamidol) or/and B_1 levels before and after the CA injection and save CEST contrast values in a matrix to construct CESTR maps (in Matlab use fnval function to evaluate interpolating cubic spline values at ω corrected for calculated B_0 shift).

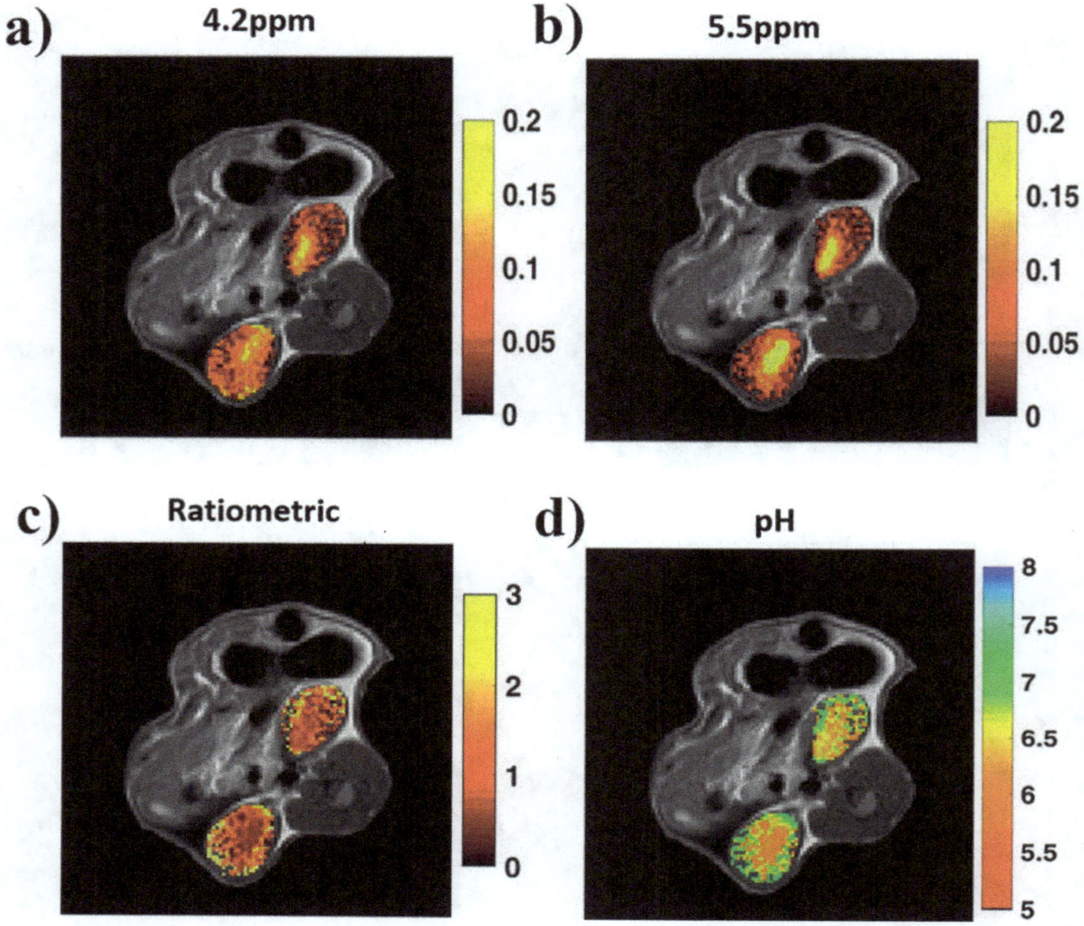

Fig. 7 Demonstration of a physiologic renal pH map from a representative mouse following lopamidol injection at 7 T. The resolved maps of ST effects at 4.2 ppm (**a**) and 5.5 ppm (**b**) were obtained with the smoothing splines algorithm, from which the ratiometric map was obtained (**c**). (**d**) pH map overlaid on the corresponding T_2-weighted anatomical image show the renal pH gradually decreasing from the cortex, medulla to calyx

4. To remove endogenous effects and to isolate contrast agent contribution, subtract postinjection CEST contrast map to preinjection CEST contrast map (Fig. 7a, b).
5. Calculate the ratio map ratioing difference CEST contrast maps obtained at different ω values (Fig. 7c) or/and B_1 levels.
6. Derive pH map from the ratio map using the experimental calibration curve calculated in Subheading 3.4, **step 6** (Fig. 7d).

3.6 Representation

The obtained Z-spectra and pH maps can be represented as averaged values in a region of interest (ROI) or as parametric pixel-by-pixel maps. Before the representation, in order to remove residual noise, contrast and pH maps can be filtered, by applying a threshold corresponding to the measured signal intensities variability of the exploited MRI scanner to discriminate between enhanced and nonenhanced voxels, following CA injection (*see* **Note 3**).

1. Select a noise threshold.
2. Set to 0 or to NaN all pixels inside the map for which the contrast increment is lower than the threshold.
3. Use the anatomical image (or alternatively the first CEST image) to identify and draw one or more ROIs (in Matlab use the `roipoly` function).
4. Create a mask from the ROI(s), a matrix that contains 1 value inside the region of interest and 0 or NaN values outside.

   For representing mean Z-spectra:

5. Calculate mean Z-spectra (pre- and postinjection), ignoring values outside the ROI.

   For representing parametric maps:

6. Represent contrast and pH maps overimposed to the anatomical image for having a morphological reference.

Representative mean spectra are shown in Fig. 8, whereas parametric images for CEST contrast quantification and pH values calculated in rat kidneys at 4.7 T and in murine kidneys at 7 T are shown in Fig. 6 and Fig. 7, respectively.

3.7 Quantitative Analysis

Statistics values as mean, median, and standard deviation can be obtained evaluating maps inside different ROI (cortex, medulla, and calyx) to have a quantitative description of the analysis results.

3.8 Results Validation

3.8.1 Evaluation of Analysis Errors

The quality of CEST fitting can be evaluated by the following three methods: (1) coefficient of variation (standard deviation/mean) within ROI, (2) contrast-to-noise ratio (CNR) between the two vials in the phantom study calculated by $\mathrm{CNR} = |S_1 - S_2| / \sqrt{(\sigma_1{}^2 + \sigma_2{}^2)}$, where $S_{1,\,2}$ are the mean values for the two ROIs and $\sigma_{1,\,2}$ are their standard deviations, and (3) goodness of fit (R^2) maps.

3.8.2 Comparison with Reference Values from the Literature

It has been documented that kidney pH values are heterogeneous, with a gradient from the cortex, medulla to calyx due to filtration and blood volume difference. MRI-based pH imaging reveals significant different pH values among the three layers, with more neutral pH values (7–7.4) for the cortex region, mild acidic pH values (6.6–7.0) for the medulla, and acidic pH values for the calyx (6.3–6.7). Please consider Table 1 for average pH values measured in specific kidney regions.

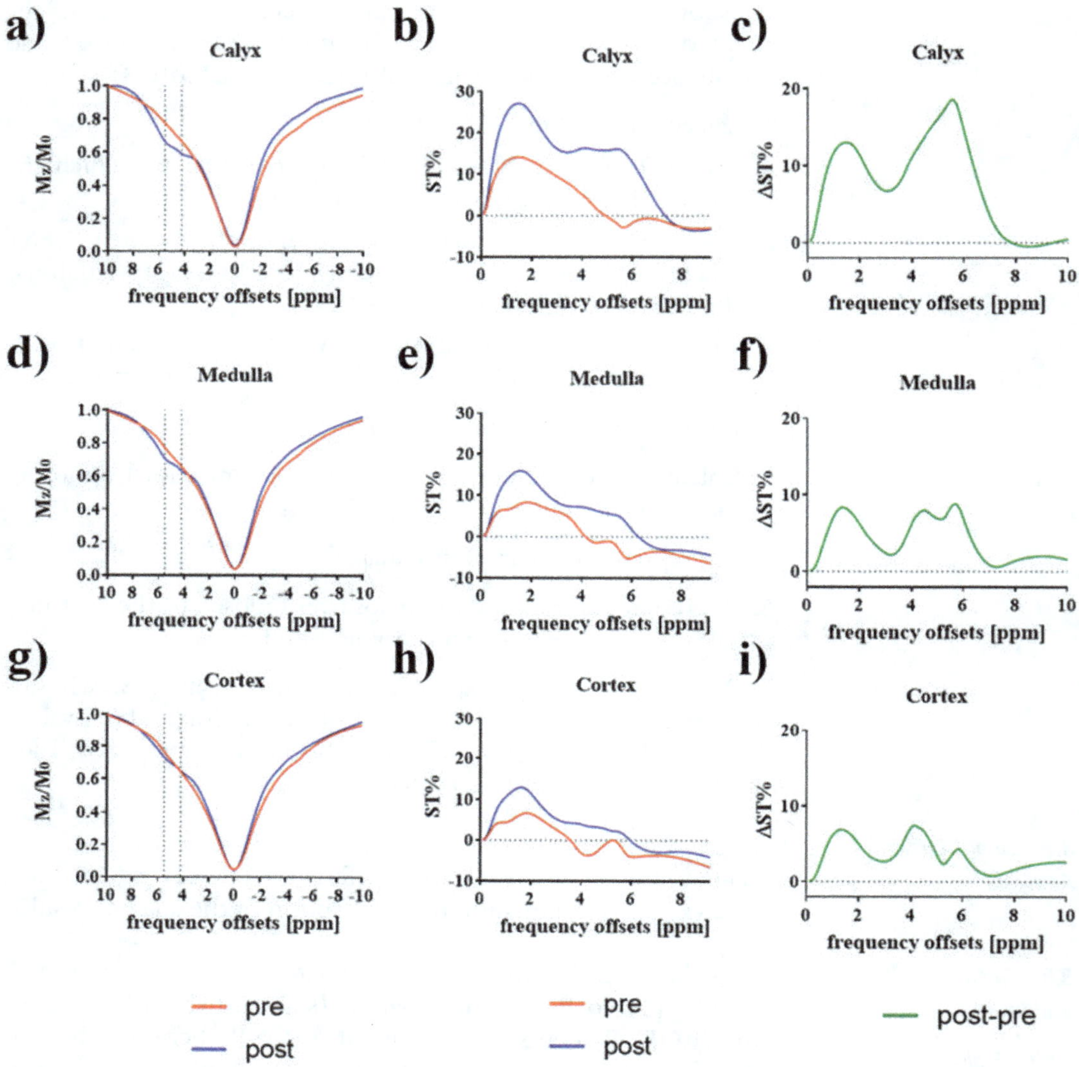

Fig. 8 Demonstration of regional CEST Z-spectra and contrast of calyx (**a**, **b**), medulla (**c**, **d**), and cortex (**e**, **f**) at 3 μT. Described CEST contrast became higher from calyx, trough medulla, to cortex, due to pH variation

Table 1
Typical pH values for each specific renal tissue for healthy mice and rats (literature values)

pH				
Inner medulla	**Outer medulla**	**Cortex**	**Field strength, T**	**Reference**
6.3 ± 0.45	7.0 ± 0.29	7.3 ± 0.13	4.7	[81]
6.6 ± 0.2	6.85 ± 0.15	7.0 ± 0.11	7	[69]
6.5 ± 0.2	6.8 ± 0.1	7.0 ± 0.1	4.7	[80]
6.6 ± 0.1	6.7 ± 0.08	6.8 ± 0.1	7	[49, 50]

4 Notes

1. Data are stored in the 2dseq file for Bruker scanners or in .img file for ASPECT MRI instrumentations. In both cases metadata files (method, acqp and reco for Bruker scanner or dat file for Aspect systems) need to be read for retrieving all the information needed to correctly read the raw binary file. Bruker import file plugins are available in ImageJ for directly opening raw Bruker files (for PV5). Matlab-based scripts for importing Bruker images and for the CEST analysis described in this chapter can be made available upon sending a request to the authors (dario.longo@unito.it; mtmcmaho@gmail.com; pzhesun@emory.edu). More information on the software can be found at the following links: http://www.cim.unito.it/website/research/research_processing.php http://godzilla.kennedykrieger.org/CEST/.
2. The choice of the regularization factor plays a key role in calculating CEST spectra and contrast; in particular, a trade-off between the "zero" estimation, noise suppression and peak identification is needed for an optimal choice [78]. Z-spectra and resulting CEST contrast obtained with different p values are shown in Fig. 9: when the regularization factor increases, the flexibility of the interpolating curve increases, yielding more evident peaks, but at the same time the smoothing of the raw data decreases. In our application p ranged between 0.90 and 0.99.
3. Signal variations (or fluctuations), as a measure of scanner instability, can be evaluated by repeating the same CEST acquisition (without saturation) several times (10–100 repetitions) and then evaluating the oscillation (or standard deviation) of

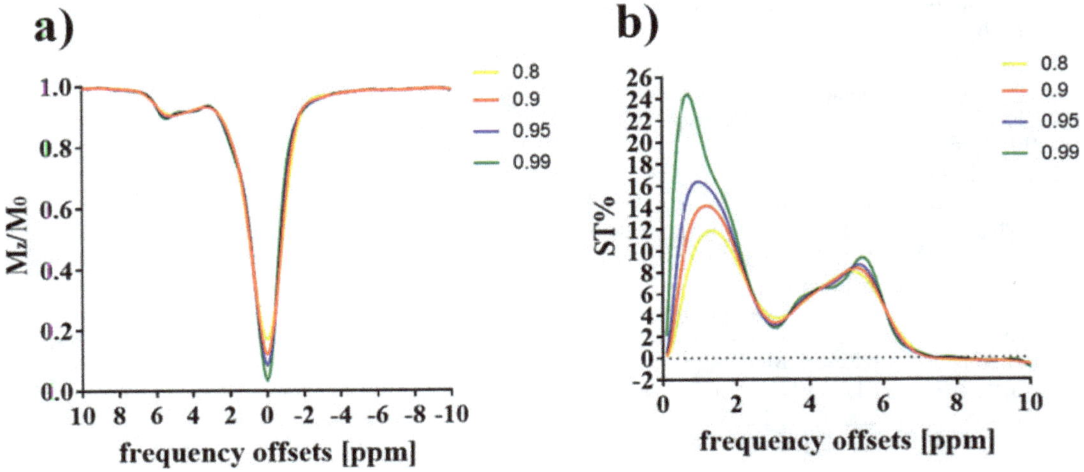

Fig. 9 Z-Spectra (**a**) and CEST contrast (**b**) obtained with different smoothing factors. The contrast decreases with a decrease of the smoothing factor value

the average signal along the repetition. Such value can be exploited to set a threshold for evaluating CEST contrast increase following contrast agent injection due to the contrast agent itself and not due to signal oscillation (i.e., it acts as a detection threshold). Signal fluctuation can be expected to be less than 0.2–1% with slight constant increase with the age of the scanner.

Acknowledgments

The Italian Ministry for Education and Research (MIUR) is gratefully acknowledged for yearly FOE funding to the Euro-BioImaging Multi-Modal Molecular Imaging Italian Node (MMMI).

This chapter is based upon work from COST Action PARENCH IMA, supported by European Cooperation in Science and Technology (COST). COST (www.cost.eu) is a funding agency for research and innovation networks. COST Actions help connect research initiatives across Europe and enable scientists to enrich their ideas by sharing them with their peers. This boosts their research, career, and innovation.

PARENCHIMA (renalmri.org) is a community-driven Action in the COST program of the European Union, which unites more than 200 experts in renal MRI from 30 countries with the aim to improve the reproducibility and standardization of renal MRI biomarkers.

References

1. Forsen S, Hoffman RA (1963) Study of moderately rapid chemical exchange reactions by means of nuclear magnetic double resonance. J Chem Phys 39(11):2892. https://doi.org/10.1063/1.1734121
2. Wolff SD, Balaban RS (1990) Nmr imaging of labile proton-exchange. J Magn Reson 86 (1):164–169. https://doi.org/10.1016/0022-2364(90)90220-4
3. Dagher AP, Aletras A, Choyke P, Balaban RS (2000) Imaging of urea using chemical exchange-dependent saturation transfer at 1.5T. J Magn Reson Imaging 12:745–748
4. Sun PZ, Zhou J, Huang J, van Zijl P (2007) Simplified quantitative description of amide proton transfer (APT) imaging during acute ischemia. Magn Reson Med 57(2):405–410. https://doi.org/10.1002/mrm.21151
5. Aime S, Delli Castelli D, Fedeli F, Terreno E (2002) A paramagnetic MRI-CEST agent responsive to lactate concentration. J Am Chem Soc 124(32):9364–9365
6. Jokivarsi KT, Grohn HI, Grohn OH, Kauppinen RA (2007) Proton transfer ratio, lactate, and intracellular pH in acute cerebral ischemia. Magn Reson Med 57(4):647–653. https://doi.org/10.1002/mrm.21181
7. Zhang L, Martins AF, Mai Y, Zhao P, Funk AM, Clavijo Jordan MV, Zhang S, Chen W, Wu Y, Sherry AD (2017) Imaging extracellular lactate in vitro and in vivo using CEST MRI and a paramagnetic shift reagent. Chemistry 23 (8):1752–1756. https://doi.org/10.1002/chem.201604558
8. Liu G, Li Y, Pagel MD (2007) Design and characterization of a new irreversible responsive PARACEST MRI contrast agent that detects nitric oxide. Magn Reson Med 58 (6):1249–1256. https://doi.org/10.1002/mrm.21428

9. Li Y, Sheth VR, Liu G, Pagel MD (2011) A self-calibrating PARACEST MRI contrast agent that detects esterase enzyme activity. Contrast Media Mol Imaging 6(4):219–228. https://doi.org/10.1002/cmmi.421
10. McVicar N, Li AX, Suchy M, Hudson RH, Menon RS, Bartha R (2013) Simultaneous in vivo pH and temperature mapping using a PARACEST-MRI contrast agent. Magn Reson Med 70(4):1016–1025. https://doi.org/10.1002/mrm.24539
11. Zhang S, Malloy CR, Sherry AD (2005) MRI thermometry based on PARACEST agents. J Am Chem Soc 127(50):17572–17573. https://doi.org/10.1021/ja053799t
12. Liu G, Li Y, Sheth VR, Pagel MD (2012) Imaging in vivo extracellular pH with a single paramagnetic chemical exchange saturation transfer magnetic resonance imaging contrast agent. Mol Imaging 11(1):47–57
13. Zhou J, Payen JF, Wilson DA, Traystman RJ, van Zijl PC (2003) Using the amide proton signals of intracellular proteins and peptides to detect pH effects in MRI. Nat Med 9 (8):1085–1090. https://doi.org/10.1038/nm907
14. Harston GW, Tee YK, Blockley N, Okell TW, Thandeswaran S, Shaya G, Sheerin F, Cellerini M, Payne S, Jezzard P, Chappell M, Kennedy J (2015) Identifying the ischaemic penumbra using pH-weighted magnetic resonance imaging. Brain 138(Pt 1):36–42. https://doi.org/10.1093/brain/awu374
15. Wang E, Wu Y, Cheung JS, Igarashi T, Wu L, Zhang X, Sun PZ (2019) Mapping tissue pH in an experimental model of acute stroke – determination of graded regional tissue pH changes with non-invasive quantitative amide proton transfer MRI. NeuroImage. https://doi.org/10.1016/j.neuroimage.2019.02.022
16. Sun PZ, Wang E, Cheung JS (2012) Imaging acute ischemic tissue acidosis with pH-sensitive endogenous amide proton transfer (APT) MRI—correction of tissue relaxation and concomitant RF irradiation effects toward mapping quantitative cerebral tissue pH. NeuroImage 60(1):1–6. https://doi.org/10.1016/j.neuroimage.2011.11.091
17. Sun PZ, Cheung JS, Wang E, Lo EH (2011) Association between pH-weighted endogenous amide proton chemical exchange saturation transfer MRI and tissue lactic acidosis during acute ischemic stroke. J Cereb Blood Flow Metab 31(8):1743–1750. https://doi.org/10.1038/jcbfm.2011.23
18. Sun PZ, Zhou J, Sun W, Huang J, van Zijl PC (2007) Detection of the ischemic penumbra using pH-weighted MRI. J Cereb Blood Flow Metab 27(6):1129–1136. https://doi.org/10.1038/sj.jcbfm.9600424
19. McVicar N, Li AX, Goncalves DF, Bellyou M, Meakin SO, Prado MA, Bartha R (2014) Quantitative tissue pH measurement during cerebral ischemia using amine and amide concentration-independent detection (AACID) with MRI. J Cereb Blood Flow Metab 34(4):690–698. https://doi.org/10.1038/jcbfm.2014.12
20. Heo HY, Zhang Y, Burton TM, Jiang S, Zhao Y, van Zijl PCM, Leigh R, Zhou J (2017) Improving the detection sensitivity of pH-weighted amide proton transfer MRI in acute stroke patients using extrapolated semisolid magnetization transfer reference signals. Magn Reson Med 78(3):871–880. https://doi.org/10.1002/mrm.26799
21. Jin T, Wang P, Hitchens TK, Kim SG (2017) Enhancing sensitivity of pH-weighted MRI with combination of amide and guanidyl CEST. NeuroImage 157:341–350. https://doi.org/10.1016/j.neuroimage.2017.06.007
22. Zhou J, van Zijl PC (2011) Defining an acidosis-based ischemic penumbra from pH-weighted MRI. Transl Stroke Res 3 (1):76–83. https://doi.org/10.1007/s12975-011-0110-4
23. Heo HY, Zhang Y, Jiang S, Lee DH, Zhou J (2016) Quantitative assessment of amide proton transfer (APT) and nuclear overhauser enhancement (NOE) imaging with extrapolated semisolid magnetization transfer reference (EMR) signals: II. Comparison of three EMR models and application to human brain glioma at 3 Tesla. Magn Reson Med 75 (4):1630–1639. https://doi.org/10.1002/mrm.25795
24. Cai K, Singh A, Poptani H, Li W, Yang S, Lu Y, Hariharan H, Zhou XJ, Reddy R (2015) CEST signal at 2ppm (CEST@2ppm) from Z-spectral fitting correlates with creatine distribution in brain tumor. NMR Biomed 28(1):1–8. https://doi.org/10.1002/nbm.3216
25. Zhou J, Tryggestad E, Wen Z, Lal B, Zhou T, Grossman R, Wang S, Yan K, Fu DX, Ford E, Tyler B, Blakeley J, Laterra J, van Zijl PC (2011) Differentiation between glioma and radiation necrosis using molecular magnetic resonance imaging of endogenous proteins and peptides. Nat Med 17(1):130–134. https://doi.org/10.1038/nm.2268
26. Zhao X, Wen Z, Huang F, Lu S, Wang X, Hu S, Zu D, Zhou J (2011) Saturation power dependence of amide proton transfer image contrasts in human brain tumors and strokes at 3 T. Magn Reson Med 66(4):1033–1041. https://doi.org/10.1002/mrm.22891

27. Zhao X, Wen Z, Zhang G, Huang F, Lu S, Wang X, Hu S, Chen M, Zhou J (2013) Three-dimensional turbo-spin-echo amide proton transfer MR imaging at 3-Tesla and its application to high-grade human brain tumors. Mol Imaging Biol 15(1):114–122. https://doi.org/10.1007/s11307-012-0563-1
28. Davis KA, Nanga RP, Das S, Chen SH, Hadar PN, Pollard JR, Lucas TH, Shinohara RT, Litt B, Hariharan H, Elliott MA, Detre JA, Reddy R (2015) Glutamate imaging (GluCEST) lateralizes epileptic foci in nonlesional temporal lobe epilepsy. Sci Transl Med 7 (309):309ra161. https://doi.org/10.1126/scitranslmed.aaa7095
29. Lee D-H, Lee D-W, Kwon J-I, Woo C-W, Kim S-T, Lee JS, Choi CG, Kim KW, Kim JK, Woo D-C (2018) In vivo mapping and quantification of creatine using chemical exchange saturation transfer imaging in rat models of epileptic seizure. Mol Imaging Biol. https://doi.org/10.1007/s11307-018-1243-6
30. Zhang S, Merritt M, Woessner DE, Lenkinski RE, Sherry AD (2003) PARACEST agents: modulating MRI contrast via water proton exchange. Acc Chem Res 36(10):783–790. https://doi.org/10.1021/ar020228m
31. Aime S, Carrera C, Delli Castelli D, Geninatti Crich S, Terreno E (2005) Tunable imaging of cells labeled with MRI-PARACEST agents. Angew Chem Int Ed Engl 44 (12):1813–1815. https://doi.org/10.1002/anie.200462566
32. Vinogradov E, Zhang S, Lubag A, Balschi JA, Sherry AD, Lenkinski RE (2005) On-resonance low B1 pulses for imaging of the effects of PARACEST agents. J Magn Reson 176(1):54–63. https://doi.org/10.1016/j.jmr.2005.05.016
33. Winter PM, Cai K, Chen J, Adair CR, Kiefer GE, Athey PS, Gaffney PJ, Buff CE, Robertson JD, Caruthers SD, Wickline SA, Lanza GM (2006) Targeted PARACEST nanoparticle contrast agent for the detection of fibrin. Magn Reson Med 56(6):1384–1388. https://doi.org/10.1002/mrm.21093
34. Yoo B, Raam MS, Rosenblum RM, Pagel MD (2007) Enzyme-responsive PARACEST MRI contrast agents: a new biomedical imaging approach for studies of the proteasome. Contrast Media Mol Imaging 2(4):189–198. https://doi.org/10.1002/cmmi.145
35. Sun PZ, van Zijl PC, Zhou J (2005) Optimization of the irradiation power in chemical exchange dependent saturation transfer experiments. J Magn Reson 175(2):193–200. https://doi.org/10.1016/j.jmr.2005.04.005
36. Woessner DE, Zhang S, Merritt ME, Sherry AD (2005) Numerical solution of the Bloch equations provides insights into the optimum design of PARACEST agents for MRI. Magn Reson Med 53(4):790–799. https://doi.org/10.1002/mrm.20408
37. Zaiss M, Bachert P (2013) Exchange-dependent relaxation in the rotating frame for slow and intermediate exchange – modeling off-resonant spin-lock and chemical exchange saturation transfer. NMR Biomed 26 (5):507–518
38. Zhou J, van Zijl PCM (2006) Chemical exchange saturation transfer imaging. Prog Nucl Magn Reson Spectrosc 48:109–136
39. Aime S, Calabi L, Biondi L, De Miranda M, Ghelli S, Paleari L, Rebaudengo C, Terreno E (2005) Iopamidol: exploring the potential use of a well-established x-ray contrast agent for MRI. Magn Reson Med 53(4):830–834. https://doi.org/10.1002/mrm.20441
40. Muller-Lutz A, Khalil N, Schmitt B, Jellus V, Pentang G, Oeltzschner G, Antoch G, Lanzman RS, Wittsack HJ (2014) Pilot study of Iopamidol-based quantitative pH imaging on a clinical 3T MR scanner. MAGMA 27 (6):477–485. https://doi.org/10.1007/s10334-014-0433-8
41. Sun PZ, Longo DL, Hu W, Xiao G, Wu R (2014) Quantification of iopamidol multi-site chemical exchange properties for ratiometric chemical exchange saturation transfer (CEST) imaging of pH. Phys Med Biol 59(16):4493
42. Longo DL, Sun PZ, Consolino L, Michelotti FC, Uggeri F, Aime S (2014) A general MRI-CEST ratiometric approach for pH imaging: demonstration of in vivo pH mapping with iobitridol. J Am Chem Soc 136 (41):14333–14336. https://doi.org/10.1021/ja5059313
43. Chen LQ, Howison CM, Jeffery JJ, Robey IF, Kuo PH, Pagel MD (2014) Evaluations of extracellular pH within in vivo tumors using acidoCEST MRI. Magn Reson Med 72 (5):1408–1417. https://doi.org/10.1002/mrm.25053
44. Randtke EA, Chen LQ, Corrales LR, Pagel MD (2014) The Hanes-Woolf linear QUESP method improves the measurements of fast chemical exchange rates with CEST MRI. Magn Reson Med 71(4):1603–1612. https://doi.org/10.1002/mrm.24792
45. Anemone A, Consolino L, Longo DL (2017) MRI-CEST assessment of tumour perfusion using X-ray iodinated agents: comparison with a conventional Gd-based agent. Eur Radiol 27 (5):2170–2179. https://doi.org/10.1007/s00330-016-4552-7

46. Longo DL, Michelotti F, Consolino L, Bardini P, Digilio G, Xiao G, Sun PZ, Aime S (2016) In vitro and in vivo assessment of nonionic iodinated radiographic molecules as chemical exchange saturation transfer magnetic resonance imaging tumor perfusion agents. Investig Radiol 51(3):155–162. https://doi.org/10.1097/RLI.0000000000000217
47. Longo DL, Bartoli A, Consolino L, Bardini P, Arena F, Schwaiger M, Aime S (2016) In vivo imaging of tumor metabolism and acidosis by combining PET and MRI-CEST pH imaging. Cancer Res 76(22):6463–6470. https://doi.org/10.1158/0008-5472.CAN-16-0825
48. Longo D, Aime S (2017) Iodinated contrast media as pH-responsive CEST agents. In: McMahon MT, Gilad AA, JBM B, PCM VZ (eds) Chemical exchange saturation transfer imaging. vol advances and applications. Pan Stanford Publishing, Singapore, pp 447–466. https://doi.org/10.1201/9781315364421-20
49. Longo DL, Busato A, Lanzardo S, Antico F, Aime S (2013) Imaging the pH evolution of an acute kidney injury model by means of iopamidol, a MRI-CEST pH-responsive contrast agent. Magn Reson Med 70(3):859–864. https://doi.org/10.1002/mrm.24513
50. Longo DL, Cutrin JC, Michelotti F, Irrera P, Aime S (2017) Noninvasive evaluation of renal pH homeostasis after ischemia reperfusion injury by CEST-MRI. NMR Biomed 30(7). https://doi.org/10.1002/nbm.3720
51. Jin T, Autio J, Obata T, Kim SG (2011) Spin-locking versus chemical exchange saturation transfer MRI for investigating chemical exchange process between water and labile metabolite protons. Magn Reson Med 65 (5):1448–1460. https://doi.org/10.1002/mrm.22721
52. Jiang W, Zhou IY, Wen L, Zhou X, Sun PZ (2016) A theoretical analysis of chemical exchange saturation transfer echo planar imaging (CEST-EPI) steady state solution and the CEST sensitivity efficiency-based optimization approach. Contrast Media Mol Imaging 11 (5):415–423. https://doi.org/10.1002/cmmi.1699
53. Ji Y, Zhou IY, Qiu BS, Sun PZ (2017) Progress toward quantitative in vivo chemical exchange saturation transfer (CEST) MRI. Israel J Chem 57(9):809–824. https://doi.org/10.1002/ijch.201700025
54. Kim J, Wu Y, Guo Y, Zheng H, Sun PZ (2015) A review of optimization and quantification techniques for chemical exchange saturation transfer MRI toward sensitive in vivo imaging. Contrast Media Mol Imaging 10(3):163–178. https://doi.org/10.1002/cmmi.1628
55. Liu G, Song X, Chan KW, McMahon MT (2013) Nuts and bolts of chemical exchange saturation transfer MRI. NMR Biomed 26 (7):810–828. https://doi.org/10.1002/nbm.2899
56. Sun PZ, Xiao G, Zhou IY, Guo Y, Wu R (2016) A method for accurate pH mapping with chemical exchange saturation transfer (CEST) MRI. Contrast Media Mol Imaging 11(3):195–202. https://doi.org/10.1002/cmmi.1680
57. Sun PZ, Sorensen AG (2008) Imaging pH using the chemical exchange saturation transfer (CEST) MRI: Correction of concomitant RF irradiation effects to quantify CEST MRI for chemical exchange rate and pH. Magn Reson Med 60(2):390–397. https://doi.org/10.1002/mrm.21653
58. Dixon WT, Ren J, Lubag AJ, Ratnakar J, Vinogradov E, Hancu I, Lenkinski RE, Sherry AD (2010) A concentration-independent method to measure exchange rates in PARACEST agents. Magn Reson Med 63 (3):625–632. https://doi.org/10.1002/mrm.22242
59. Yang X, Song X, Ray Banerjee S, Li Y, Byun Y, Liu G, Bhujwalla ZM, Pomper MG, McMahon MT (2016) Developing imidazoles as CEST MRI pH sensors. Contrast Media Mol Imaging 11(4):304–312. https://doi.org/10.1002/cmmi.1693
60. Kujawa A, Kim M, Demetriou E, Anemone A, Livio Longo D, Zaiss M, Golay X (2019) Assessment of a clinically feasible Bayesian fitting algorithm using a simplified description of Chemical Exchange Saturation Transfer (CEST) imaging. J Magn Reson 300:120–134. https://doi.org/10.1016/j.jmr.2019.01.006
61. Pavuluri K, Manoli I, Pass A, Li Y, Vernon HJ, Venditti CP, McMahon MT (2019) Noninvasive monitoring of chronic kidney disease using pH and perfusion imaging. Sci Adv. https://doi.org/10.1126/sciadv.aaw8357
62. Sun PZ (2012) Simplified quantification of labile proton concentration-weighted chemical exchange rate (kws) with RF saturation time dependent ratiometric analysis (QUESTRA): normalization of relaxation and RF irradiation spillover effects for improved quantitative chemical exchange saturation transfer (CEST) MRI. Magn Reson Med 67(4):936–942

63. Ward KM, Balaban RS (2000) Determination of pH using water protons and chemical exchange dependent saturation transfer (CEST). Magn Reson Med 44(5):799–802
64. Wu R, Longo DL, Aime S, Sun PZ (2015) Quantitative description of radiofrequency (RF) power-based ratiometric chemical exchange saturation transfer (CEST) pH imaging. NMR Biomed 28(5):555–565. https://doi.org/10.1002/nbm.3284
65. Arena F, Irrera P, Consolino L, Colombo Serra S, Zaiss M, Longo DL (2018) Flip-angle based ratiometric approach for pulsed CEST-MRI pH imaging. J Magn Reson 287:1–9. https://doi.org/10.1016/j.jmr.2017.12.007
66. Anemone A, Consolino L, Arena F, Capozza M, Longo DL (2019) Imaging tumor acidosis: a survey of the available techniques for mapping in vivo tumor pH. Cancer Metastasis Rev. https://doi.org/10.1007/s10555-019-09782-9
67. Anemone A, Consolino L, Conti L, Reineri F, Cavallo F, Aime S, Longo DL (2017) In vivo evaluation of tumour acidosis for assessing the early metabolic response and onset of resistance to dichloroacetate by using magnetic resonance pH imaging. Int J Oncol 51(2):498–506. https://doi.org/10.3892/ijo.2017.4029
68. Sheth VR, Li Y, Chen LQ, Howison CM, Flask CA, Pagel MD (2012) Measuring in vivo tumor pHe with CEST-FISP MRI. Magn Reson Med 67(3):760–768. https://doi.org/10.1002/mrm.23038
69. Longo DL, Dastru W, Digilio G, Keupp J, Langereis S, Lanzardo S, Prestigio S, Steinbach O, Terreno E, Uggeri F, Aime S (2011) Iopamidol as a responsive MRI-chemical exchange saturation transfer contrast agent for pH mapping of kidneys: in vivo studies in mice at 7 T. Magn Reson Med 65(1):202–211. https://doi.org/10.1002/mrm.22608
70. Zhou IY, Wang E, Cheung JS, Zhang X, Fulci G, Sun PZ (2017) Quantitative chemical exchange saturation transfer (CEST) MRI of glioma using Image Downsampling Expedited Adaptive Least-squares (IDEAL) fitting. Sci Rep 7(1):84. https://doi.org/10.1038/s41598-017-00167-y
71. Li AX, Hudson RH, Barrett JW, Jones CK, Pasternak SH, Bartha R (2008) Four-pool modeling of proton exchange processes in biological systems in the presence of MRI-paramagnetic chemical exchange saturation transfer (PARACEST) agents. Magn Reson Med 60(5):1197–1206. https://doi.org/10.1002/mrm.21752
72. Zhou IY, Fuss TL, Igarashi T, Jiang W, Zhou X, Cheng LL, Sun PZ (2016) Tissue characterization with quantitative high-resolution magic angle spinning chemical exchange saturation transfer Z-spectroscopy. Anal Chem 88(21):10379–10383. https://doi.org/10.1021/acs.analchem.6b03137
73. Xu J, Zaiss M, Zu Z, Li H, Xie J, Gochberg DF, Bachert P, Gore JC (2014) On the origins of chemical exchange saturation transfer (CEST) contrast in tumors at 9.4 T. NMR Biomed 27(4):406–416
74. Zaiss M, Xu J, Goerke S, Khan IS, Singer RJ, Gore JC, Gochberg DF, Bachert P (2014) Inverse Z-spectrum analysis for spillover-, MT-, and T1-corrected steady-state pulsed CEST-MRI—application to pH-weighted MRI of acute stroke. NMR Biomed 27(3):240–252. https://doi.org/10.1002/nbm.3054
75. Kim M, Gillen J, Landman BA, Zhou J, van Zijl PC (2009) Water saturation shift referencing (WASSR) for chemical exchange saturation transfer (CEST) experiments. Magn Reson Med 61(6):1441–1450. https://doi.org/10.1002/mrm.21873
76. Wei W, Jia G, Flanigan D, Zhou J, Knopp MV (2014) Chemical exchange saturation transfer MR imaging of articular cartilage glycosaminoglycans at 3 T: accuracy of B0 field inhomogeneity corrections with gradient echo method. Magn Reson Imaging 32(1):41–47. https://doi.org/10.1016/j.mri.2013.07.009
77. Sun PZ, Farrar CT, Sorensen AG (2007) Correction for artifacts induced by B(0) and B(1) field inhomogeneities in pH-sensitive chemical exchange saturation transfer (CEST) imaging. Magn Reson Med 58(6):1207–1215. https://doi.org/10.1002/mrm.21398
78. Stancanello J, Terreno E, Castelli DD, Cabella C, Uggeri F, Aime S (2008) Development and validation of a smoothing-splines-based correction method for improving the analysis of CEST-MR images. Contrast Media Mol Imaging 3(4):136–149. https://doi.org/10.1002/cmmi.240
79. Terreno E, Stancanello J, Longo D, Castelli DD, Milone L, Sanders HM, Kok MB, Uggeri F, Aime S (2009) Methods for an improved detection of the MRI-CEST effect.

Contrast Media Mol Imaging 4(5):237–247. https://doi.org/10.1002/cmmi.290

80. Wu Y, Zhou IY, Igarashi T, Longo DL, Aime S, Sun PZ (2018) A generalized ratiometric chemical exchange saturation transfer (CEST) MRI approach for mapping renal pH using iopamidol. Magn Reson Med 79(3):1553–1558. https://doi.org/10.1002/mrm.26817
81. Raghunand N, Howison C, Sherry AD, Zhang S, Gillies RJ (2003) Renal and systemic pH imaging by contrast-enhanced MRI. Magn Reson Med 49(2):249–257. https://doi.org/10.1002/mrm.10347

14

Subsegmentation of the Kidney in Experimental MR Images using Morphology-Based Regions-of-Interest or Multiple-Layer Concentric Objects

Leili Riazy, Bastien Milani, João S. Periquito, Kathleen Cantow, Thoralf Niendorf, Menno Pruijm, Erdmann Seeliger, and Andreas Pohlmann

Abstract

Functional renal MRI promises access to a wide range of physiologically relevant parameters such as blood oxygenation, perfusion, tissue microstructure, pH, and sodium concentration. For quantitative comparison of results, representative values must be extracted from the parametric maps obtained with these different MRI techniques. To improve reproducibility of results this should be done based on regions-of-interest (ROIs) that are clearly and objectively defined.

Semiautomated subsegmentation of the kidney in magnetic resonance images represents a simple but very valuable approach for the quantitative analysis of imaging parameters in multiple ROIs that are associated with specific anatomic locations. Thereby, it facilitates comparing MR parameters between different kidney regions, as well as tracking changes over time.

Here we provide detailed step-by-step instructions for two recently developed subsegmentation techniques that are suitable for kidneys of small rodents: i) the placement of ROIs in cortex, outer and the inner medulla based on typical kidney morphology and ii) the division of the kidney into concentrically oriented layers.

This chapter is based upon work from the COST Action PARENCHIMA, a community-driven network funded by the European Cooperation in Science and Technology (COST) program of the European Union, which aims to improve the reproducibility and standardization of renal MRI biomarkers.

Key words Magnetic resonance imaging (MRI), Kidney, Mice, Rats, Segmentation, ROI

1 Introduction

The potential of magnetic resonance imaging (MRI) for the diagnosis and monitoring of renal disease remains largely untapped. Functional renal MRI promises access to a wide range of (patho)-physiologically relevant parameters via techniques such as blood oxygenation sensitive T_2*-mapping (aka blood oxygenation level-dependent MRI, BOLD), perfusion measurement by arterial spin labeling (ASL), and diffusion weighted imaging (DWI). Insights into microstructural changes can be obtained with DWI and T_1-mapping, for example to probe for renal fibrosis. Emerging techniques including pH-mapping via chemical exchange saturation transfer (CEST) and sodium (^{23}Na) imaging complement the renal MRI portfolio. For quantitative comparison of results, representative values must be extracted from the parametric maps obtained with any of these MRI techniques. To improve reproducibility of results this should be done based on regions-of-interest (ROIs) that are clearly and objectively defined.

Semiautomated subsegmentation of the kidney in MRI represents a simple but very valuable approach for the quantitative analysis of imaging parameters in multiple ROIs that are associated with specific anatomic locations, for example, the distinct layers: cortex, outer medulla, and inner medulla. Thereby, it facilitates comparing MR parameters between different kidney regions, as well as tracking changes over time. Here we use the term *subsegmentation* in order to make a clear distinction between segmenting the kidney into smaller subregions and the identification of the kidney organ borders within an image, for which commonly the term *segmentation* is used.

In this chapter we provide detailed step-by-step instructions for two recently proposed subsegmentation techniques [1, 2], which are suitable for kidneys of small rodents: (1) the placement of ROIs in cortex, outer and the inner medulla based on typical kidney morphology (used in [1, 3–8]) and (2) the division of the kidney into concentrically oriented layers (used in [2, 9–13]). They work independent of the actual image contrasts or parameter map values and hence are well suited for a wide range of MRI mapping techniques. Both techniques allow for the exclusion of one or several regions in the kidney from the analysis, for example regions that show obvious image artefacts. Changes in kidney size are accommodated for by both techniques, but results should be treated with due caution if the relative sizes of the renal layers are significantly different from naive healthy kidneys or change throughout the experiment.

The first method described here is the *Segmentation of Morphology-Based Renal Regions-of-Interest* (SOMBRERO) [1]. Quantitative histomorphological data on the dimensions of the renal layers were obtained from a number of freshly excised kidneys of adult male rats, where anatomical structures were identified to be distributed in certain proportions. The percentages referring to the corresponding locations exclude the rather broad (and in case of the cortical–medullary border zone undulating) transition regions among the layers that are prone to partial volume effects. The percentages are adapted to MRI images by determining a standardized location, length, width and angle of the kidney in the image. Subsequently, ROIs at anatomical locations such as the cortex, outer medulla, and inner medulla are returned automatically in form of masks. These masks can then easily be applied to the user's parameter maps.

The strength of this technique is that it creates ROIs whose positions have been carefully chosen to provide representative values for the renal cortex, outer medulla and inner medulla, leaving a generous "buffer zone" at the transition regions between the renal layers. Also, access to five (or three) ROIs in each layer allow assessment of inter-layer and intra-layer variability. Differences between the parameters in the three renal layers can be expressed as ratios, such as $T_2*(cortex)/T_2*(outer\ medulla)$. The transition regions between the renal layers are not accessible with this approach at present, but such a feature could be included without difficulty in the future, even by the user. ROI locations have been defined for rat kidneys in coronal view (with respect to the kidney). However, this method is in principle applicable to mouse and rat kidneys in axial, sagittal, and coronal view. An extension to other orientations or mice would only require some additional careful morphometric measurements to define the relative ROI positions.

The second technique is the *multiple-layer concentric objects* segmentation (MLCO; for human MRI proposed as 12-layer concentric objects, TLCO) [2, 9]. A series of concentrically oriented layers is generated after a manual retracing of the outline of the kidney in the respective MR image. The desired number of concentric objects (COs) can be freely chosen by the user, although most publications have used twelve layers in humans thus far.

This technique was developed for human kidney MRI; although the COs do not refer to specific anatomic locations, they approximately reflect the layered structure of the kidney through their concentric nature. This makes it suited for MRI of rodent kidneys, whose simpler anatomic structure is better represented by the concentric layers than that of the human kidney. While the outermost and innermost COs are straightforward to interpret and are generally considered as a proxy of respectively cortex and medulla, a clear association of the intermediate concentric objects with the renal layers remains challenging, in particular, because the broad transition zones and, thereby, probable partial volume effects are neglected. Differences between the parameters in the three renal layers can only be indirectly expressed by the slope of the curve when plotting the COs' mean values against their position. This technique is applicable to mouse and rat kidneys in axial, sagittal, and coronal view (with respect to the kidney). One of its strengths is its applicability to human kidneys. A direct comparison between human results and those from rodent kidneys would, however, require a carefully calibrated conversion, due to the morphological differences.

Notwithstanding their limitations, both kidney subsegmentation techniques are very valuable semiautomated tools for the quantitative analysis of imaging parameters, specifically for comparing MR parameters between groups, between different kidney regions and monitoring changes over time. Use of these objectively defined ROIs (rather than manually drawn ROIs) should help to improve reproducibility and comparability of results in future studies.

This chapter is part of the book Pohlmann A, Niendorf T (eds) (2020) Preclinical MRI of the Kidney—Methods and Protocols. Springer, New York.

2 Materials

2.1 Software Requirements

2.1.1 Essential Tools

The SOMBRERO method is provided in Python (3.6) programming language. It has been implemented and tested using the following software, which is available for macOS 10.14.5 (used for development), Windows and Linux operating systems.

1. Spyder 3.2.4, installed through Anaconda (https://www.anaconda.com), which is open-source.

   The MLCO method requires the following software:

2. The MATLAB® programming environment (MathWorks, Natick, MA, USA, https://www.mathworks.com/products/matlab.html). It may also be possible to use the open-source alternative Octave (https://www.gnu.org/software/octave/), but this has not been tested and may require some adaptations in the MLCO toolbox.

2.1.2 Toolboxes

The provided software for SOMBRERO requires the installation of the following packages: *numpy*, *matplotlib*, *cv2*, *math*, *pydicom*, *os*, and *pickle*.

These can be conveniently installed one-by-one through the *Anaconda Navigator* for Windows. For Linux or MacOS the following line in the terminal will install all them at once:

```
pip install numpy matplotlib cv2 math pydicom os pickle
```

2.1.3 Software

SOMBRERO: The software is provided online at GitHub: https://github.com/lriazy/sombrero/

MLCO: The software is provided online at GitHub: https://github.com/bmilani/conObj

2.2 Source Data: Format Requirements

2.2.1 Imaging Planes

Common MRI imaging planes are sagittal, coronal, and axial slices as displayed in Fig. 1. For the sake of this tutorial we will focus on coronal slices. Other imaging planes are possible for these segmentations as well (*see* **Note 1**).

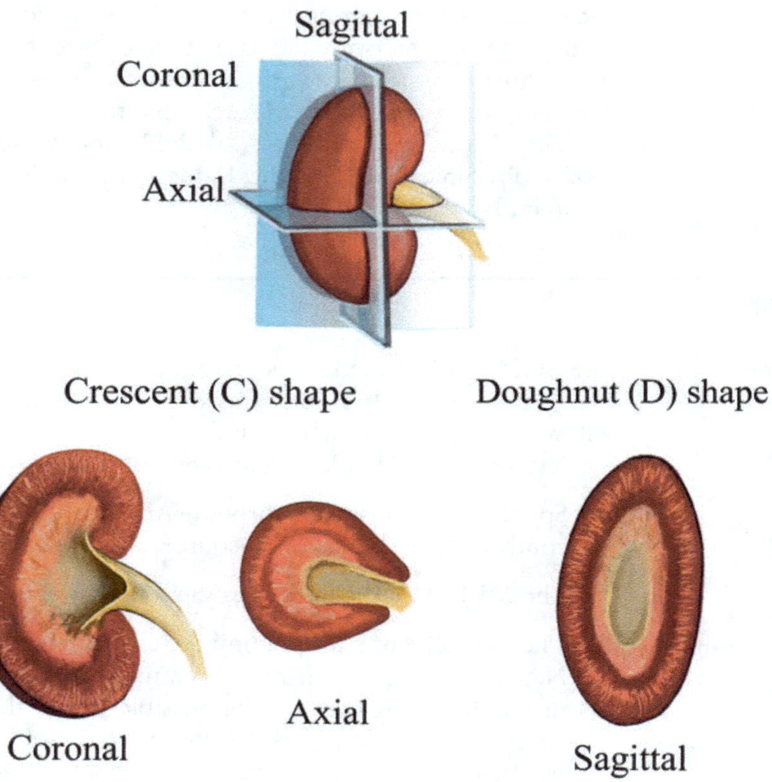

Fig. 1 Typical MR imaging planes and their resulting kidney shapes. The coronal, axial, and sagittal planes do not correspond to the scanner coordinate system, but instead are defined with respect to the double-oblique spatial orientation of the kidney. "C" stands for crescent and "D" doughnut

2.2.2 Input Requirements

In this chapter, all input files are assumed to be Dicoms. However, any way to import an image as a matrix to Matlab or NumPy array to Python will work equivalently.

3 Methods

3.1 Segmentation of Morphology-Based Renal Regions-of-Interest (SOMBRERO)

3.1.1 Settings

In order to display interactive plots, make sure your graphics backend is set on "automatic."

This can be looked up in Preferences > IPython console > Graphics > Graphics backend.

3.1.2 Loading Images

1. Open the script roirect.py, which is executed cell-by-cell. Running a cell can be done by a button or by pressing CTRL + ENTER.
2. The images are loaded by the line:

```
im = pydicom.dcmread('EnIm1.dcm')
```

in the script. Modify 'EnIm1.dcm' to be the path to your dicom file. In this case, the file is located in the same directory as the script. Therefore the filename is sufficient.

3.1.3 Definition of Bounding Box

1. Execute the first cell in `roirect.py`.
2. Drag on the image to draw a new rectangle (Fig. 2a).
3. Use the edge markers to adjust the height and width of the rectangle
4. Shift the rectangle using the central marker.

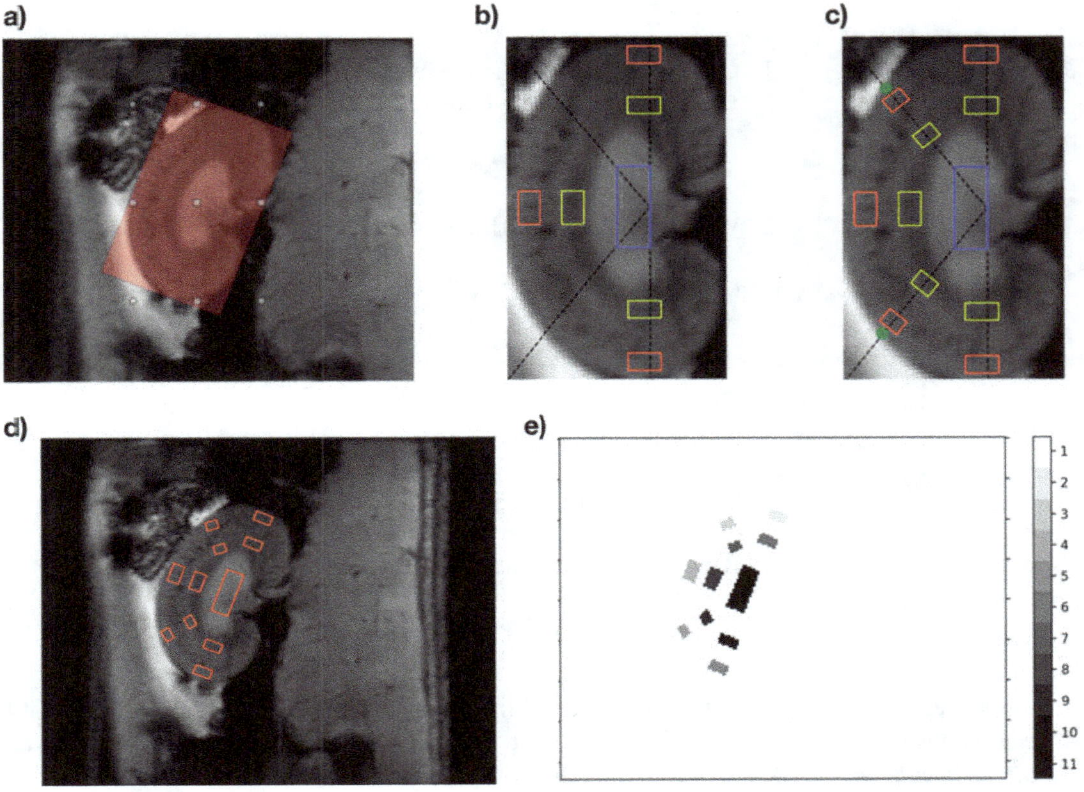

Fig. 2 (**a**) Manual selection of the kidney with the rectangle tool. (**b**) Cropped and straightened kidney image with reference lines. The red boxes are located in the cortex, the yellow box in the outer medulla and the blue box in the inner medulla. (**c**) Display of the successful selection of two border points (in green) at the intersection of the kidney border and the diagonal line. (**d**) The ROIs after transformation to the locations in the original image (without cropping or other processing). (**e**) The final mask of ROIs as an image of the same size as the original image with coded regional masks

5. Tip the rectangle using one of the edge markers (Note: A finer adjustment of the angle can be done by pressing the UP and DOWN buttons).
6. Press ENTER to end the adjustments and proceed.

3.1.4 Diagonal Boundary Selection

1. A new window opens up automatically (Fig. 2b).
2. Mark two points marking the end of the kidney on the black diagonal lines.
3. The resulting image should look like Fig. 2c).

3.1.5 Generation of Mask for Imaging Series

1. Execute the next section to transform the morphologic ROIs back to their locations in the original image (Fig. 2d).
2. Execute the next section to generate and visualize the variable roimask, which contains numbered masks for each ROI (Fig. 2e).

3.1.6 Saving Mask

1. Generate a path to the file by connecting the path (`path=''` and `filename=1` will save the file `1.pickle` in the current folder).

```
pfile = os.path.join(path,filename+'pickle')
```

2. Write the file using the following commands:

```
with open(pfile,'wb') as f:
pickle.dump([S, roimask], f)
```

3.1.7 Loading Mask

1. Generate a path to the file by connecting the path just as in saving the file:

```
pfile = os.path.join(path,filename+'pickle')
```

2. Read the file into the variables `S` and `roimask`:

```
S, roimask = pickle.load(open(pfile,"rb"))
```

3.2 Multilayer Concentric Objects (MLCO) Segmentation

Given the character of in-house developed programs, the MLCO toolbox allows the user the freedom and obligation to specify all details exactly. Subheadings 3.2.1–3.2.4 describe essential steps, where any of the proposed options have to be chosen. Finally, Subheading 3.2.5 shows an example for each choice made as in the preceding sections and composes a script, which is ready to run.

3.2.1 Load an Image or a List of Images in a Matlab Array

1. Open the matlab script called demo_script.m.
2. Note that you can execute a cell of a matlab script by pressing CTRL + ENTER.

3. Load a list of images by executing for example the following line:

```
myImageList=conObjDicomRead('Dir','C:\Users\conObj\myGRE\');
```

4. This loads the image list stored in C:\Users\conObj\myGRE\.
5. The variable `myImageList`, is now a three-dimensional array containing a list of matrices that each corresponds to a gray scale image.
6. You can visualize this image list by executing the line

```
conObjImage(myImageList);
```

This function plots the first image in the image stack. If you would like to display the mean of all images. The file has to be opened and modified. Line 41 has to be modified from

```
imagesc(argIm(:,:,curImNum));
```

to

```
imagesc(mean(argIm(:,:,:),3))
```

7. You can navigate through the images with the up and down arrow of your keyboard.

3.2.2 Defining the Number of Layers

In order to realize the concentric object technique, you have to choose a mask-number, which is the number of masks that will patch the chosen segmented area of you images. We also call this number the "number of layers" and we gave the name `nLayers` to this number in our script (*see* **Note 2**). If you want 9 layers, execute the line

```
nLayers=9;
```

The number of layers is inevitably limited by the image resolution. For experimental MR, 9 layers are recommended, whereas MR images of human kidneys were usually divided into 12 layers.

3.2.3 Segmenting the Area of Your Choice in the Image

In the following, the segmentation of "C"-shaped kidney slices from MR images will be described. This applies to coronal (Fig. 3) and axial (Fig. 4) slices as shown in Fig. 1.

1. Execute the line

```
[myBound_ext,myBound_int]=conObjBound_C(myImageList);
```

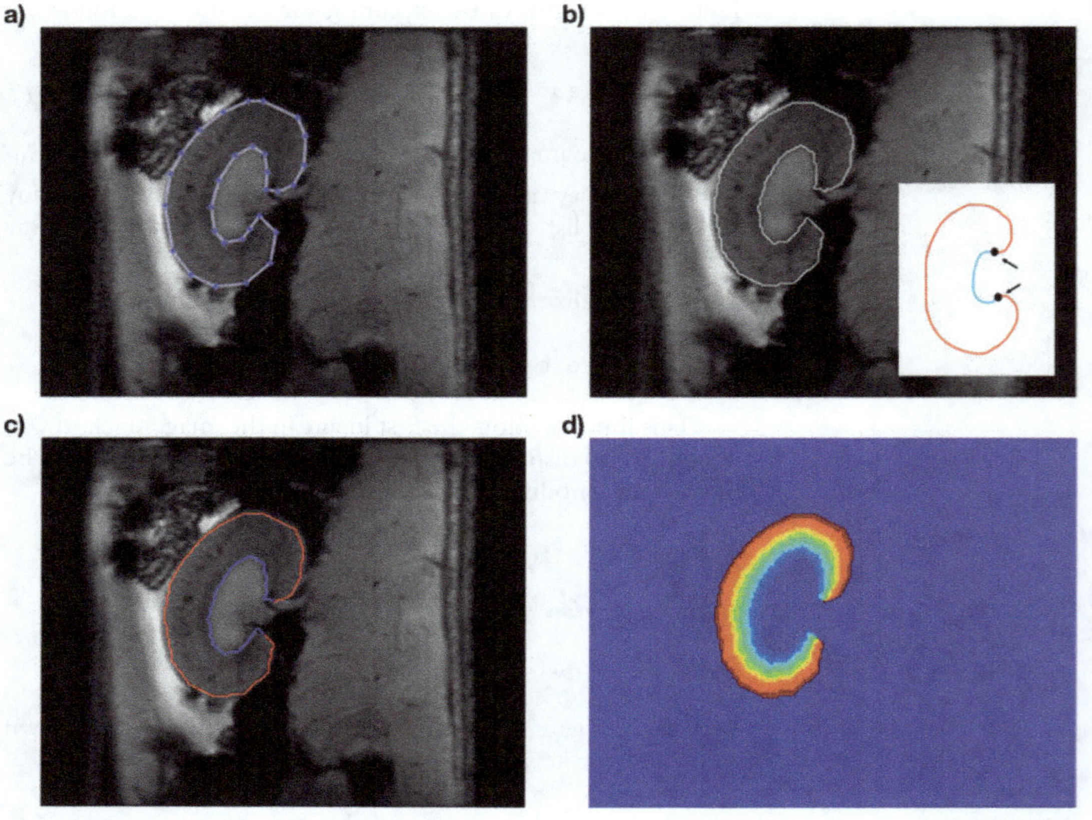

Fig. 3 (**a**) Closed manual contour of the kidney. Modification of the contour at the blue points is still possible at this stage. (**b**) The contour of the kidney turns white, after the contour is finished. The required input of two points describe the inner and outer borders. (**c**) After the two points have been entered, the inner and outer contour can be automatically separated into blue and red contours. (**d**) Output of the finished MLCO procedure

2. A matlab figure appears displaying the first image stored in myImageList.
3. Navigate through the images with the up and down arrow of your keyboard.
4. Adjust the contrast by pressing on CTRL+D and fix the change by pressing on CTRL+F.
5. By clicking on the picture, you can manually segment the area of your choice (Fig. 3a).
6. Note that pressing the key ESC allows you to reset your selection. You can also zoom in the picture with the available Matlab tools. If any problem appears during this manual segmentation, pressing the key ESC often solves the problem!
7. Double click on the picture to close the polygon. You can still modify the position of its vertices interactively on the picture (Fig. 3a).

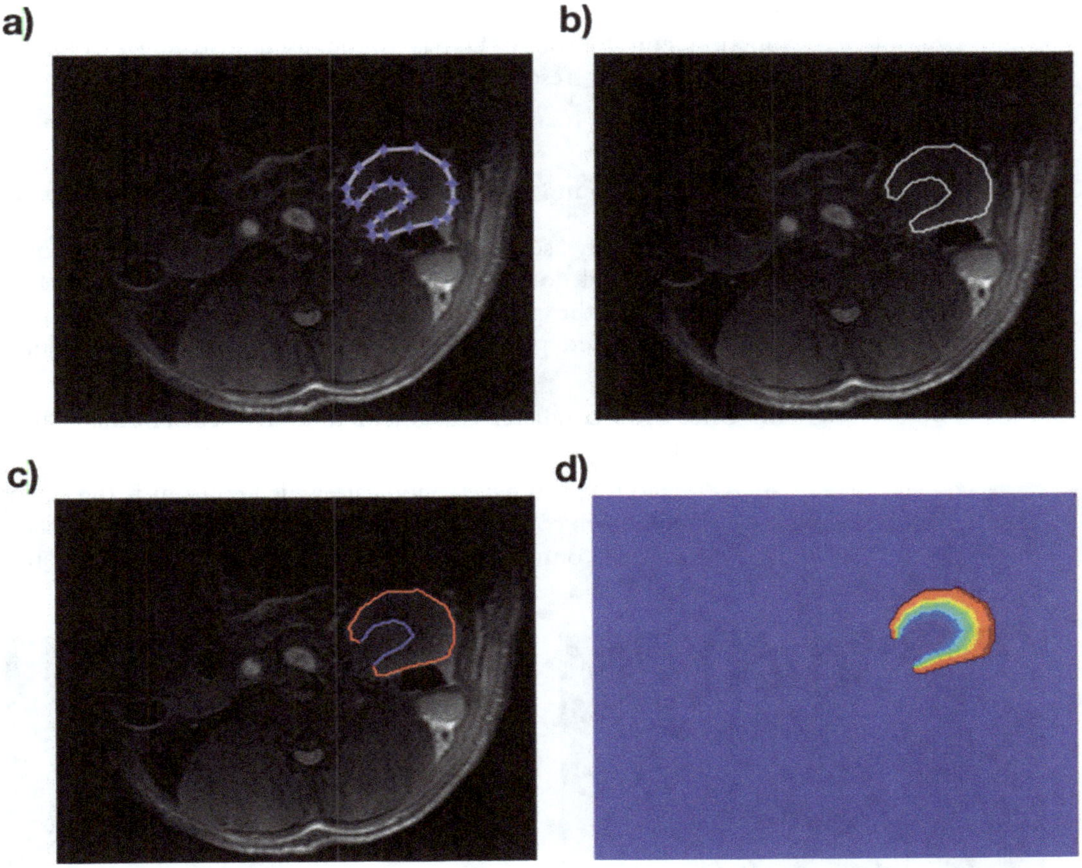

Fig. 4 (**a**) Manual contouring of the outer kidney boundary in the MLCO method. (**b**) The contour of the kidney turns white, after the contour is finished. (**c**) After the two points have been entered, the inner and outer contour can be automatically separated into blue and red contours. (**d**) Output of the finished MLCO procedure

8. When you are finished, double-click inside the polygon.
9. The contour of your segmentation will now appear in white (Fig. 3b).
10. Click near the white line at two different locations to indicate where the separation between the inner part and the outer part of the contour should occur. (Note: You do not need to press exactly on the white line because the program will choose the location on the white line that is the closest to your click.) (Fig. 3b)
11. The inner and outer part of the contour appear now in blue and red respectively (Fig. 3c).
12. You can now close the figure. The polygon of the outer contour is now stored in the variable myBound_ext and the polygon of the inner contour is now stored in myBound_int.

The same procedure can be applied for axial slices (Fig. 4). We describe in the following how to segment an area that contains a hole. The procedure is very similar to the previous one but the function conObjBound_D has to be used instead of conObjBound_C (C for crescent and D for doughnut).

1. First execute the line

```
[myBound_ext,myBound_int] = conObjBound_D(myImageList);
```

2. As previously, segment manually the area of your choice (Fig. 5a) and double-click in the polygon to validate it. The contour of the polygon is now white and you can choose another closed polygon that has to lie inside the first one (Fig. 5b).
3. Once the second area is segmented, double-click inside it such that its polygon also appears in white (Fig. 5c).
4. As previously, you have to indicate which contour is the outer one and which contour is the inner one. For that purpose, click first near the outer contour and then click near the inner one.

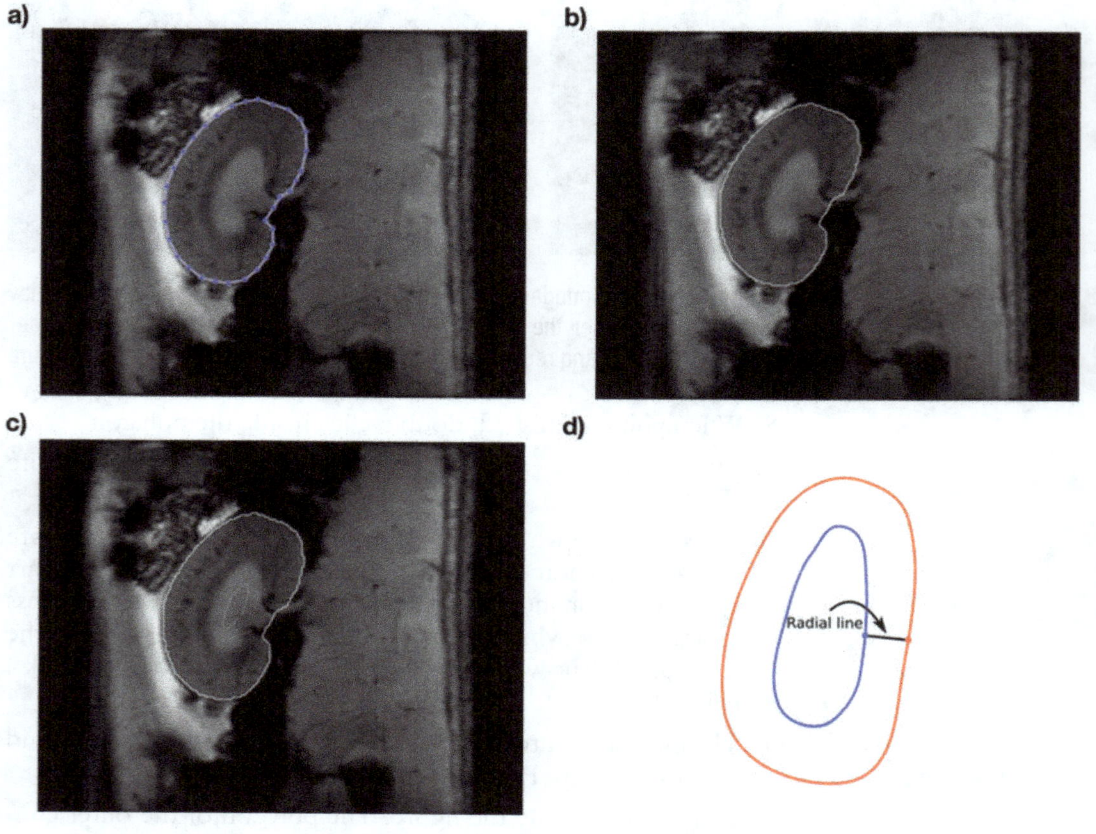

Fig. 5 (**a**) Outer contour for the "D"-shaped kidneys. (**b**) Entered contour in white. (**c**) Inner contour added manually, which is different from the previous "C"-shape procedure. (**d**) The required input of two points describe a radial line

But the two location you click on must be approximately on the same radial line (as on Fig. 5d) to allow the algorithm to work correctly.

5. Once the two location are chosen, the outer and inner contour appear in red and blue respectively (Fig. 6a). This closes the step of the segmentation.

3.2.4 Build the List of Masks That Realizes the Concentric Object Technique

1. Execute the following line:

```
myCO_mask = conObjMask(myImageList, myBound_ext ,
myBound_int,.nLayers);
```

2. You can visualize the masks with the command

```
conObjImage(myCO_mask);
```

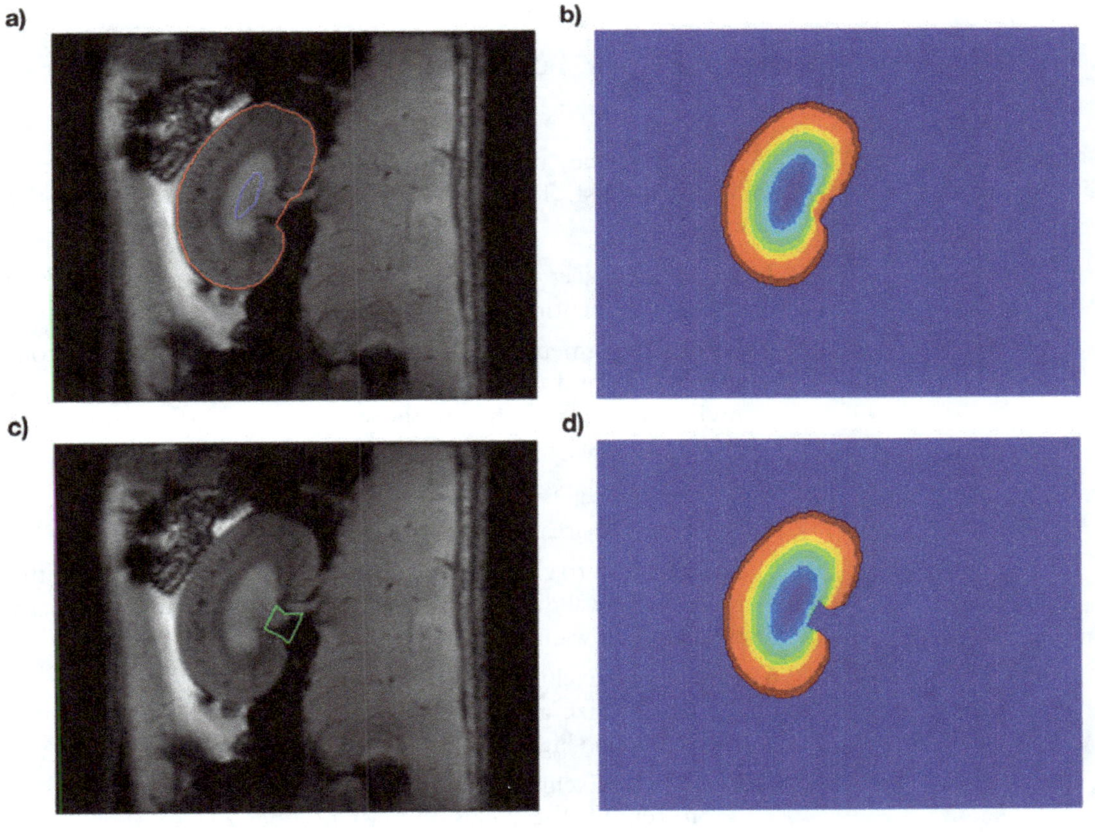

Fig. 6 (**a**) Inner and outer contour can again be identified after two points are entered. (**b**) The finished output from the MLCO method for "D"-shaped kidneys. (**c**) Exclusion of regions. (**d**) Result from MLCO method after excluding the regions specified in (**c**)

3. Browse through the different masks with the up and down arrow of the keyboard. Alternatively, you can visualize the list of masks by executing

```
conObjMaskImage(myCO_mask)
```

or

```
conObjMaskImage(myCO_mask,'jet')
```

The last line results for example in Figs. 3d and 4d for the segmentation in the crescent shape and in Fig. 6b) for the segmentation in the doughnut shape.

3.2.5 Basic Script for Applying the Concentric Object Technique

Assuming the location of the images to be in the folder 'C:\Users\conObj\myGRE\', a basic script could look as follows:

```
myImageList = conObjDicomRead('Dir' ,'C:\Users\con-Obj\myGRE\');

[myBound_ext,myBound_int] = conObjBound_C(myImageList);

myCO_mask = conObjMask(myImageList, myBound_ext ,
myBound_int,... nLayers);
```

3.2.6 Exclusion of Regions

This part describes multiple possibilities, which are optional for modifying the list. The only steps required are the first and the second.

1. Create an object of the class conObjExclusion.m in the *conObj* folder by executing: myExclusion = conObjExclusion;
2. Manually segment some region of the image to exclude from the analysis and to store these exclusion regions in the object myExclusion. For that purpose, execute: myExclusion.stack (myImageList);
3. A figure appears.
4. Segment the area of your choice.
5. Double-click to close the polygon and double-click again in the polygon to validate it. (You can execute **steps 2–5** as many times as you want to add new exclusion regions.)
6. Execute myExclusion.show(myImageList);
   to visualize all the exclusion mask that are in the object myExclusion (Fig. 6c).
7. Execute myExclusion.remove[2];
   to remove the exclusion mask number 2.
8. Execute myExclusion.clear;
   to empty the object `myExclusion`.

9. To construct a new list of masks from the previous list of masks myCO_mask but excluding the region stored in the object myExclusion, simply execute

```
myCO_mask_new=myExclusion.crop(myCO_mask);
```

10. The new list of masks myCO_mask_new can be displayed by executing the following line

```
conObjMaskImage(myCO_mask_new);
```

which results in Fig. 6d.

4 Notes

1. The orientation of the kidney was assumed to be coronal throughout this chapter. However, the MLCO method does not refer to specific anatomical locations and can therefore be used in any of the cases displayed in Fig. 1. The SOMBRERO method can potentially be used in other planes as well but would need new percentage values from kidney histology as a reference.
2. For human renal MRI the use of 12 layers was proposed [2]. For rats and mice another number of layers may be more suitable. This also depends on the spatial resolution that can be achieved with that particular MRI technique and available hardware, because it would probably not make much sense to have layers with a width of less than one (noninterpolated) pixel. As a default we recommend to use the proposed number of 12 layers.

Acknowledgments

This work was funded in part (Kathleen Cantow, Erdmann Seeliger, Thoralf Niendorf, Andreas Pohlmann, Joao Periquito) by the German Research Foundation (Gefoerdert durch die Deutsche Forschungsgemeinschaft (DFG), Projektnummer 394046635, SFB 1365, RENOPROTECTION . Funded by the Deutsche Forschungsgemeinschaft (DFG, German Research Foundation), Project number 394046635, SFB 1365, RENOPROTECTION).
This chapter is based upon work from COST Action PARENCH IMA, supported by European Cooperation in Science and Technology (COST). COST (www.cost.eu) is a funding agency for research and innovation networks. COST Actions help connect research initiatives across Europe and enable scientists to enrich their ideas by sharing them with their peers. This boosts their research, career, and innovation.

PARENCHIMA (renalmri.org) is a community-driven Action in the COST program of the European Union, which unites more than 200 experts in renal MRI from 30 countries with the aim to improve the reproducibility and standardization of renal MRI biomarkers.

References

1. Pohlmann A, Cantow K, Huelnhagen T, Grosenick D, Periquito S, Boehmert L, Gladytz T, Waiczies S, Flemming B, Seeliger E, Niendorf T (2017) Experimental MRI monitoring of renal blood volume fraction variations en route to renal magnetic resonance oximetry. Tomography 3:188–200. https://doi.org/10.18383/j.tom.2017.00012
2. Milani B, Ansaloni A, Sousa-Guimaraes S, Vakilzadeh N, Piskunowicz M, Vogt B, Stuber M, Burnier M, Pruijm M (2016) Reduction of cortical oxygenation in chronic kidney disease: evidence obtained with a new analysis method of blood oxygenation level-dependent magnetic resonance imaging. Nephrol Dial Transplant 32:2097–2105. https://doi.org/10.1093/ndt/gfw362
3. Pohlmann A, Hentschel J, Fechner M, Hoff U, Bubalo G, Arakelyan K, Cantow K, Seeliger E, Flemming B, Waiczies H (2013) High temporal resolution parametric MRI monitoring of the initial ischemia/reperfusion phase in experimental acute kidney injury. PLoS One 8: e57411
4. Arakelyan K, Cantow K, Hentschel J, Flemming B, Pohlmann A, Ladwig M, Niendorf T, Seeliger E (2013) Early effects of an x-ray contrast medium on renal T2*/T2 MRI as compared to short-term hyperoxia, hypoxia and aortic occlusion in rats. Acta Physiol 208:202–213
5. Pohlmann A, Arakelyan K, Hentschel J, Cantow K, Flemming B, Ladwig M, Waiczies S, Seeliger E, Niendorf T (2014) Detailing the relation between renal T2* and renal tissue pO2 using an integrated approach of parametric magnetic resonance imaging and invasive physiological measurements. Invest Radiol 49:547–560
6. Pohlmann A, Arakelyan K, Seeliger E, Niendorf T (2016) Magnetic resonance imaging (MRI) analysis of ischemia/reperfusion in experimental acute renal injury. In: Kidney research. Springer, New York, NY, pp 113–127
7. Cantow K, Arakelyan K, Seeliger E, Niendorf T, Pohlmann A (2016) Assessment of renal hemodynamics and oxygenation by simultaneous magnetic resonance imaging (MRI) and quantitative invasive physiological measurements. In: Kidney research. Springer, New York, NY, pp 129–154
8. Hoff U, Bubalo G, Fechner M, Blum M, Zhu Y, Pohlmann A, Hentschel J, Arakelyan K, Seeliger E, Flemming B (2019) A synthetic epoxyeicosatrienoic acid analogue prevents the initiation of ischemic acute kidney injury. Acta Physiol 227(2):e13297
9. Piskunowicz M, Hofmann L, Zuercher E, Bassi I, Milani B, Stuber M, Narkiewicz K, Vogt B, Burnier M, Pruijm M (2015) A new technique with high reproducibility to estimate renal oxygenation using BOLD-MRI in chronic kidney disease. Magn Reson Imaging 33:253–261. https://doi.org/10.1016/j.mri.2014.12.002
10. Ponikowski P, Voors AA, Anker SD, Bueno H, Cleland JGF, Coats AJS, Falk V, González-Juanatey JR, Harjola V-P, Jankowska EA, Jessup M, Linde C, Nihoyannopoulos P, Parissis JT, Pieske B, Riley JP, Rosano GMC, Ruilope LM, Ruschitzka F et al (2016) 2016 ESC guidelines for the diagnosis and treatment of acute and chronic heart failure. Eur J Heart Fail 18:891–975. https://doi.org/10.1002/ejhf.592
11. Vakilzadeh N, Muller M-E, Forni V, Milani B, Hoffman L, Piskunowicz M, Maillard M, Zweiacker C, Pruijm M, Burnier M (2015) Comparative effect of a renin inhibitor and a thiazide diuretic on renal tissue oxygenation in hypertensive patients. Kidney Blood Press Res 40:542–554. https://doi.org/10.1159/000368530
12. Pruijm M, Milani B, Pivin E, Podhajska A, Vogt B, Stuber M, Burnier M (2018) Reduced cortical oxygenation predicts a progressive decline of renal function in patients with chronic kidney disease. Kidney Int

93:932–940. https://doi.org/10.1016/j.kint.2017.10.020

13. Vakilzadeh N, Zanchi A, Milani B, Ledoux J-B, Braconnier P, Burnier M, Pruijm M (2019) Acute hyperglycemia increases renal tissue oxygenation as measured by BOLD-MRI in healthy overweight volunteers. Diabetes Res Clin Pract 150:138–143. https://doi.org/10.1016/j.diabres.2019.03.009

15

Analysis Protocols for MRI Mapping of Renal T_1

Philippe Garteiser, Gwenaël Pagé, Sabrina Doblas, Octavia Bane, Stefanie Hectors, Iris Friedli, Bernard E. Van Beers, and John C. Waterton

Abstract

The computation of T_1 maps from MR datasets represents an important step toward the precise characterization of kidney disease models in small animals. Here the main strategies to analyze renal T_1 mapping datasets derived from small rodents are presented. Suggestions are provided with respect to essential software requirements, and advice is provided as to how dataset completeness and quality may be evaluated. The various fitting models applicable to T_1 mapping are presented and discussed. Finally, some methods are proposed for validating the obtained results.

This chapter is based upon work from the COST Action PARENCHIMA, a community-driven network funded by the European Cooperation in Science and Technology (COST) program of the European Union, which aims to improve the reproducibility and standardization of renal MRI biomarkers. This analysis protocol chapter is complemented by two separate chapters describing the basic concept and experimental procedure.

Key words Magnetic resonance imaging (MRI), Kidney, Mice, Rats, T_1 mapping, Processing, Fitting

1 Introduction

The computation of T_1 maps from MR datasets represents an important step towards the precise characterization of kidney disease models in the small animal. Although some concepts pertaining to T_1 mapping are relatively general, there are some important points that need to be observed specifically for each different acquisition strategy. In this section we will describe in more detail the three main classes of data fitting procedures corresponding to saturation recovery, inversion recovery, and variable flip angle protocols.

This analysis protocol chapter is complemented by two separate chapters describing the basic concept and experimental procedure, which are part of this book.

This chapter is part of the book Pohlmann A, Niendorf T (eds) (2020) Preclinical MRI of the Kidney—Methods and Protocols. Springer, New York.

2 Materials

2.1 Software Requirements

The method described in this chapter does require the following software tools:

1. For Bruker users, the availability of a Bruker post-processing station with Bruker Paravision fitting tools ("ISA Tools") installed, or if an independent console is not available, the scanner console. It may not always be possible or practical to alter the vendor-proposed routines to adapt to a particular use case.
2. A programming environment capable of applying fitting models, such as MATLAB® including the curve fitting toolbox (MathWorks, https://www.mathworks.com/products/matlab.html), Octave (https://www.gnu.org/software/octave/), ...
3. An image processing software (e.g., Image J, we recommend using Fiji, which is ImageJ with a wide range of plugins already included, https://fiji.sc/, open source), as a practical tool for the image quality check or for measuring the SNR.
4. For region based approaches, analysis can be done in the R language [1].
5. To speed up computation time, it may be necessary to use optimized compiled code executables or to take advantage of parallel computing.

2.2 Source Data: Format Requirements and Quality Check

2.2.1 Input Requirements

To be able to calculate T_1 maps, multiple images with different repetition times, inversion times or flip angles are needed. It is necessary to have access to some scan parameters, including matrix size and number of slices, scaling information (offset and slope), and the values of the repetition times, inversion times or flip angle. Additional time delays may also be required. In the case of protocols with multiple acquisitions, the receiver gain should also be accessible. Consistency in the acquisition parameters is paramount, especially the parameter that is varied, which should sample the same interval for each animal in the study. The completeness of the data needs to be verified ahead of the processing, by checking that the matrices have the expected size and dimensionality, or in the case of multiple protocols datasets, by ensuring that each expected protocol has indeed been acquired.

2.2.2 Physiologic Motion Check

Physiological motion is an important source of image error. Because it is difficult to avoid entirely in vivo, even in the presence of triggered acquisitions, it represents an important determinant of the dataset quality. The amount of physiologic motion can be assessed visually or via quantitative estimators (see below). Frames displaying high respiratory motion may be either discarded altogether, or they may be weighted differently in the fitting procedure.

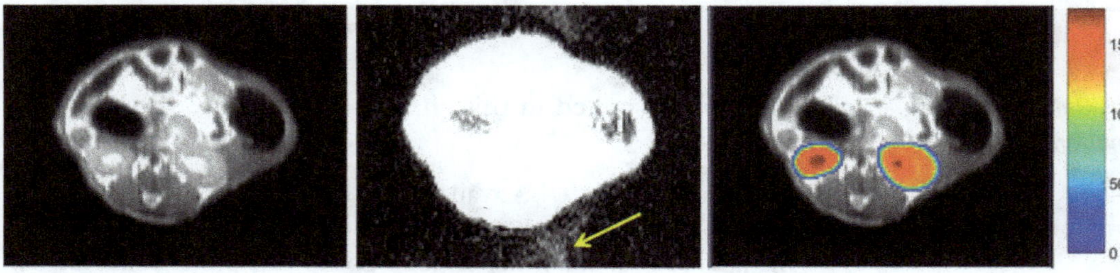

Fig. 1 Illustration of physiologic respiration-based noise. Left: original image. Middle: same image with a different windowing applied. Respiratory noise is evident as a signal smeared in the phase-encoding direction (vertical) only in the image with a strong windowing applied. Different amounts of noise may be tolerated depending on the final intended use of the data. Right: image with T_1 map overlay on the kidneys (color scale in ms)

In the simplest cases (especially with cartesian sampling schemes), respiratory motion can be identified as high intensity regions in the air surrounding the animal, corresponding to smeared projection of the signal along the phase-encoding direction (Fig. 1). Such motion may not be immediately visible and instead require to enhance the image windowing. Varying degrees of physiologic motion may be tolerated depending on the application. Automated methods can be put in place, to selectively remove frames where the noise level in the air region surrounding the animal exceeds a certain limit, in a retrospective fashion [2].

2.2.3 Acquisition Geometry Check

The geometry of the acquisition also needs to be set and verified prior to processing.

1. Verify the slice position and orientation to ensure that an optimal delineation of the kidneys is possible. A coronal orientation is often chosen, because it enables to have large regions of interest that depict all the anatomical regions of the kidney in a single image.
2. Visually check image centering to ensure that the dataset can be exploited.

2.2.4 Acquisition Parameters Consistency Check (Multiple Scans Case Only)

Regardless of the technique which is applied, it is preferable to acquire a single protocol where the parameter of interest varies.

1. Assume that the acquisition parameters are the same for all acquired images and move on to the next step.

If such a protocol is not available on the system, the same scan has to be acquired several times while varying the parameter of interest. This is the case typically for T_1 mapping with variable flip angle approach.

2. Check that all parameters (other than the varied parameter of interest) have stayed the same.

2.2.5 Receiver Gain Consistency Check (Multiple Scans Case Only)

1. Check that the receiver gain setting is identical for each scan when merging data from separate protocols.
2. If the receiver gain is not the same: contact the manufacturer to obtain receiver gain amplification tables.
3. Use the receiver gain amplification tables to calculate correcting factors.
4. Apply the correction factors to set each image at a common amplification level.

This exposes the user to noise compression or amplification and should only be used as a last resort.

2.2.6 Data Intensity Scaling Consistency Check (Multiple Scans Case Only)

The data should also be rescaled to the same intensity mapping. This ensures comparability of data coming from different datasets. For Bruker-generated data, it is recommended to use the absolute mapping option in the reconstruction options. If this has not been done during acquisition, additionally for Bruker-generated data, at the console, the user must:

1. Duplicate the processing.
2. Activate “Prototype Reconstruction”.
3. Set output mapping to “User Scale”.
4. Set parameters “Output Slope/Output Offset” accordingly to the setting of the first scan of the series. The setting of the first scan of the series can be checked in the “Single Parameter” parameter editor.

3 Methods

3.1 Data Exclusion

1. Check that all data points have sufficient signal to noise (SNR of 5 or higher).
2. If not all data points have high SNR then consider the necessity to only use data points with sufficient signal to noise (see next two steps).
3. For variable repetition time protocols, eliminate the data points at low repetition times (TR) that have insufficient SNR.
4. For inversion recovery protocols eliminate the data points close to the zero-crossing that have sufficient signal to noise.

3.2 Data Coregistration

To improve dataset quality, coregistration of images can be implemented to correct for respiratory motion, if such tools are available. The elastix package [3], MATLAB’s built-in imregtform function, SPM [4], or AIR [5] (among others) can be used toward that objective.

3.3 Model Fitting

With contemporary computing hardware, fast fitting of the model to the signal intensity magnitude images can be performed on each pixel of the initial dataset. A region-based approach (wherein the fitting procedure is applied to ROI averages), can also be applied, but by construction it will lack the ability to examine the local spatial variations of tissue T_1.

3.3.1 Fitting Data for Saturation Recovery Experiments

1. Select an appropriate fitting equation. For the VTR protocol, the following equation is applicable (under the assumption of a perfect pulse) [6]:

$$S = S_0\left(1 - e^{-\mathrm{TR}/T_1}\right) + \varepsilon \tag{1}$$

   where S is the signal magnitude, S_0 is the maximal available signal magnitude (including amplification factors), TR is the repetition time, T_1 is the longitudinal relaxation time, and ε is an additive noise component with Rician distribution.
2. If S_0 is known, linearize the fitting equation. A plot of $\ln(1 - S/S_0)$ against TR yields a straight line of slope $-1/T_1$ from which T_1 can be extracted with linear regression (*see* **Note 1**).
3. If the longest TR is significantly longer than T_1, please refer to **Note 3**.
4. If S_0 is not known, Eq. 1 can be fitted with nonlinear regression.
5. Initialize the fit with appropriate starting values for S_0 (*see* **Note 2**), using the signal obtained at the longest TR (*see* **Notes 3** and **4**).
6. Initialize the fit with appropriate starting values for T_1 (*see* **Note 2)** using the value obtained by linear regression if applicable (*see* **item 2**).
7. Perform the fit with the Levenberg-Marquardt, the trust region or the maximum likelihood algorithms (*see* **Note 5**).

3.3.2 Fitting Data for Inversion Recovery Experiments

1. Select an appropriate fitting equation. For the inversion-recovery protocol, the following equation is applicable (assuming perfect pulses and absence of relaxation during pulses) [6, 7]:

$$S = \left|S_0\left(1 - 2e^{-\mathrm{TI}/T_1}\right) + \varepsilon\right| \tag{2}$$

   where S is the signal magnitude, S_0 is the maximal available signal magnitude (including amplification factors), TI is the inversion time, T_1 is the longitudinal relaxation time, and ε is an additive noise component with Rician distribution.
2. If S_0 is known, linearize the fitting equation. A plot of $\ln((S_0 - S)/(2 \cdot S_0))$ against TI yields a straight line of slope $-1/T_1$ from which T_1 can be extracted with linear regression (*see* **Note 1**).

3. Optionally, apply a corrective formula to account for the perturbation in recovery caused by the small angle imaging pulses (*see* **Note 6**):

$$\frac{1}{T_1} = \frac{1}{T_1^*} + \frac{\ln(\cos(\theta))}{\tau} \tag{3}$$

4. Optionally, the following equation is also applicable (assuming perfect pulses and absence of relaxation during pulses) [2, 8–11] and adds a saturation-correcting factor (*see* **Notes 7** and **8**):

$$S = S_0\left(1 - \beta \cdot e^{-TI/T_1^*}\right) \tag{4}$$

5. If S_0 is known, linearize fitting Eq. 4. A plot of $\ln(1 - S/S_0)$ against TI yields a straight line of intercept $\ln(\beta)$ and of slope $-1/T_1$ from which $T_1{}^*$ can be extracted with linear regression. The actual T_1 is subsequently recovered from the values of T_1^* and β as follows:

$$T_1 = T_1^* \cdot (\beta - 1) \tag{5}$$

6. If S_0 is not known, Eqs. 2 and 4 can be fitted with nonlinear regression using S_0, T_1 and β as adjustable parameters and if applicable the correction of Eq. 5.
7. Initialize the fit with appropriate starting values (*see* **Note 2**) for S_0, using the signal obtained at the longest TI (*see* **Notes 3** and **4**).
8. Initialize the fit with appropriate starting values (*see* **Note 2**) for T_1 using the value obtained by linear regression if applicable (*see* **Note 4**), or using the graphical procedure outlined in **Note 9**.
9. If the longest TR is significantly longer than T_1, please refer to **Note 10**.
10. Perform the fit with the Levenberg-Marquardt, the trust region or the maximum likelihood algorithms (*see* **Note 5**).

3.3.3 Fitting Data for Variable Flip Angle Experiments

1. If only two flip angles are available, use the following simplified equation involving α_1 and α_2 the two flip angles used, β the ratio image obtained between the two flip angles, and TR the repetition time TR [12] to compute the T_1:

$$T_1 = \frac{TR}{\ln\left(\frac{\beta \cdot \sin(\alpha_2) \cdot \cos(\alpha_1) - \sin(\alpha_1) \cdot \cos(\alpha_2)}{\beta \cdot \sin(\alpha_2) - \sin(\alpha_1)}\right)} \tag{6}$$

2. In the more general case, the following equation is applicable (*see* **Notes 11** and **12**):

$$S(\theta) = S_0 \cdot \sin(\theta) \cdot ((1 - E_1)/(1 - E_1 \cdot \cos(\theta))) \tag{7a}$$

where

$$E_1 = exp(-TR/T_1) \tag{7b}$$

3. Determine T_1 using linear regression on the linear form of Eqs. 7a and 7b [13]:
   Plot $S(\theta)/\sin(\theta)$ against $S(\theta)/\tan(\theta)$.
4. Retrieve the slope of the plot from the linear regression. This is E_1 (definition in Eq. 7b).
5. Compute the T_1 estimate directly as $-1/\ln(E_1)$.
6. Retrieve the intercept of the plot from the linear regression. This is $S_0(1 - E_1)$. The S_0 value is estimated by dividing the intercept value that was found by $1 - E_1$ (using for E_1 the value obtained previously).
7. Alternately, determine T_1 using a nonlinear fitting procedure.
8. Initialize the fit with starting values (*see* **Note 2**) for S_0 and T_1 obtained using the linearization described previously (*see* **Note 4**).
9. Perform the fit with the Levenberg-Marquardt, the trust region or the maximum likelihood algorithms (*see* **Note 5**).

3.4 Visual Display

T_1 maps can be shown as gray-scaled or color-coded maps. T_1 maps from the region of interest can be superimposed after coregistration on a morphological image or on an image acquired with the T_1 mapping protocol to better illustrate anatomical location. Window scales, usually run from $T_1 = 0$ to $T_1 = 3000$ ms, should be provided with the map and should be kept constant between figures.

3.5 Quantification

The fitting algorithm is usually applied on a voxel-by-voxel basis to yield a T_1 map. Mean T_1 is then calculated by averaging T_1 values within a region of interest. It is recommended to define a region of interest for each anatomical subregion of the kidney, as the pathology of interest can affect differently these subregions [14]. Typical ROIs are cortex, outer medulla and inner medulla, using morphological images as references to draw these ROIs. Provided sufficient spatial resolution is available, finer structures such as the outer and inner stripes of the outer medulla [15], or the corticomedullary junction [7], may be distinguished. It is also common to report T_1 changes relative to baseline or to the contralateral kidney.

3.6 Results Validation

3.6.1 Evaluation of Analysis Errors and Variability Using Synthetic Data

Synthetic datasets of various complexities should be generated to test the validity of the processing solution. Artificial noise can be added to assess the stability of the fitting procedure. T_1 of the numeric phantom should match the expected T_1. This approach is, however, limited by the signal equation, which may or may not recapitulate the real situation complexity. Hence, the use of physical phantoms can also be recommended (*see* procedure outlines in the chapter by Irrera P et al. "Dynamic Contrast Enhanced (DCE) MRI-Derived Renal Perfusion and Filtration: Experimental Protocol").

3.6.2 Comparison with Reference Values from the Literature

Relatively few studies have reported T_1 values for kidney acquired in animal models at high magnetic fields (4.7 T and higher). Typical ranges for normal kidney tissue are T_1 = 1000–1700 ms at magnetic field strengths of 7 or 9.4 T [14–16], with significant differences reported between mouse strains [16]. Acute kidney injury and unilateral nephrectomy have been reported to increase T_1 values in kidney, up to T_1 = 1944 ms at 7 T for severe acute injury [15] and well above T_1 = 2000 ms at 9.4 T for unilateral nephrectomy [14].

4 Notes

1. The accurate estimation of S_0 is, not trivial. Indeed, in Eqs. 1 and 2, signal evolution is asymptotic and even at very high TR or TI values, the signal only approaches the actual S_0 value. Furthermore, in these protocols, TR or TI directly affect the acquisition duration. Hence, the precision of the estimation of S_0 directly affects scan duration. In the linearization approach, the available precision on S_0 dictates the precision with which T_1 is recovered (error propagation). Hence with this approach, increased acquisition time is needed to improve the precision of the measurement. If the duration of the experiment is a concern (dynamic studies, animal models of severe diseases, difficult anesthesia), it may be preferable to leave S_0 as free parameter and to use a nonlinear fitting procedure.
2. In nonlinear fitting algorithms it can be advantageous to provide starting points that are close to the final values. Indeed, this allows to decrease the number of iterations required to reach convergence, and hence can limit the computation time. Furthermore, using starting values close to the true values also helps identifying the global minimum rather than a distant local minimum. Hence, strategies can be adopted to provide as accurate as possible initial estimates for the free parameters of the nonlinear fitting procedure.

3. In some cases, an initial S_0 estimate for fitting initialization can be obtained from the highest signal available (at the latest saturation or inversion recovery delays for instance). This estimate will only be precise if the longest delay that is sampled is sufficiently long.
4. The outlined strategies for determining reasonable starting values may not work in all cases. For instance, in the presence of high experimental noise or in the case of poorly controlled acquisition conditions, the initial estimates may prove unreliable. In this case, reasonable starting values for the T_1 may be alternately obtained from the literature. Special care should be taken to select literature reference values from studies where similar magnetic field strength, protocol type and experimental disease models were used.
5. Careful comparison of the performance of the fitting algorithms should be conducted on datasets obtained on the disease model and hardware setup used in the study. The various algorithms may be compared in terms of computation speed and goodness-of-fit figures of merit such as the root-mean-squared error before a final choice is made.
6. In inversion recovery protocols, the T_1 relaxation process is sampled several times after an inversion RF pulse using small gradient echo shots, EPI readouts or FISP readouts. Thus, the natural longitudinal recovery is perturbed by the application of the imaging RF pulses of flip angle θ and separated by a repetition interval τ. The effect can be accounted for by correcting T_1^*, the apparent T_1 resulting from the fit, using the expression given in Eq. 3 [17–19].
7. With inversion-recovery protocols followed by multiple shots, it would be preferable to use long delays between the imaging RF pulses, to drive down the saturation effect of the fast repeating gradient echo excitation RF pulses. This is not always practical, since short delays are required to fit a large number of imaging shots within a single inversion recovery interval. This is linked to the requirement that no transverse magnetization remains at the end of an imaging shot once the subsequent imaging shot is acquired, that is, that the condition of spoiled magnetization is applicable. The generally accepted condition is thus to ensure that $\tau \gg T_2^*$. Thus, although not ideal, it is acceptable to shorten the repetition time between imaging RF pulses, to reach an optimal situation where the two conflicting constraints of having both a large number of imaging shots per inversion recovery and a sufficiently good spoiling of magnetization between consecutive imaging shots are met. Similarly, it can be advantageous to work at low flip angle, to minimize the perturbation to the natural magnetization recovery relative to

the ideal case when no imaging RF pulses are applied after the inversion RF pulse. This comes at a disadvantage of having a smaller signal to noise ratio. However, this may be preferable when exactness of the recovered T_1 is important. In conclusion, the selection of the most appropriate fitting equation should be guided by careful examination of the specific acquisition protocol that was used, and of values of the imaging delays, flip angles, and typical expected tissue magnetic properties in the disease model at hand.

8. More complete correction schemes can be applied in the case of Look–Locker protocols. In particular, the delay between the inversion RF pulse and the first imaging RF pulse may be different than the delay between subsequent sequential imaging RF pulses. The imperfections in the inversion profile may also be modelled in the equation. Expressions taking this delay into account are available. Furthermore, in inversion recovery protocols, some variants may be segmented. For instance, partial k-space segments can be acquired by groups of imaging shots at several times post inversion. The various individual shots in a segment are used to reconstruct an image at a single inversion delay (the delay between the inversion RF pulse and the half of the imaging segment). Imaging segments may be separated by arbitrary delays. Expressions are available to take into account these delays [20–22].

9. In the case of inversion recovery protocols, a simpler method may be used to provide a reasonable estimate of T_1 to be used as starting point. Indeed, the signal has the typical shape where the image magnitude first drops down to zero, then comes back up (*see* Fig. 2). This is due to the fact that the image magnitude is gotten from the transverse component of the magnetization, without discerning whether the magnetization is below or above the transverse plane. This offers a graphical way to determine rapidly the T_1 by identifying the point at which the signal is minimal. The recovery delay at which this condition is verified is an approximation of the time when the longitudinal magnetization crosses the transverse plane. The precision of this estimate will be improved if the sampling of inversion times is dense around this point. The delay of the zero-crossing is equal to $T_1 \times \ln(2)$. Hence the true T_1 can be identified by dividing the zero crossing delay by $\ln(2)$. This can be useful to obtain a rapid estimate of the T_1 during parameter optimization. This computation can be performed very simply at each voxel by identifying the index of the signal vector where the smallest signal intensity is obtained. This strategy is, however, limited when only few points are available along the regrowth or when the signal to noise is low. Both cases can

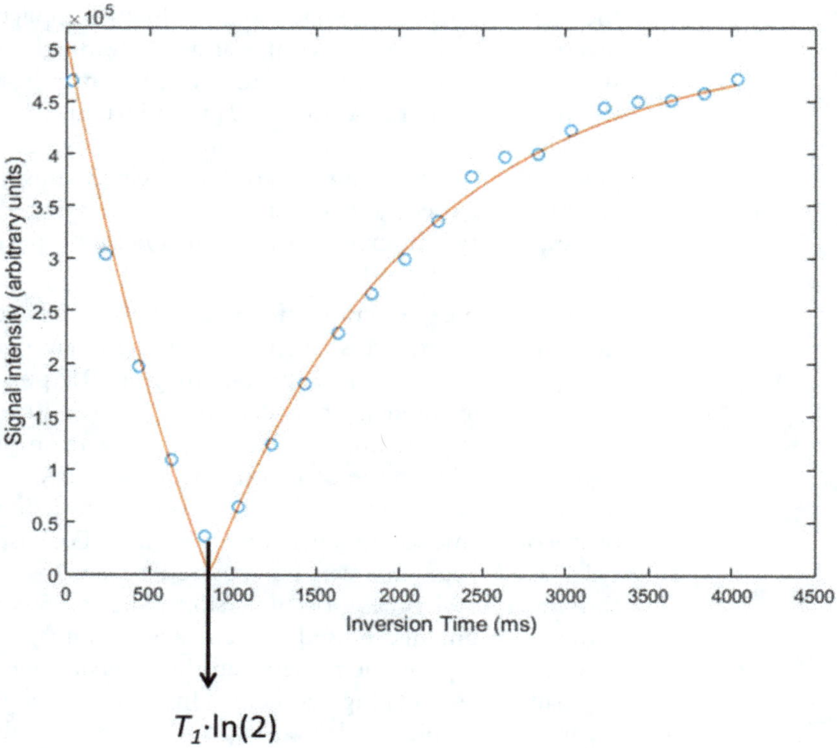

Fig. 2 Inversion recovery plot depicting the graphical method to identify T_1. An estimate of T_1 is obtained by identification of the inversion time yielding the smallest available signal, and dividing this value by ln(2). Although this quantification is not optimally accurate, it may prove useful in determining sufficiently close values to serve as a good initialization point for nonlinear fitting procedures

alter the accuracy of the estimation of the delay time yielding zero crossing.

10. Depending on the acquisition conditions, images are available at TI (or TR) $\gg T_1$. In that case, Eqs. 1 and 2 collapse to $S = S_0$. Such images can be used to normalize the data, and the nonlinear fitting procedure can be carried out on S/S_0 rather than S. By suppressing the free parameter S_0 from the fitting procedure, the numeric stability of the fit is improved, at the expense of the longer acquisition time required for the acquisition of the TI $\gg T_1$ protocol. This approach is also subject to the problem of error propagation from the S_0 estimation into the T_1 term exposed previously.

11. The true signal behavior may differ significantly from this expression, especially if the applied flip angle is not homogeneous. In that case, a corrective, smoothly spatial-varying $\zeta(B_1^+)$ term may need to be applied to account for excitation radiofrequency field heterogeneity. The effectively obtained flip angles, θ_{eff}, are in that case a modulation of the prescribed

flip angle series, θ, such that $\theta_{\mathrm{eff}} = \zeta(B_1^+) \cdot \theta$. The evaluation of the ζ field is not trivial, and becomes especially important at higher field strengths. Post-processing methods based on large scale features in the image such as low pass filtering, or fitting of slowly spatially varying functions, can be proposed, but only extract the combined effects of transmit (B_1^+) and receive (B_1^-) heterogeneities [23]. The modulation fields can be subtracted out before performing the fit, provided that the reception field is sufficiently homogeneous. Of note, this assumption is quite difficult to validate, especially at high field strengths or when single receive RF coil elements are used as the detection circuitry.

12. Alternately, a reference T_1 map acquired with a Look–Locker protocol at lower spatial resolution and short acquisition time can be used to correct B_1 heterogeneity. Indeed, such protocol is much less prone to B_1 heterogeneity artifacts, hence the T_1 it provides can be assumed to be precise [19]. This low spatial resolution reference T_1 map is fed into a separate fit of Eq. 7a expressed as function of $\theta_{\mathrm{eff}} = \zeta(B_1^+) \cdot \theta$ rather than merely θ, and letting ζ as free parameter. Finally, the modulation map ζ determined in that way can be injected back into Eq. 7a, this time letting T_1 and S_0 as free parameters to be determined, and operating at the full spatial resolution of the VFA dataset. This approach enables a more precise quantification of T_1 because the ${B_1}^+$ and ${B_1}^-$ effects are effectively separated out into the ζ and the S_0 maps, respectively. However, this approach is more complex and requires to acquire separate reference T_1 map, increasing the overall scan time duration.

Acknowledgments

This chapter is based upon work from COST Action PARENCH IMA, supported by European Cooperation in Science and Technology (COST). COST (www.cost.eu) is a funding agency for research and innovation networks. COST Actions help connect research initiatives across Europe and enable scientists to enrich their ideas by sharing them with their peers. This boosts their research, career, and innovation.

PARENCHIMA (renalmri.org) is a community-driven Action in the COST program of the European Union, which unites more than 200 experts in renal MRI from 30 countries with the aim to improve the reproducibility and standardization of renal MRI biomarkers.

References

1. Team RC (2015) R: a language and environment for statistical computing. R Foundation for Statistical Computing, Vienna
2. Ramaswamy R, Campbell-Washburn AE, Wells JA, Johnson SP, Pedley RB, Walker-Samuel S et al (2015) Hepatic arterial spin labelling MRI: an initial evaluation in mice. NMR Biomed 28(2):272–280
3. Klein S, Staring M, Murphy K, Viergever MA, Pluim JP (2010) elastix: a toolbox for intensity-based medical image registration. IEEE Trans Med Imaging 29(1):196–205
4. Huhdanpaa H, Hwang DH, Gasparian GG, Booker MT, Cen Y, Lerner A et al (2014) Image coregistration: quantitative processing framework for the assessment of brain lesions. J Digit Imaging 27(3):369–379
5. Woods RP, Grafton ST, Holmes CJ, Cherry SR, Mazziotta JC (1998) Automated image registration: I. General methods and intrasubject, intramodality validation. J Comput Assist Tomogr 22(1):139–152
6. Haacke EM, Brown RW, Thompson MR, Venkatesan R (2014) Magneticresonance imaging, physical principles and sequence design. Wiley, Hoboken, NJ
7. Bosch CS, Ackerman JJ, Tilton RG, Shalwitz RA (1993) In vivo NMR imaging and spectroscopic investigation of renal pathology in lean and obese rat kidneys. Magn Reson Med 29 (3):335–344
8. Jiang K, Tang H, Mishra PK, Macura SI, Lerman LO (2018) A rapid T1 mapping method for assessment of murine kidney viability using dynamic manganese-enhanced magnetic resonance imaging. Magn Reson Med 80 (1):190–199
9. Pastor G, Jimenez-Gonzalez M, Plaza-Garcia S, Beraza M, Reese T (2017) Fast T1 and T2 mapping methods: the zoomed U-FLARE sequence compared with EPI and snapshot-FLASH for abdominal imaging at 11.7 Tesla. MAGMA 30(3):299–307
10. Rajendran R, Lew SK, Yong CX, Tan J, Wang DJ, Chuang KH (2013) Quantitative mouse renal perfusion using arterial spin labeling. NMR Biomed 26(10):1225–1232
11. Wang JJ, Hendrich KS, Jackson EK, Ildstad ST, Williams DS, Ho C (1998) Perfusion quantitation in transplanted rat kidney by MRI with arterial spin labeling. Kidney Int 53 (6):1783–1791
12. Ko SF, Yip HK, Zhen YY, Lee CC, Lee CC, Huang SJ et al (2017) Severe bilateral ischemic-reperfusion renal injury: hyperacute and acute changes in apparent diffusion coefficient, T1, and T2 mapping with immunohistochemical correlations. Sci Rep 7 (1):1725
13. Cheng HL, Wright GA (2006) Rapid high-resolution T(1) mapping by variable flip angles: accurate and precise measurements in the presence of radiofrequency field inhomogeneity. Magn Reson Med 55(3):566–574
14. Kierulf-Lassen C, Nielsen PM, Qi H, Damgaard M, Laustsen C, Pedersen M et al (2017) Unilateral nephrectomy diminishes ischemic acute kidney injury through enhanced perfusion and reduced pro-inflammatory and pro-fibrotic responses. PLoS One 12(12): e0190009
15. Hueper K, Peperhove M, Rong S, Gerstenberg J, Mengel M, Meier M et al (2014) T1-mapping for assessment of ischemia-induced acute kidney injury and prediction of chronic kidney disease in mice. Eur Radiol 24(9):2252–2260
16. Tewes S, Gueler F, Chen R, Gutberlet M, Jang MS, Meier M et al (2017) Functional MRI for characterization of renal perfusion impairment and edema formation due to acute kidney injury in different mouse strains. PLoS One 12(3):e0173248
17. De Graaf R (2007) In vivo NMR spectroscopy, principles and techniques, 2nd edn. Wiley-Interscience, Hoboken, NJ
18. van Schie JJ, Lavini C, van Vliet LJ, Vos FM (2015) Feasibility of a fast method for B1-inhomogeneity correction for FSPGR sequences. Magn Reson Imaging 33 (3):312–318
19. Zhang J, Chamberlain R, Etheridge M, Idiyatullin D, Corum C, Bischof J et al (2014) Quantifying iron-oxide nanoparticles at high concentration based on longitudinal

relaxation using a three-dimensional SWIFT Look-Locker sequence. Magn Reson Med 71 (6):1982–1988

20. Nkongchu K, Santyr G (2005) An improved 3-D Look-Locker imaging method for T (1) parameter estimation. Magn Reson Imaging 23(7):801–807
21. Henderson E, McKinnon G, Lee TY, Rutt BK (1999) A fast 3D Look-Locker method for volumetric T1 mapping. Magn Reson Imaging 17(8):1163–1171
22. Nkongchu K, Santyr G (2007) Phase-encoding strategies for optimal spatial resolution and T1 accuracy in 3D Look-Locker imaging. Magn Reson Imaging 25(8):1203–1214
23. Marques JP, Kober T, Krueger G, van der Zwaag W, Van de Moortele PF, Gruetter R (2010) MP2RAGE, a self bias-field corrected sequence for improved segmentation and T1-mapping at high field. NeuroImage 49 (2):1271–1281

Permissions

All chapters in this book were first published in PMKMP, by Springer; hereby published with permission under the Creative Commons Attribution License or equivalent. Every chapter published in this book has been scrutinized by our experts. Their significance has been extensively debated. The topics covered herein carry significant findings which will fuel the growth of the discipline. They may even be implemented as practical applications or may be referred to as a beginning point for another development.

The contributors of this book come from diverse backgrounds, making this book a truly international effort. This book will bring forth new frontiers with its revolutionizing research information and detailed analysis of the nascent developments around the world.

We would like to thank all the contributing authors for lending their expertise to make the book truly unique. They have played a crucial role in the development of this book. Without their invaluable contributions this book wouldn't have been possible. They have made vital efforts to compile up to date information on the varied aspects of this subject to make this book a valuable addition to the collection of many professionals and students.

This book was conceptualized with the vision of imparting up-to-date information and advanced data in this field. To ensure the same, a matchless editorial board was set up. Every individual on the board went through rigorous rounds of assessment to prove their worth. After which they invested a large part of their time researching and compiling the most relevant data for our readers.

The editorial board has been involved in producing this book since its inception. They have spent rigorous hours researching and exploring the diverse topics which have resulted in the successful publishing of this book. They have passed on their knowledge of decades through this book. To expedite this challenging task, the publisher supported the team at every step. A small team of assistant editors was also appointed to further simplify the editing procedure and attain best results for the readers.

Apart from the editorial board, the designing team has also invested a significant amount of their time in understanding the subject and creating the most relevant covers. They scrutinized every image to scout for the most suitable representation of the subject and create an appropriate cover for the book.

The publishing team has been an ardent support to the editorial, designing and production team. Their endless efforts to recruit the best for this project, has resulted in the accomplishment of this book. They are a veteran in the field of academics and their pool of knowledge is as vast as their experience in printing. Their expertise and guidance has proved useful at every step. Their uncompromising quality standards have made this book an exceptional effort. Their encouragement from time to time has been an inspiration for everyone.

The publisher and the editorial board hope that this book will prove to be a valuable piece of knowledge for researchers, students, practitioners and scholars across the globe.

List of Contributors

James T. Grist, Esben Søvsø Szocska Hansen, Frank G. Zöllner, and Christoffer Laustsen

Ludger Starke, Karsten Tabelow, Thoralf Niendorf and Andreas Pohlmann

Frank G. Zöllner, Walter Dastrù, Pietro Irrera, Dario Livio Longo, Kevin M. Bennett, Scott C. Beeman, G. Larry Bretthorst and Joel R. Garbow

Galen D. Reed, Natalie J. Korn, Christoffer Laustsen and Cornelius von Morze

Lingzhi Hu, Hua Pan and Samuel A. Wickline

João S. Periquito, Ludger Starke, Carlota M. Santos, Andreia C. Freitas, Nuno Loução, Pablo García Polo, Rita G. Nunes, Thoralf Niendorf and Andreas Pohlmann

Neil Peter Jerome and João S. Periquito

João S. Periquito, Martin Meier, Thoralf Niendorf, Andreas Pohlmann and Neil Peter Jerome

Paula Ramos Delgado, Ekkehard Küstermann, André Kühne, Jason M. Millward, Thoralf Niendorf, Andreas Pohlmann and Martin Meier

Suraj D. Serai and Meng Yin

Kai-Hsiang Chuang, Frank Kober and Min-Chi Ku

Ludger Starke, Thoralf Niendorf and Sonia Waiczies

Hahnsung Kim, Yin Wu, Daisy Villano, Dario Livio Longo, Michael T. McMahon and Phillip Zhe Sun

Leili Riazy, Bastien Milani, João S. Periquito, Kathleen Cantow, Thoralf Niendorf, Menno Pruijm, Erdmann Seeliger and Andreas Pohlmann

Philippe Garteiser, Gwenaël Pagé, Sabrina Doblas, Octavia Bane, Stefanie Hectors, Iris Friedli, Bernard E. Van Beers and John C. Waterton

Index

www.ingramcontent.com/pod-product-compliance
Lightning Source LLC
LaVergne TN
LVHW080637210926
848485LV00003B/280